Diagnosis and Control of Diseases of Fish and Shellfish

Diagnosis and Control of Diseases of Fish and Shellfish

Edited by
Brian Austin
Professor Emeritus, University of Stirling, Scotland, UK

Aweeda Newaj-Fyzul
University of the West Indies
Trinidad and Agriquatics, Chaguanas, Trinidad

WILEY

This edition first published 2017

Registered Offices
John Wiley & Sons, Inc., 111 River Street, Hoboken, NJ 07030, USA
John Wiley & Sons Ltd, The Atrium, Southern Gate, Chichester, West Sussex, PO19 8SQ, UK

Editorial Office
The Atrium, Southern Gate, Chichester, West Sussex, PO19 8SQ, UK

For details of our global editorial offices, customer services, and more information about Wiley products visit us at www.wiley.com.

Wiley also publishes its books in a variety of electronic formats and by print-on-demand. Some content that appears in standard print versions of this book may not be available in other formats.

Library of Congress Cataloging-in-Publication data applied for

ISBN - 9781119152101

Cover Design: Wiley
Cover Image: ©teaa1946/Gettyimages

Set in 10/12pt Warnock by SPi Global, Chennai, India

Printed and Bound in Singapore by Markono Print Media Pte Ltd

10 9 8 7 6 5 4 3 2 1

Contents

List of Contributors

Brian Austin
University of Stirling
Scotland
UK

Mags Crumlish
Institute of Aquaculture
University of Stirling
Scotland
UK

Andrea Gustinelli
Department of Veterinary Medical Sciences
Alma Mater Studiorum
University of Bologna
Bologna
Italy

Seyed Hossein Hoseinifar
Department of Fisheries
Gorgan University of Agricultural Sciences and Natural Resources
Gorgan
Iran

Ahran Kim
Department of Aquatic Life Medicine
Pukyong National University
Busan
Republic of Korea

Do-Hyung Kim
Department of Aquatic Life Medicine
Pukyong National University
Busan
Republic of Korea

Matt Longshaw
Benchmark Animal Health Ltd
Edinburgh Technopole
Scotland
UK

Thanh Luan Nguyen
Department of Aquatic Life Medicine
Pukyong National University
Busan
Republic of Korea

Simon MacKenzie
Institute of Aquaculture
University of Stirling
Scotland
UK

Aweeda Newaj-Fyzul
University of the West Indies
Trinidad

and

Agriquatics
Chaguanas
Trinidad

Giuseppe Paladini
Institute of Aquaculture
University of Stirling
Scotland
UK

Miriam Reverter
CRIOBE, Paris Sciences et Lettres (PSL)
University of Perpignan Via Domitia

Perpignan
France

and

Laboratoire d'Excellence "CORAIL"
Moorea
French Polynesia

Felipe Reyes-López
Department of Cell Biology
Physiology and Immunology
Universitat Autonoma de Barcelona
Bellaterra
Spain

Pierre Sasal
CRIOBE, Paris Sciences et Lettres (PSL)
University of Perpignan Via Domitia
Perpignan
France

and

Laboratoire d'Excellence "CORAIL"
Moorea
French Polynesia

Denis Saulnier
Laboratoire d'Excellence "CORAIL"
Moorea
French Polynesia

and

Ifremer
Taravao
Tahiti
French Polynesia

S.M. Sharifuzzaman
Institute of Marine Sciences and Fisheries
University of Chittagong
Bangladesh

Andrew P. Shinn
Benchmark Animal Health Ltd
Edinburgh Technopole
Scotland
UK

and

Fish Vet Group Asia Ltd
Chonburi
Thailand

Yun-Zhang Sun
Key Laboratory of Healthy Mariculture for the East China Sea
Ministry of Agriculture
Fisheries College
Jimei University
Xiamen
China

Nathalie Tapissier-Bontemps
CRIOBE, Paris Sciences et Lettres (PSL)
University of Perpignan Via Domitia
Perpignan
France

and

Laboratoire d'Excellence "CORAIL"
Moorea
French Polynesia

Eva Vallejos-Vidal
Institut de Biotecnologia i Biomedicina
Universitat Autonoma de Barcelona
Bellaterra
Spain

Manfred Weidmann
Virology Unit
Institute of Aquaculture
University of Stirling
Scotland
UK

Zhigzhang Zhou
Key Laboratory for Feed Biotechnology of the Ministry of Agriculture
Feed Research Institute
Chinese Academy of Agricultural Sciences
Beijing
China

Preface

There has been continual expansion in aquaculture since the end of the Second World War, and currently total production is approximately equal to that of wild-caught fisheries. Yet, this expansion is marred by continued problems of disease. New pathogens emerge, and others become associated with new conditions. Some of these pathogens become well established and develop into major killers of aquatic species. Examples include infectious salmon anaemia virus, francisellosis and amoebic gill disease. Research has seen significant developments in diagnostics and disease control. The former has progressed from the descriptive, through serological to molecular methods. This progression has led to greater sensitivity, specificity and reliability. However, it is not always clear what a positive result means in the absence of clinical disease manifestations. Developments in disease control have encompassed therapy (disinfectants, antibiotics) and prophylaxis (vaccines, probiotics, prebiotics, immunostimulants). There is a trend away from the use of chemicals because of issues with the development and spread of resistance, tissue residues and environmental concerns. Interest in disease prevention has soared, from the development of vaccines to interest in probiotics, and now to the use of medicinal plant products.

The primary aim of this book is to focus on developments in the diagnosis and control of diseases of fish and shellfish, notably those affecting aquaculture. The book is primarily targeted at research workers, including postgraduate students, diagnosticians and individuals concerned with the management of diseases of fish and shellfish. It is anticipated that the readership will include veterinarians, fish pathologists, microbiologists, public health scientists and microbial ecologists.

Brian Austin and Aweeda Newaj-Fyzul
2017

1

Introduction

Brian Austin[1] *and Aweeda Newaj-Fyzul*[2]

[1] *Institute of Aquaculture, University of Stirling, Stirling, Scotland, UK*
[2] *University of the West Indies, Trinidad and Agriquatics, Chaguanas, Trinidad*

There is confusion over the meaning of the term 'disease'. A definition from an article in the *British Medical Journal* is as follows:

> … a disease is the sum of the abnormal phenomena displayed by a group of living organisms in association with a specified common characteristic or set of characteristics by which they differ from the norm of their species in such a way as to place them at a biological disadvantage. (Campbell *et al.*, 1979)

According to these authors, a disease is something that occurs to a group of organisms rather than to an individual. Also, the definition is far reaching and reflects the complex relationship between the disease-causing situation (not necessarily a micro-organism) and the host. However, there is more to disease than the interaction of a pathogen (dictionary definition is of a disease-causing organism) and the host. According to Kinne (1980), who was writing about diseases of marine animals, diseases could be caused by genetic disorders, nutritional imbalance, pathogens, physical injury and pollution. Thus, disease could be attributed to biological (*biotic*) as well as non-biological (*abiotic*) causes. Kinne (1980) described diseases in terms of epidemiology (*epizootiology* for animal diseases), as follows.

- *Sporadic* diseases, which occur sporadically in comparatively small numbers of individuals in a population.
- *Epidemics/Epizootics*, which are large-scale outbreaks of communicable disease occurring temporarily in limited areas.
- *Pandemics/Panzootics*, which are large-scale outbreaks of communicable disease occurring over large areas.
- *Endemics/Enzootics*, which are diseases persisting or reoccurring as low-level outbreaks in defined areas.

The interest in diseases of aquatic organisms is primarily directed towards aquaculture which, to paraphrase definitions, is the rearing of aquatic species in controlled conditions. Here, disease may be of sudden onset with rapid progression to high mortalities, with an equally quick decline (*acute* disease). Conversely, there may be cases where the disease develops more slowly, with less severity but longer persistence (*chronic* disease).

Diagnosis and Control of Diseases of Fish and Shellfish, First Edition. Edited by Brian Austin and Aweeda Newaj-Fyzul.

It is apparent that as society moves through the twenty-first century, aquatic animals continue to suffer the vagaries of disease, especially as new diseases continue to occur, e.g. acute hepatopancreatic necrosis disease syndrome (AHPND), which is attributed to infection of the shrimp with *Vibrio parahaemolyticus.* However, the study of aquatic pathobiology is largely an aerobic affair as most laboratories do not consider the possible role of anaerobes or microaerophiles. It would be interesting to determine if this reflects a lack of expertise, interest or suitable methods rather than the absence of occurrence of anaerobic or microaerophilic pathogens/parasites. The majority of literature points to a single species of pathogen as the main cause of disease situations but there are reports of sequential viral and bacterial as well as parasitic and opportunistic bacterial combinations. Certainly, it is appreciated that there have been important developments in disease diagnosis, with progression from traditional phenotyping to the use of newly developed molecular techniques. In many modern laboratories, identification is now routinely accomplished by sequencing of the 16S rRNA gene, a move that has led to greater confidence in the outputs although this will reflect the accuracy of the data in the databases.

However, whereas the use of new technologies is to be encouraged, an ongoing dilemma remains about the authenticity of isolates studied. Also, many studies are based on the examination of single isolates, the relevance of which to fish pathology or science in general is not always clear. Certainly, too many conclusions result from the examination of too few isolates. Nevertheless, the study of pathogenicity mechanisms, diagnostics and disease control by means of vaccines has benefited from molecular approaches. Yet it is appreciated that many laboratories still rely on conventional methods for achieving disease diagnoses, and it is unlikely that this situation will change in the foreseeable future. However, it is pertinent to enquire what diagnosis is supposed to achieve. If the underlying aim is to underpin efforts at disease control, then it is unclear whether detailed and time-consuming work resulting in identifying a pathogen to species level would necessarily help disease control strategies.

The use of pathological specimens taken from advanced cases of disease would be unlikely to reveal species succession, which could occur throughout a disease cycle. Also, we focus on pure cultures, and are generally uncomfortable with the notion that two or more organisms could be associated with a single disease condition. Diagnostic microbiology aims to isolate the dominant organism, as a single pure culture, from pathological material. It is speculative how often the wrong organism may be chosen, as the true pathogen becomes overwhelmed by contaminants. Yet laboratory cultures are used extensively for associated studies of pathogenicity mechanism and disease control. Unfortunately, all too often, cultures lose some of their characteristics in the laboratory which may reflect loss of DNA – and therefore ensuing data need not reflect the true role of the culture with its host.

Histological examination of diseased tissue may be invaluable in recognizing cases where organisms, presumed to the pathogen, may be observed but culturing not achieved. The uncultured *Candidatus* have become associated with some diseases. It is unclear if such organisms are incapable of growing *in vitro* or if suitable media have not been developed. It is unknown how many more of these unculturable organisms remain to be recognized. Could such uncultured organisms be dormant, damaged or senescent, a concept which has been put forward for some water-borne organisms by Stevenson (1978)? Then there are situations where there is pathology, for example red mark syndrome of rainbow trout, for which the cause is uncertain but may reflect infection with a rickettsia (Metselaar *et al.*, 2010).

It is interesting to note that Al Gore, when Vice President of the USA, suggested that diseases (of humans) would be controlled within our lifetimes. Since then, human society has suffered from the emergence of new diseases (e.g. Middle East respiratory syndrome (MERS) coronavirus) and the recurrence of others (e.g. Ebola, H1N1 and Zika). The use of medically important antibiotics in any non-medical situation, including aquaculture, is fraught with problems, of which the development and spread of resistance, and issues with tissue level, top the list of concerns. The result is that there is a deliberate move away from the use of antibiotics in many countries. Certainly, control of diseases of aquatic organisms has undergone dramatic improvements from the initial emphasis on control (therapy) to prevention (prophylaxis). Unfortunately, the dramatic progress in human vaccinology has not been reflected in the number of commercial products available to aquaculture. However, there is no shortage of ingenuity in the development of disease control strategies, as illustrated by the growing interest in non-specific immunostimulants, prebiotics, probiotics and plant products.

This text will focus on the diagnosis and control of infectious diseases of farmed aquatic animals.

Conclusion

- The list of parasitic, bacterial and viral pathogens continues to grow, although the significance of some organisms to pathology is difficult to ascertain – are they truly parasite/pathogens, secondary invaders or contaminants?
- There has been considerable improvement in the taxonomy and hence diagnosis (accuracy and sensitivity) of many pathogens, particularly involving the sequencing of the 16S rRNA gene.
- Disease control has progressed from therapeutic to prophylactic, and now involves a wide range of approaches including vaccines, non-specific immunostimulants, prebiotics, probiotics and plant products.

References

Campbell, E.J.M., Scadding, J.G. and Roberts, M.S. (1979) The concept of disease. *British Medical Journal*, **2**, 757–762.

Kinne, O. (1980) Diseases of Marine Animals, vol 1. General Aspects, Protozoa to Gastropoda, John Wiley & Sons, Chichester.

Metselaar, M., Thompson, K.D., Gratacap, R.M.L., *et al.* (2010) Association of red-mark syndrome with a *Rickettsia*-like organism and its connection with strawberry disease in the USA. *Journal of Fish Diseases*, **33**, 849–858.

Stevenson, L.H. (1978) A case for bacterial dormancy in aquatic systems. *Microbial Ecology*, **4**, 127–133.

2

Bacterial Diagnosis and Control in Fish and Shellfish

Mags Crumlish

Institute of Aquaculture, University of Stirling, Stirling, Scotland, UK

Introduction

Aquaculture is described as an 'organised production of the crop in the aquatic medium' (FAO, 1987) and while this might be considered a very generic description, it is actually quite accurate given the diversity in production and range of species farmed. These systems are often categorized as either intensive, semi-intensive or extensive which is more a reflection of the production levels in these types of systems as the boundaries between each category are not well defined. Aquaculture is practised in all parts of the world and farms may be located in coastal areas, open marine water and inland in earthen ponds or river-based cages. Given the ubiquitous presence of bacteria within the environment, disease outbreaks can occur in each of these production types and locations.

Global aquaculture production has continued to expand at approximately 9% per year since the 1970s, with Asia dominating the production levels, particularly in finfish (FAO, 2014). It is in Asia that we see the largest and most rapid expansion. The growth of Asian aquaculture has outstripped that of European and North American production, which remains high but with limited capacity for significant growth compared with Asian aquaculture (Bostock *et al.*, 2010). This is primarily due to the increasing desire for intensification but also the availability of the more diverse species range suitable for farming in Asia. At present, it is estimated that more than 600 aquatic species are raised in freshwater, brackish and marine farms of varied intensity (FAO, 2014). These 600 species include both vertebrate and invertebrate animal species as well as plants, but for the purposes of this chapter, we will focus our attention on the most intensive farmed species that are traded globally for human food and include examples from finfish and crustaceans only. From this point onwards, the use of the term 'fish' includes finfish and shrimp unless otherwise stated.

Bacterial Infections in Aquaculture

Bacteria are described as single-celled organisms that have a rather simple cellular structure, lacking membrane-bound organelles. They are found ubiquitously in all habitats, including

Diagnosis and Control of Diseases of Fish and Shellfish, First Edition. Edited by Brian Austin and Aweeda Newaj-Fyzul.

fresh and sea water, and display a range of cellular morphologies. Bacterial classification relies on identification of phenotypic and genotypic characteristics and the relatively simple Gram stain reaction remains the most reliable method allowing species to be separated into either Gram-positive or Gram-negative groups. It is the chemical and physical properties of the bacterial cell wall that allow the retention of the coloured dye used during the Gram stain reaction. In aquaculture, disease outbreaks occur from both Gram-negative and Gram-positive bacterial species, which may be rod-like or spherical cocci in shape. It is not the purpose of this chapter to discuss in detail the varied bacterial species; the reader is referred to Austin and Austin (2016) for more in-depth detail on specific aquatic bacterial pathogens. A list of the commonly reported bacterial diseases that affect intensive monoculture systems is provided in Table 2.1.

The bacterial pathogens that have been identified and characterized the most are those that cause greater economic impact as determined through high mortalities or morbidity at the farm. At present, it is fair to say that we see more infections from Gram-negative than Gram-positive species (see Table 2.1). However, further intensification and introduction of novel host species combined with increasing consumer demand for non-local or exotic food types may change this in the future. Furthermore, bacterial identification and taxonomy is a rapidly developing area (Austin and Austin, 2016) as we move away from phenotypic-only tests and rely more on molecular tools for pathogen identification. This will not only result in taxonomic changes but with appropriate development, such methods may provide additional diagnostic tools leading to the production of novel control strategies applicable within aquaculture.

Bacterial Disease Diagnostics and Control of Infections

The principles behind aquatic bacterial diagnostics are similar to those practised in human clinical and terrestrial veterinary medicine. While the methods and approaches are similar, the type of samples and the diagnostic tests used will depend on the reason for the initial investigation. In aquaculture, diagnostic samples are provided to the laboratory to determine the health status of animals prior to transportation of live shipments or used to confirm that animals are specific pathogen free (SPF). However, like other farming sectors, the most common use of diagnostics in aquaculture is investigation of an unexpected mortality or morbidity within the farmed stocks from a suspected disease. Not all causes of mortality are infectious and so disease outbreaks can only be confirmed using a diagnostic approach. This means that to perform the diagnosis, we need to have a combination of information which includes the farm history and outbreak or event history, followed by a visual examination of the animals with and without clinical signs prior to taking samples for the laboratory tests.

Disease outbreaks are multifactorial, where the clinical outcome is dependent on the interaction between the host and the pathogen. To be more accurate, it is the interaction of the host immune response with the virulence factors produced by the pathogen that provides the range of clinical signs observed. Disease outbreaks in aquatic farms are often described as either acute or chronic, which is a reflection of the onset of the disease condition rather than an accurate description of the infection itself.

Reliance on observations of gross clinical signs of disease in aquaculture is limited, as the clinical presentation can vary tremendously and not all clinical signs have a microbial

Table 2.1 Bacterial pathogens commonly reported in intensive production systems.

Disease	Pathogen	Comments
Gram-negative bacteria		
Skin ulcers	*Aliivibrio logei*	
Cold water vibriosis or Hitra disease	*Aliivibrio salmonicida*	
Septicaemia or motile *Aeromonas* septicaemia (MAS)	*Aeromonas hydrophila* *Aeromonas sobria* *Aeromonas caviae*	Taxonomically difficult to identify at times, usually a complex
Furunculosis	*Aeromonas salmonicida*	
Enteric septicaemia of catfish (ESC) and bacillary necrosis of pangasius (BNP)	*Edwardsiella ictaluri*	
Edwardsiellosis	*Edwardsiella tarda*	
Edwardsiellosis	*Edwardsiella piscicida*	
Rainbow trout fry syndrome (RTFS) or cold water disease	*Flavobacterium psychrophilum*	Formerly *Cytophaga psychrophila*
Columnaris or saddleback	*Flavobacterium columnare*	Formerly *Flexibacter/Cytophaga columnaris*
Gill disease or gill rot	*Flavobacterium branchiophilum*	
Francisellosis	*Francisella asiatica* *Francisella noatunensis*	Warm-water species Cold-water species
Winter ulcer disease	*Moritella viscosa*	
Septicaemia	*Pseudomonas fluorescens*	
Red spot or winter disease	*Pseudomonas anguilliseptica*	
Pasteurellosis	*Photobacterium damselae* subsp. *piscicida*	Formerly *Pasteurella piscicida*
Marine columnaris	*Tenacibaculum maritimum*	Formerly *Flexibacter maritimus*
Septicaemia	*Vibrio alginolyticus*	
Vibriosis	*Vibrio anguillarum*	Also known as *Listonella anguillarum*
Vibriosis	*Vibrio ordalii*	
Enteric red mouth disease (ERM)	*Yersinia ruckeri*	
Gram-positive bacteria		
Streptococcosis	*Streptococcus agalactiae* *Streptococcus iniae*	Formerly *S. difficilis*
Lactococcosis	*Lactococcus garvieae*	
Bacterial kidney disease (BKD)	*Renibacterium salmoninarum*	
Mycobacteriosis 'fish tuberculosis'	*Mycobacterium* spp.	

aetiology. Infections due to the Gram-negative bacterium *Edwardsiella ictaluri* in Asian catfish species *Pangasianodon hypophthalmus* provide few if any external clinical signs (Ferguson *et al.*, 2001). It is only upon internal examination of these fish that the clinical signs may become more apparent. However, the clinical signs associated with infections due to *Aeromonas hydrophila* in many freshwater farmed fish species can be grossly similar to pathology arising from poor handling or grading stress. Identification of the cause of the disease problem is not simple as many factors, including both biotic and abiotic, can contribute to the disease process. It is fair to say that we are still scratching the surface of knowledge about the disease dynamics involved in an infectious disease outbreak within the aquatic farming environment.

In aquaculture, like other disciplines, the role of the bacteriology laboratory is to screen samples provided and identify the aetiological agent causing the disease under investigation. Most samples submitted to the laboratory are in the form of inoculated media plates which are incubated at an appropriate temperature and examined for colony growth and purity of culture. Given that recovery of a single bacterial species is rare from farmed aquatic animals, especially those that are sick, care must be taken during sampling to control unwanted contamination. The purpose of the initial colony morphology screening on the agar plates is to support the diagnosis of an infectious aetiology and not to identify every single organism that is recovered on the media. There is also a need to ensure that all sampling and subsequent investigations are performed aseptically to avoid unwanted contamination.

Species identification has traditionally relied on phenotypic tests to provide the identification of the suspected pathogen (Frerichs and Millar, 1993). It is the prerogative of each individual laboratory to decide on the number of samples to process and the range of assays to include during pathogen identification. This will depend on the capacity and capabilities of the laboratory. Primary identification tests often include Gram stain, a motility test, identification of either oxidase and/or catalase enzyme reaction and determination of oxidation or fermentation of a carbohydrate substrate such as glucose (Frerichs and Millar, 1993). This is usually sufficient to identify the bacterial species to genus if not species level and further testing can include biochemical profiling using one of the many commercially available kits.

The value of such traditional primary bacterial identification assays has been reduced over time as we include more molecular tools and yet, in many cases, they can provide immediate results and are cheap to perform. The cost-effectiveness of any test is important within any diagnostic service. Several biochemical kits are commercially available which are not specifically designed for use with aquatic pathogens but several authors have found them useful after minor adaptations. There are several types of kits available but the most frequently used include the API 20E, API ZYM, API 20NE, API 50 CH, Vitek® system (bioMérieux) and Biolog MicroPlates (Biolog, Inc.) (Popovic *et al.*, 2007).

All identification tests take place in the laboratory under controlled conditions following standard procedures as provided by the diagnostic staff and facility. Such protocols would be tested for sensitivity and specificity prior to implementation and should be reviewed regularly to ensure the most suitable methods are being applied. As in other animal production sectors, we have seen a move away from the more traditional bacterial identification methods towards the application of molecular-based probes, using nucleotide sequence analysis (Austin and Austin, 2016). The development of new technologies within aquatic diagnostics has relied on adaptations of techniques applied within human clinical and veterinary medicine (Adams and Thompson, 2011) and has led to the development of 'rapid diagnostics'.

Modern Approaches in Bacterial Diagnostics

Conventionally, most bacterial diagnostic assays are laboratory based but there is a move towards the production of more rapid diagnostic tools that can be applied directly at the farm site. The on-farm application is attractive within aquaculture, particularly in intensive farming practices where there are thousands of animals in a single farm. Therefore, one of the strengths of the pond or cageside diagnostic kits may lie in the ability to screen large populations for the presence of specific pathogens or the more rapid identification of fastidious organisms such as *Flavobacterium psychrophilum*, the aetiological agent of bacterial cold-water disease and rainbow trout fry syndrome (Davis, 1946; Madsen and Dalsgaard, 1998). Before moving away from centralized laboratories, first we need to develop a robust and reliable kit that is easy to use and provides rapid results at the farm. This might be considered the Holy Grail of aquatic bacterial infections.

Traditional laboratory-based identification tests are often considered time consuming and labour intensive. This is not productive within a diagnostic service where the emphasis lies on the ability to confirm the diagnosis in a timely manner. This has led to the development and uptake of molecular probes within aquatic disease diagnosis. Most bacteriology laboratories will use or have access to polymerase chain reaction (PCR) assays to help in the identification of specific bacterial pathogens. The PCR-based technologies rely on the detection of a common target specific to the bacterial species. This is normally within the conserved genes present on the bacterial ribosomal RNA or it may be detection of a specific housekeeping gene (Frans *et al.*, 2008). Over the last 20 years, numerous 16S rRNA assays have been developed and can be used for the identification or confirmation of a bacterial species within a sample. The obvious benefit of molecular tools is time reduction, especially as these assays are not reliant on the recovery of viable cultures.

The trend in application of nucleic acid assays within aquatic diagnosis has led to the development of multiplex PCR which allows the detection of multiple targets (pathogens) in a single sample. These are more advantageous as detection of more than one target in a single sample can significantly reduce the amount of time and consumables used when processing, thus reducing the overall assay costs. The lack of commercially available vaccines to control aquatic diseases is one of the key drivers in the development of rapid diagnostic kits.

Multiplex PCR assays have almost become routine within aquatic animal health research, with many providing simultaneous detection of three or more major pathogens within the sample. These have been developed for freshwater bacterial pathogens (del Cerro *et al.*, 2002; Panangala *et al.*, 2007), marine bacterial species (Gonzalez *et al.*, 2004) and several species of Gram-positive cocci causing streptococcosis in farmed fish (Mata *et al.*, 2004). Of course, all bacterial strains are not equally pathogenic, which led to the implementation of gene-specific DNA microarray assays that differentiated pathogenic strains. This was particularly useful in the detection of pathogenic *Vibrio* species within shellfish studies as the microbial community is likely to consist of a combination of pathogenic and non-pathogenic strains present within the sample (Panicker *et al.*, 2004).

Microbial epidemiology studies have applied the varied bacterial DNA fingerprinting methods, such as multilocus sequence typing (MLST) or pulsefield gel electrophoresis (PFGE), to promote rapid identification of infectious bacterial strains. Such assays have often relied on the presence of several 'housekeeping' genes and compared large numbers of strains from varied clinical outbreaks (Delannoy *et al.*, 2013). Screening large numbers of clinically distinct isolates provides the most robust data in understanding the incidence and prevalence of disease outbreaks. While such approaches have been used in aquatic pathogen studies, they remain expensive and time consuming and hence are not readily applicable for rapid diagnosis as yet. Whole genome sequencing was once considered prohibitively expensive but the costs are rapidly reducing and this is becoming a more attractive tool to support advances in aquatic bacterial disease investigation. It is in the field of proteomic research that perhaps we see the future of bacterial identification and disease diagnosis. The use of matrix-assisted laser desorption ionization-time of flight mass spectrometry (MALDI-TOF MS) allows the identification of bacteria using either intact cells or cell extracts. It is described as rapid, highly sensitive and economically cost-effective in terms of labour and running costs (Singhal *et al.*, 2015). The application of MALDI-TOF MS within the fields of clinical medicine and food microbiology is rapidly advancing (Pavlovic *et al.*, 2013) although uptake within aquatic bacterial studies is more limited.

Most aquaculture is performed in rural locations which is why the move towards pondside or on-farm rapid diagnostic kits is particularly attractive, as they can be applied on site. Lateral flow kits are good examples of the novel methods being developed in aquaculture. In the field of human medicine, such assays can be widely implemented, give a rapid response and support healthcare and diagnostics. The reader is directed to a review by Sajid *et al.* (2015) which provides excellent detail on the varied designs, formats and potential applications of lateral flow assays generally.

There are several research papers which advocate the use of rapid diagnostic kits in aquaculture and yet industry uptake has been poor. Technology transfer from the laboratory to the field has been a much more arduous process. Prior to implementation within routine diagnostics, more evidence is needed on how such methods might advantage the diagnosis where the clear benefit would be in early detection of disease outbreaks leading to measurable reduction in animal losses. There is a recognized need to ensure accuracy, specificity and sensitivity of the particular assay or kit but, perhaps more importantly, in aquaculture there is the cost-benefit analysis to consider.

Control Strategies Against Bacterial Diseases

Intensive farming systems have a health management plan which is embedded within the farming practice and will encompasses optimal nutritional, water quality and husbandry to ensure the health and welfare of the animals during production. Broadly, the health management plan will include prevention of disease outbreaks and treatment regimes during infections. Vaccination is now considered routine practice for many intensive finfish aquaculture systems where greater development of attenuated and DNA vaccines is predicted (Brudeseth *et al.*, 2013). However, the lack of commercially available vaccines for the global finfish culture as a whole means that there is a perpetual reliance on antibiotics to treat bacterial infections. Furthermore, farmed shrimp species cannot be conventionally vaccinated as they lack the appropriate immune system (Xiong *et al.*, 2016). This leads to greater reliance on biosecurity and alternative chemotherapeutants.

Biosecurity can be considered as a set of criteria, which may include physical, chemical or biological variables designed to protect against the entry and spread of pathogens within the farming system. As aquaculture has grown and intensified, we have seen a shift away from a comprehensive biosecure plan towards a more pathogen-specific approach. In some aquaculture sectors, this may be economically beneficial but the lack of a comprehensive biosecurity plan can leave the farming sector vulnerable to emerging aquatic diseases. A good example of this is the recent outbreak of acute hepatopancreatic necrosis disease, also called early mortality syndrome, due to specific strains of the bacterium *Vibrio parahaemolyticus* (Tran *et al.*, 2013). This disease was first reported in warm-water shrimp farms in China in 2009 and quickly spread to other countries which were intensively farming the warm-water shrimp (Zorriehzahra and Banaederakhshan, 2015). The impact of this disease heavily affected the global supply of warm-water farmed shrimp species (*Penaeus monodon* and *Litopenaeus vannamei*) where at the peak of the outbreak in 2013, global annual losses of more than US$1 billion were reported (GAA, 2013). Over-reliance on a single biosecurity practice such as only stocking with specific pathogen-free shrimp may weaken the overall biosecurity practices on the farm, leaving the sector vulnerable to the emergence of new pathogens or diseases.

By following a therapeutic regime, we can use antibiotics to effectively treat a bacterial infection in aquatic farming systems. Unfortunately, the concept of therapeutic antibiotic treatments has not been widely used outside the intensive salmon sector. There are many reasons for this but the lack of rigour and frequent misuse of antibiotics in aquaculture have promoted the spread of antibiotic resistance (Defoirdt *et al.*, 2011). Alternatives are actively being sought which has reignited the interest in bacteriophage therapy and probiotics (Newaj-Fyzul and Austin, 2015) in aquaculture.

Emerging Bacterial Diseases

Previously we have mentioned the growth and intensification of the global aquaculture sector and highlighted these strengths in enabling farmed aquatic food to become a significant contributor within global food security. However, without proper vigilance, these strengths may become opportunities for future disease outbreaks and certainly we are seeing a worrying trend in new and emerging diseases in aquaculture. Emerging diseases are not limited to the presence of novel pathogens but can also be applied more widely to mean appearance of an existing disease in a new geographical location or increased incidence of the disease. While new diseases continue to emerge, there are those that have had a more immediate impact in the global aquaculture sector. Outbreaks of francisellosis have caused significant mortalities in both warm- and cold-water fish farming sectors. These bacteria are described as intracellular Gram-negative coccobacilli causing high numbers of mortalities during outbreaks in the cod sector in Norway (Olsen *et al.*, 2006). This was due to *Francisella noatunensis* (Mikalsen and Colqhoun, 2010). Another species, *Francisella asiatica*, is the aetiological agent of warm-water francisellosis affecting farmed tilapia (Jeffrey *et al.*, 2010).

Previously, only two species of *Edwardsiella* were thought to cause disease in farmed fish species but comparative phylogenetic studies performed on *E. tarda* isolates have identified a new species called *E. piscicida* (Abayneh *et al.*, 2013). Outbreaks of disease from *E. piscicida* in farmed whitefish (*Coregonus lavaretus*) were reported recently in Finland (Shafiei *et al.*, 2016). In the last 10 years, the rainbow trout sector has suffered from emerging diseases with a suspected bacterial aetiology, including red mark syndrome (Ferguson *et al.*, 2006; Metselaar *et al.*, 2010) and rainbow trout gastroenteritis (Del-Pozo *et al.*, 2010). It is hoped that further analysis will assist in clarifying the role of bacteria recovered from these infections but both continue to cause significant economic losses for the farmed trout sector.

Climate Change and Aquatic Bacterial Disease

Descriptions of climate change impacting aquaculture are often separated into direct, for example water availability, water temperature, extreme climatic events, and indirect challenges, such as transport costs, aquafeed production and costs. Of these challenges, the most significant impact on aquatic bacterial infections is temperature. All bacterial species thrive at their optimal growth temperature. Most will survive within a temperature tolerance range, where their growth may be compromised but they remain viable. Sometimes we use thermal ranges to describe bacterial pathogens as cold water (psychotrophic) or warm water (mesophiles), but the reality is often that aquatic bacteria may survive in quite large thermal ranges.

It is not unusual to see the terms pathogen/pathogenicity/virulence used interchangeably when describing a bacterial disease and yet they have very specific meanings. So, before moving on to discuss the effect of temperature on bacterial disease, let's first agree on what these terms mean. The *pathogen* is the organisms or bacteria which are able to cause disease in a susceptible host species under the right conditions. *Pathogenicity* is the ability of the bacterium to cause disease and *virulence* is a way to measure how it might cause disease. We might think about virulence as the tools that the pathogen has to allow it to cause the disease. Specific bacterial pathogens possess a wide range of virulence tools (sometimes called factors) which may be intrinsic to the bacterial species and found on the chromosome, such as the presence of capsules and production of endotoxins. Or they may be acquired through mobile genetic elements such as plasmids and bacteriophages. The production and secretion of the virulence factors allow the pathogen to attach, survive, reproduce and colonize the host, thus causing an infection. As we will see, aquatic pathogenicity and infectivity are directly influenced by environmental temperatures.

Climate change resulting in elevated water temperatures will alter the incidence and prevalence of the bacterial diseases currently present in our global aquaculture systems. As a direct result of rising water temperature, we may see changes in the seasonality patterns associated with some bacterial infections, such as furunculosis due to *Aeromonas salmonicida* or bacterial kidney disease (BKD) from *Renibacterium salmoninarum*. These bacterial infections often occur during rising water temperatures (Gubbins *et al.*, 2013) as altered water temperatures will affect their incidence and prevalence.

Another outcome of climate change is the spread of bacterial pathogens into new geographical areas, resulting in emerging infections. Marcos-Lopez *et al.* (2010) reported that the Gram-positive *Lactococcus garvieae* may spread northwards within Europe due to climate change, thus directly changing the disease occurrence from this organism within aquaculture. The reported increase in *Vibrio*-related diseases is thought to be due to elevated sea surface temperatures again driven by climate change (Harvell *et al.*, 2002). *Vibrio* species are dominant in the marine ecosystem where they can cause disease in molluscs (Paillard *et al.*, 2004) and fish (Austin and Austin, 2016). Baker-Austin *et al.* (2013) correlated warming water temperatures with the increased emergence of *Vibrio* disease outbreaks observed in northern Europe. Such changes in water-borne infections are perhaps more of an immediate threat for shellfish farms as these production systems are located in coastal regions and already suffer from economically devastating disease outbreaks, commonly due to *Vibrio vulnificus*, *V. anguillarum*, *V. tapetis* and *V. splendidus* (Rowley *et al.*, 2014). While water temperature will certainly affect the growth and physiological response of the host, including immune activity (Langston *et al.*, 2002; Le Morvan *et al.*, 1998), it will also impact on the pathogenicity of the bacterium.

Ishiguro *et al.* (1981) demonstrated that incubating the bacterial species *Aeromonas salmonicida* at higher than optimal temperatures produced spontaneous mutants with lower virulence compared with the parent strains. There are several examples of thermal restriction influencing virulence expression in aquatic pathogens. Disease outbreaks in rainbow trout fry due to *Flavobacterium psychrophilum* are often reported when the water temperature is between 12 °C and 14 °C (Austin and Austin, 2012) where the lower temperature of 12 °C preferentially promoted upregulation of the *gfp* reported gene (Gomez *et al.*, 2012). This gene regulates proteolytic activity expressed by the bacterium, causing the degradation of the host tissues as seen in the typical presentation of external lesions (Ostland *et al.*, 2000) during disease outbreaks. Perhaps more work is required to determine the thermosensing properties of aquatic bacterial pathogens and their influence on virulence expression. Such data would significantly improve our understanding of bacterial disease dynamics in our aquatic farming systems.

Polymicrobial and Concurrent Infections

The concept of concurrent, simultaneous and polymicrobial infections in terrestrial animal farming practice is well established and yet this is only recently being considered in aquatic disease investigation. Given that bacteria and other microbes are ubiquitous in our farming waters and our knowledge of host–pathogen interactions is still developing, it is fair to say that this is an area of future research for aquatic bacterial diseases, particularly as the trend for intensive monoculture continues.

Experimental studies have explored the impact of polymicrobial outbreaks leading to increased mortalities in aquaculture systems. Parasitic infection in rainbow trout with *Myxobolus cerebralis* was found to impair the fishes' immune response, leaving them susceptible to infection with the bacterium *Yersinia ruckeri* (Densmore *et al.*, 2004). Increased mortality was reported in farmed Atlantic salmon that were exposed to sea lice (*Caligus rogercresseyi*) and then the bacterium *Piscirickettsia salmonis* (Lhorente *et al.*, 2014). Phuoc *et al.* (2008) showed that previous exposure to the viral pathogen resulting in the disease white spot syndrome, not only impairing the shrimp immune response but also increasing the growth and establishment of a subsequent *Vibrio* infection in shrimp. Further experimental studies have shown that co-infections can alter the pathogenicity of bacteria, resulting in higher mortality rates (Oh *et al.*, 2008) than those observed for single microbial infections (Dong *et al.*, 2015).

There is therefore a need to develop more robust experimental infectivity models which include polymicrobial and concurrent infections as this reflects more accurately the real-world situation in aquaculture sites. These new experimental models should also include the role of thermal preference in disease outbreaks. This would directly support the development of novel disease control strategies and reduce production losses.

Public Health and Aquaculture

The expansion of global aquaculture will place more demands on our natural water resources and increase the contact with and consumption of farmed aquatic animals. There is a concern that as a consequence, we may see increased incidence of fish-borne zoonoses

(Haenen *et al.*, 2013). While many aquatic bacterial pathogens have been suggested as zoonotic, the evidence is often lacking outside single case reports. In many cases of reported bacterial zoonosis from aquaculture, the patient had a pre-existing medical condition which left them immunocompromised and vulnerable to infection. As stated previously, given the thermal activity of aquatic pathogens, few are able to cause true zoonosis and so the current risk of bacterial zoonosis from aquaculture is low. Presently, true aquatic zoonosis is restricted to members of *Mycobacterium* species, *Streptococcus iniae, Clostridium botulinum* and *Vibrio vulnificus* (Gauthier, 2015). The bacterium *Erysipelothrix rhusiopathiae* is considered zoonotic yet it does not cause disease in fish (Gauthier, 2015). As described by Haenen *et al.* (2013), perhaps the perceived greater risk from aquatic zoonotic infections is through topical transmission.

Several *Vibrio* species can cause disease in both humans and aquatic animals although outbreaks remain low and exposure is often through wound infections. Baker-Austin *et al.* (2010) reported that although low in incidence, there is good evidence supporting zoonosis from aquatic *V. vulnificus* compared with other marine *Vibrio* species. Previously *V. vulnificus* was considered more of a threat to human health through consumption of infected seafood, particularly shrimp, oysters and clams sourced from either farmed or capture fisheries (Jones and Oliver, 2009). However, there is concern that people are suffering from serious wound infections from handling contaminated seafood or through increased exposure from infected waters where levels of *V. vulnificus* are high (Jones and Oliver, 2009).

Aquatic bacterial zoonosis is an area of developing research which would benefit from the use of genomic, especially transcriptomic technology to confirm pathogenic status and route of transmission. Combining the laboratory identification results with active epidemiological surveillance and risk analysis will help tremendously in confirming true zoonotic status (Gauthier, 2015).

Conclusion

The aim of this chapter was to describe the existing and emerging bacterial disease outbreaks that threaten the sustainable intensification of global aquaculture. Infectious disease outbreaks in aquaculture systems are complex and the application of modern diagnostic tools is helping to advance our knowledge of the bacterial infectivity process within the wide range of aquatic farming systems globally. Gaps in our knowledge are being addressed through the use of 'omics' technology which, given time, should provide tools to enable the rapid identification of pathogens and differentiation between pathogenic and commensal organisms. Global warming is an important ecological driver affecting all food production systems and climate-driven changes is likely to be the biggest challenge to how we cope with existing and emerging bacterial infections in our aquaculture farming systems.

References

Abayneh, T., Colquhoun, D.J. and Sorum, H. (2013) *Edwardsiella piscicida* sp. nov., a novel species pathogenic to fish. *Journal of Applied Microbiology*, **114**(3), 644–654.

Adams, A. and Thompson, K.D. (2011) Development of diagnostics for aquaculture: challenges and opportunities. *Aquaculture Research*, **42**(s1), 93–102.

Austin, B. and Austin, D. (2016) *Bacterial Fish Pathogens: Disease of Farmed and Wild Fish*, 6th edn, Springer Science, New York.

Baker-Austin, C., Stockley, L., Rangdale, R. and Martinez-Urtaza, J. (2010) Environmental occurrence and clinical impact of *Vibrio vulnificus* and *Vibrio parahaemolyticus:* a European perspective. *Environmental Microbiology Reports*, **2**(1), 7–18.

Baker-Austin, C., Trinanes, J.A., Taylor, N.G.H., Hartnell, R., Siitonen, A. and Martinez-Urtaza, J. (2013) Emerging *Vibrio* risk at high latitudes in response to ocean warming. *Nature Climate Change*, **3**, 73–77.

Bostock, J., McAndrew, B., Richards, R., *et al.* (2010) Aquaculture: global status and trends. Philosophical Transactions of the Royal Society B. Available at: http://rstb.royalsocietypublishing.org/content/365/1554/2897 (accessed 28 November 2016).

Brudeseth, B.E., Wiulsrod, R., Fredriksen, B.N., *et al.* (2013) Status and future perspectives of vaccines for industrialised fin-fish farming. *Fish and Shellfish Immunology*, **35**(6), 1759–1768.

Davis, H.S. (1946) Care and Diseases of Trout. US Department of Interior Research Report No. 12. US Government Printing Office Washington DC.

Defoirdt, T., Sorgeloos. P/ and Bossier. P. (2011) Alternatives to antibiotics for control of bacteria disease in aquaculture. *Current Opinion in Microbiology*, **14**(3), 251–258.

Delannoy, C.M.J., Crumlish, M., Fontaine, M.C., *et al.* (2013) Human *Streptococcus agalactiae* strain in aquatic mammals and fish. *BMC Microbiology*, **13**, 41.

del Cerro, A., Marquez, I. and Guijarro, J.A. (2002) Simultaneous detection of *Aeromonas salmonicida, Flavobacteium psychrophilum* and *Yersinia ruckeri*, three major fish pathogens, by multiplex PCR. *Applied and Environmental Microbiology*, **68**(10), 5177–5180.

Del-Pozo, J., Crumlish, M., Ferguson, H.W., Green, D.M. and Turnbull, J.F. (2010) A prospective longitudinal study of '*Candidatus* arthromitus'-associated rainbow trout gastroenteritis in the UK. *Preventive Veterinary Medicine*, **94**(3-4), 289–300.

Densmore, C.L., Ottinger, C.A. Blazer, V.S. and Iwanowicz, L.R. (2004) Immunomodulation and disease resistance in postyearling rainbow trout infected with *Myxobolus cerebralis*, the causative agent of whirling disease. *Journal of Aquatic Animal Health*, **16**, 73–82.

Dong, H.T., Nguyen, V.V., Phiwsaiya, K., *et al.* (2015) Concurrent infections of *Flavobacterium columnare* and *Edwardsiella ictaluri* in striped catfish, *Pangasiandon hypophthalmus* in Thailand. *Aquaculture*, **448**, 142–150.

Food and Agriculture Organization (FAO). (1987) Introduction to Aquaculture. Project Report RAF/82/009. Available at: www.fao/org (accessed 28 November 2016).

Food and Agriculture Organization (FAO). (2014) *The State of World Fisheries and Aquaculture*, Food and Agriculture Organization, Rome.

Ferguson, H.W., Turnbull, J.T., Shinn, A., Thompson, K., Dung, T.T. and Crumlish, M. (2001) Bacillary necrosis in farmed *Pangasius hypophthalmus* (Sauvage) from the Mekong Delta, Vietnam. *Journal of Fish Diseases*, **24**, 509–513.

Ferguson, H.W., Girons, A., Rizgalla, G., *et al.* (2006) Strawberry disease in rainbow trout in Scotland: pathology and association with *Flavobacterium psychrophilum. Veterinary Record*, **158**(18), 630–632.

Frans, I., Lievens, B., Heusdens, C. and Willems, K.A. (2008) Detection and identification of fish pathogens: what is the future? *Israeli Journal of Aquaculture- Bamidgeh*, **60**(4), 213–229.

Frerichs, G.N. and Millar, S.D. (1993) *Manual for the Isolation and Identification of Fish Bacterial Pathogens*, Pisces Press, Virginia Beach.

Gauthier, D.T. (2015) Bacterial zoonoses of fishes: a review and appraisal of evidence for linkages between fish and human infections. *Veterinary Journal*, **203**(1), 27–35.

Global Aquaculture Alliance (GAA). Available at: www.Gaalliance.org (accessed 28 November 2016).

Gomez, E., Perez-Pascual, D., Fernandez, L., *et al.* (2012) Construction and validation of a GFP-based vector for promoter expression analysis in the fish pathogen *Flavobacterium psychrophilum*. *Gene*, **497**(2), 263–268.

Gonzalez, S.F., Krun, M.J., Nielsen, M.E., Santos, Y. and Call, D.R. (2004) Simultaneous detection of marine fish pathogens by using multiplex PCR and a DNA microarray. *Journal of Clinical Microbiology*, **42**(2), 1414–1419.

Gubbins, M., Bricknell, I. and Service, M. (2013) Impacts of climate change on aquaculture. *MCCIP Science Review*, 318–327.

Haenen, O.L., Evans, J.J. and Berthe, F. (2013) Bacterial infections from aquatic species: potential for and prevention of contact zoonoses. *Revue Scientifique et Technique*, **32**(2), 497–507.

Harvell, C.D., Mitchel, C.E., Ward, J.R., *et al.* (2002) Climate warming and disease risks for terrestrial and marine biota. *Science*, **296**, 2158–2162.

Ishiguro, E.E., Kay, W.W., Ainsworth, T, *et al.* (1981) Loss of virulence during culture of *Aeromonas salmonicida* at high temperature. *Journal of Bacteriology*, **148**(1), 333–340.

Jeffrey, K.R., Stone, D., Feist, S.W. and Verner-Jeffrey, D.W. (2010) An outbreak of disease caused by *Francisella* sp. in Nile tilapia *Oreochromis niloticus* at a recirculation fish farm in the UK. *Diseases of Aquatic Organisms*, **91**, 161–165.

Jones, M.K. and Oliver, J.D. (2009) *Vibrio vulnificus*: disease and pathogenesis. *Infection and Immunity*, **77**(5), 1723–1733.

Langston, A.L., Hoare, R., Stefansson, M., Fitzgerald, R., Wergeland, H. and Mulchay, M. (2002) The effect of temperature on non-specific defence parameters of three strains of juvenile Atlantic halibut (*Hippoglossus hippoglossus* L.). *Fish and Shellfish Immunology*, **12**(1), 61–67.

Le Morvan, C., Troutaud, D. and Deschaux, P. (1998) Differential effects of temperature on specific and nonspecific immune defences in fish. *Journal of Experimental Biology*, **201**(Pt 2), 165–168.

Lhorente, J.P., Gallardo, J.A., Villanueva, B., Carabano, M.J. and Neira, R. (2014) Disease resistance in Atlantic Salmon (*Salmo salar*): coinfection of the intracellular bacterial pathogen *Piscirikettsia salmonis* and the sealouse *Caligus rogercresseyi*. *PLoS One* **9**(4), e95397.

Madsen, L. and Dalsgaard, I. (1998) Characterisation of *Flavobacterium psychrophilum*: comparison of proteolytic activity and virulence of strains isolated from rainbow trout (*Oncorhynchus mykiss*), in *Methodology in Fish Diseases Research* (eds A.C. Barnes, G.A. Davidson, M. P. Hiney and D. McIntosh) Fisheries Research Services, Aberdeen, pp. 45–52.

Marcos-Lopez, M., Gale, P., Oidtmann, B.C. and Peeler, E.J. (2010) Assessing the impact of climate change on disease emergence in freshwater fish in the United Kingdom. *Transboundary and Emerging Diseases*, **57**(5), 293–304.

Mata, A.I., Gibello, A., Casamayor, A., Blanco, M.M., Dominguez, L. and Fernandez-Garayzabal, J.F. (2004) Multiplex PCR assay for detection of bacterial pathogens associated with warm-water streptococcosis in fish. *Applied and Environmental Microbiology*, **70**(5), 3183–3187.

Metselaar, M., Thompson, K.D., Gratacap, R.M., *et al.* (2010) Association of red-mark syndrome with a Rickettsia-like organism and its connection with strawberry disease in the USA. *Journal of Fish Diseases*, **33**(10), 849–858.

Mikalsen, J. and Colqhoun, D.J. (2010) *Francisella asiatica* sp. nov. isolated from farmed tilapia (*Oreochromis* sp.) and elevation of *Francisella philomiragia* subsp. *noatunensis* to species ran as *Francisella noatunensis* comb. no., sp. nov. *International Journal of Systematic and Evolutionary Microbiology*, **59**. DOI:ijs.0.002139-0.

Newaj-Fyzul, A. and Austin. B. (2015) Probiotics, immunostimulants, plant products and oral vaccines and their role as feed supplements in the control of bacterial fish diseases. *Journal of Fish Diseases*, **38**(11), 937–955.

Oh, M.J., Kim, W.S., Kitamura, A.I., Lee, H.K., Son, B.W., Jung, T.S. and Jung, S.J. (2008) Change of pathogenicity in Olive flounder *Paralichthys olivaceus* by co-infection of *Vibrio harveyi*, *Edwardsiella tarda* and marine birnavirus. *Aquaculture*, **257**, 156–160.

Olsen, A.B., Mikalsen, J., Rode, M., *et al.* (2006) A novel systemic granulomatous inflammatory disease in farmed Atlantic cod, *Gadus morhua* L., associated with a bacterium belonging to the genus *Francisella*. *Journal of Fish Diseases*, **29**, 307–311.

Ostland, V.E., Byrne, P.J., Hoover, G. and Ferguson, H.W. (2000) Necrotic myositis of rainbow trout, *Oncorhynchus mykiss* (Walbaum): proteolytic characteristics of a crude extracellular preparation from *Flavobacterium psychrophilum*. *Journal of Fish Diseases*, **23**, 329–336.

Paillard, C., Le Roux, F. and Borrego, J.J. (2004) Bacterial disease in marine bivalves, a review of recent studies: trends and evolution. *Aquatic Living Resource*, **17**, 477–498.

Panangala, V.S., Shoemaker, C.A., van Santen, V.L., Dybvig, K. and Klesius, P.H. (2007) Multiplex-PCR for simultaneous detection of 3 bacterial fish pathogens, *Flavobacterium columnare*, *Edwardsiella ictaluri* and *Aeromonas hydrophila*. *Diseases of Aquatic Organisms*, **74**, 199–208.

Panicker, G., Myers, M.L. and Bej, A.K. (2004) Rapid detection of *Vibrio vulnificus* in shellfish and Gulf of Mexico water by real-time PCR. *Applied and Environmental Microbiology*, **70**(12), 7436–7444.

Pavlovic, M., Huber, I., Konrad, R. and Busch, U. (2013) Application of MALDI-TOF MS for the identification of food borne bacteria. *Open Microbiology Journal*, **7**, 135–141.

Phuoc, L.H., Corteel, M., Nauwynck, H.J., *et* al. (2008) Increased susceptibility of white spot syndrome virus-infected *Litopenaeus vannamei* to *Vibrio campbellii*. *Environmental Microbiology*, **10**(10), 2718–2727.

Popovic, N.T., Coz-Rakovac, R. and Strunjak-Perovic, I. (2007) Commercial phenotypic tests (API 20E) in diagnosis of fish bacteria: a review. *Veterinarni Medicina*, **52**(2), 49–53.

Rowley, A.F., Cross, M.E., Culloty, S.C., *et al.* (2014) Potential impact of climate change on the infectious diseases of commercially important shellfish populations in the Irish Sea – a review. *ICES Journal of Marine Science*, **71**(4), 741–759.

Sajid, M., Kawdw, A.N. and Daud, M. (2015) Designs, formats and applications of lateral flow assay: a literature review. *Journal of Saudi Chemical Society*, **19**, 689–705.

Shafiei, S., Viljamaa-Dirks, S., Sundell, K., Heinikainen, S., Abayneh, T. and Wilkund, T. (2016) Recovery of *Edwardsiella piscicida* from farmed whitefish, *Coregonus lavaretus* (L.), in Finland. *Aquaculture*, **454**, 19–26.

Singhal, N., Kumar, M., Kanaujia, P.K. and Virdi, J.S. (2015) MALDI-TOF mass spectrometry: an emerging technology for microbial identification and diagnosis. *Frontiers in Microbiology*, **6**, 791.

Tran, L., Nunan, L., Redman, R.M., *et al.* (2013) Determination of the infectious nature of the agent of acute hepatopancreatic necrosis syndrome affecting penaeid shrimp. *Diseases of Aquatic Organisms*, **105**(1), 45–55.

Xiong, J., Dai, W. and Li, C. (2016) Advances, challenges and directions in shrimp disease control: the guidelines from an ecological perspective. *Applied Microbiology and Biotechnology*, **100**(16), 6947–6954.

Zorriehzahra, M.J. and Banaederakshan, R. (2015) Early mortality syndrome (EMS), a new emerging threat in shrimp industry. *Advances in Animal and Veterinary Sciences*, **3**(2s), 64–72.

3

Complexities of Diagnostics of Viruses Affecting Farmed Aquatic Species

Manfred Weidmann

Virology Unit, Institute of Aquaculture, University of Stirling, Scotland, UK

According to the 2015 FAO report on aquaculture, there are 530 species of finfish, molluscs, crustaceans and other organisms used in aquafarming around the world. Thus there is the potential for a multitude of viruses to affect these species and a requirement for diagnostic tools to detect these. The implications are that virus diagnostics services will always be specialized for certain major (local) aquaculture species with an economic impact, since the whole variety of viruses affecting farmed species could never be handled by one single diagnostics provider.

Aquatic viruses (Box 3.1) drift through the water passively and their chance of hitting something in which to amplify is very low. Therefore, not surprisingly, aquatic viruses are very promiscuous with a huge host range. Infectious pancreatic necrosis virus (IPNV), for example, replicates in about 50 finfish species. A penned-in finfish shoal in a cage is an ideal situation for an aquatic virus. Once the infection establishes a hold, the basic reproduction number (R_0) of virus infection amongst the fish in the cage easily shoots beyond the threshold where only the host number can limit R_0.

Box 3.1 Virus abbreviations used in alphabetical order

Host Pisces

ENV	Erythrocytic necrosis virus	Iridoviridae
EHNV	Haematopoietic necrosis virus	Iridoviridae
IHNV	Infectious hematopoietic necrosis virus	Rhabdoviridae
IPNV	Infectious pancreatic necrosis virus	Birnaviridae
ISAV	Infectious salmon anaemia virus	Orthomyxoviridae
ISKN	Infectious spleen and kidney necrosis virus	Iridoviridae
KHV[a]	Koi herpes virus	Herpesviridae
NNV[b]	Nervous necrosis virus	Nodaviridae
OMV[c]	*Oncorhynchus masou* virus	Herpesviridae
PMCV	Piscine myocarditis virus	Totiviridae
PRV	Piscine orthoreovirus	Reoviridae

(Continued)

Diagnosis and Control of Diseases of Fish and Shellfish, First Edition. Edited by Brian Austin and Aweeda Newaj-Fyzul.

Box 3.1 (Continued)

RSIV	Red sea bream iridovirus	Iridoviridae
SAV	Salmonid alphavirus	Togaviridae
SGPV	Salmon gill poxvirus	Poxviridae
SVCV	Spring viraemia of carp virus	Rhabdoviridae
VHSV	Viral haemorrhagic septicaemia virus	Rhabdoviridae

Host Crustacea

CMNV	Covert mortality nodavirus	Nodaviridae
HPV[d]	Hepatopancreatic parvovirus	Parvoviridae
IHHNV[e]	Infectious hypodermal and haematopoietic necrosis virus	Parvoviridae
IMNV	Infectious myonecrosis virus	Totivirida
LSNV	Laem–Singh virus	Luteoviridae-like
MrNV	*Macrobrachium rosenbergii* nodavirus	Nodaviridae
PvNV[f]	*Penaeus vannamei* nodavirus	Nodaviridae
PmNV	*Penaeus monodon* nudivirus	Nudiviridae
PvSNP[g]	*Penaeus vannamei* singly enveloped nucleopolyhedrovirus	Baculoviridae
TSV	Taura syndrome virus	Picornaviridae
WSSV	White spot syndrome virus	Nimaviridae
YHV	Yellow head virus	Roniviridae

Host Mollusca

AbHV	Abalone herpes virus	Herpesviridae
OsHV-1 μVar	Microvariant of Oyster herpes virus	Herpesviridae

a) Synonym: Cyprinid herpesvirus 3 CyHV-3.
b) Nervous necrosis virus is a summary designation for betanodaviruses causing nervous necrosis in finfish. NNV isolates are grouped into four genotypes (SJMMV, TGNNV, BFNNV, RGNNV) and have been described from 24 finfish species (*Chelidonichthys lucernus* betanodavirus, *Dicentrarchus labrax* betanodavirus, *Diplodus vulgaris* betanodavirus, *Epinephelus costae* betanodavirus, Giant grouper nervous necrosis virus, Grouper betanodavirus, *Halobatrachus didactylus* betanodavirus, *Lates calcarifer* nervous necrosis virus, *Mullus barbatus* betanodavirus, Pacific cod betanodavirus, *Pagellus acarne* betanodavirus, *Paralichthys olivaceus* nervous necrosis virus, *Parapercis sexfasciata* nervous necrosis virus, *Priacanthus macracanthus* nervous necrosis virus, *Pterygotrigla hemisticta* nervous necrosis virus, Red spotted grouper nervous necrosis virus, Senegalese sole Iberian betanodavirus, Sevenband grouper nervous necrosis virus, *Sparus aurata* betanodavirus, *Spondyliosoma cantharus* betanodavirus, Striped Jack nervous necrosis virus, *Upeneus japonicus* nervous necrosis virus).
c) Synonym: Coho salmon herpesvirus (CHV).
d) Synonym: *Penaeus monodon* densovirus (*Pmo*DNV).
e) Synonym: *Penaeus stylirostris* densovirus (PstDV).
f) Synonyms: Monodon baculovirus (MBV), singly enveloped nuclear polyhedrosis virus from *P. monodon* (PmSNPV), *Penaeus monodon* nucleopolyhedrovirus (PemoNPV).
g) Synonym: *Baculovirus penaei* (BPV).

Diagnostics in aquaculture to date have focused on detecting virus usually when clinical signs are already apparent. However, too little is understood about how to detect an initial infection in a shoal and how to predict outcome. There are no concepts of clinical threshold. So the detection of a virus in a farmed finfish shoal actually comes down to throwing a dice to determine whether virus-positive fish are suffering from disease which will spread, or if they are just infected with no apparent disease which will not spread. Should an alarm be raised if the virus can be detected in the water? What is the indicative concentration threshold of virus from which such a warning should be translated into husbandry and management decisions? How many of the fish in a farmed shoal are infected and how many should be sampled to obtain a representative result? What are the factors that threaten the whole shoal, demanding management or control measures, and why are some shoals not affected by disease, even though viruses can be detected in some of the fish?

The picture can be complicated. For pancreatic disease (PD) caused by salmonid alphavirus (SAV), farmers describe that although SAV may be detected in fish in two out of 10 pens at one site, 95% of the fish will succumb to disease in one of the two pens whereas only a few will die in the second pen. Clearly genetic background, vaccination coverage, vaccine efficacy and possibly even behaviour patterns of the fish play a role.

Table 3.1 gives an overview of approved diagnostic tests as listed in the *Manual of Diagnostic Tests for Aquatic Animals* (Aquatic Manual) of the OIE. Virus isolation can only be performed by laboratories with virus culture facilities. For finfish, there are several recommended antigen detection methods, some relying on cell culture lysates, some on stamp smears from infected tissues. These tests vary in level of complexity and detection sensitivity and can essentially only be performed by specialized laboratories. Only polymerase chain reaction (PCR) is used at the same level as virus isolation and it has been shown that real-time (RT)-PCR is as sensitive as virus isolation for the detection of rhabdoviruses (Knusel *et al.*, 2007). Reflecting discussions in medical virology, RT-PCR is a very good tool to compensate for missing virus isolation facilities but it cannot replace basic virological, sequencing and epidemiological work as virus isolates are still the basis of all research and development (Carman, 2001).

The profit-oriented aquaculture industry needs to be aware that minimizing virus identification for fear of detecting notifiable viruses, and thus facing economic loss, will inevitably lead to missing emerging virus threats which have the potential to cause even more damage than any response to an isolated identification in one region. Unfortunately, short-sighted secretive avoidance strategies seem to prevail over far-sighted improvement.

Surprisingly, real time RT-PCR protocols are recommended for only 4/10 finfish-infecting viruses notifiable to the OIE and clearly more work needs to be done here to include this much better PCR method which is more specific (probes), less prone to carry over contamination (closed tube system) and adaptable to high throughput (robotic systems).

Some of the recommended RT-PCR protocols do not use specific probes for verification of the amplificate. SYBR Green-based RT-PCR with melting curve analysis has not survived in medical virus diagnostics as the melting curve peaks were shown to be subject to too much variation and therefore not reliable in a diagnostic setting. The specificity control provided by the probe is regarded as essential and given that decisions in aquaculture always entail commercial implications, non-probe formats are not appropriate.

Since a molecular test can be only as good as the sequence database it was designed from, sequencing efforts are essential. A review of sequences deposited in Genbank for finfish viruses relevant for European finfish aquaculture reveals that more effort is needed (Table 3.2). The majority of sequence entries for finfish are only partial and the impact of next-generation

Table 3.1 Tests recommended by the OIE for notifiable virus infections of farmed aquatic species.

Virus	VI	NT	Ag. detection Misc.	IFAT	Antigen capture ELISA	PCR	Real -time PCR	LAMP	ISH	DPH	Aquaculture species
EHNV	+		+		+	+					
RSIV	+		+	+		+					Pisces
ISAV	+			+		+	+				
SAV	+	+				+	+				
OMV	+	+				+					
KHV	+					+					
SVCV	+	+		+	+	+					
VHSV	+	+		+	+	+	+				
IHNV	+		+	+	+	+					
NNV*	+			+		+	+				
IHHNV						+	+		+	+	Crustacea
IMNV						+	+		+		
TSV			+			+	+		+		
WSSV						+	+	+	+		
MrNV			+		+	+	+	+	+		
YHV						+			+		
PmNV[a]						+			+	+	
PvSNPV[b]						+			+		
AbHV						+	+		+		Mollusca
OsHV-1 μVar						+	+		+		

Not detailed are EM, Immuno-EM and IHC techniques.
DPH, dot plot hybridization; ELISA, enzyme-linked immunosorbent assay; EM, electron microscopy; IHC, immunohistochemistry; IFAT, indirect fluorescent antibody test; ISH, *in situ* hybridization; LAMP, loop-mediated amplification; NT, neutralization test; PCR, polymerase chain reaction; VI, virus isolation.

sequencing (NGS) cannot yet be seen as the number of sequences deposited in the last three years (2013–2016) is not very high and the number of complete genomes or segments as a whole is very low indeed.

It is unclear how many sequences are withheld from publication as some of the aquafarming industry is loath to release information on virus detection and virus sequences. At the same time, profit-oriented thinking has led to the patenting of particular viruses in order to reserve the right to develop and commercialize the use of SAV-2 (WO2014041189 A12014 Norvartis Ag) and more recently efforts are under way to do the same for SGPV. These approaches inhibit free diagnostic test development and the advancement of diagnostics in aquaculture, to the detriment of the whole industry.

The availability of sequences is not much different for viruses affecting shrimp (see Table 3.2). However, since real time PCR is the best option for diagnostics in shrimp,

Table 3.2 Selection of sequences available for viruses infecting farmed aquatic species

Virus	Virus type	Segments	Sequences deposited in Genebank	Deposited 07-2013 and 07-2016	Complete segments	Aquaculture species
IPNV	ds RNA	2	776	29%	40 (5%)	
ISAV	-ss RNA	8	1568	12%	78 (4.9%)	
SAV	ss RNA	1	300	28%	14 (4.6%)	Salmonids
PMCV	ds RNA	1	152	10%	2 (1.3%)	
PRV	ds RNA	11	482	91%	141 (29%)	
NNV	ssRNA	2	953	12%	45 (4.7%)	Serranids
SVCV	-ss RNA	1	281	1%	11 (3.9%)	
VHSV	-ss RNA	1	890	6%	26 (2.9%)	Cyprinids
IHNV	-ss RNA	1	546	21%	7 (1.2%)	
WSSV	dsDNA	1	755	22%	0 (1.3%)	
YHV	ssRNA	1	86	20%	7 (8.1%)	
TSV	ssRNA	1	332	0%	6 (1.8%)	Penaeid shrimp
IMNV	dsRNA	1	27	77%	8 (30%)	
IHHNV	ssDNA	1	185	9%	14 (7.5%)	

companies (predominantly Asian) have real time PCR kits on offer for almost all the viral agents that affect panaeid shrimp (Table 3.3). This is in contrast to what is commercially available for molecular detection of viruses in finfish. There seems to be little demand for diagnostic kits for commercial finfish farming although a major impact has been reported from Europe for NNV on sea bream and sea bass in the Mediterranean (Vendramin *et al.*, 2016) and SAV on salmon (Kilburn *et al.*, 2012). This is a strong indicator that many centralized diagnostic services appear to be using in-house tests.

There have been calls to improve reporting of the performance of detection assays used in aquaculture (Gardner *et al.*, 2014) but there are no external quality assessement (EQA) panels available for OIE-recommended or in-house molecular tests to improve standardization of test results, as happened in medical virus diagnostics (Wallace and MacKay, 2013).

In general, the diagnostic scene seems to operate very much in an experience-based mode. However, in-house tests, even if used by government bodies, can fail. Infectious salmon anaemia virus (ISAV), an orthomyxovirus with eight negative sense RNA segments, occurs in a non-pathogenic and a pathogenic form which carries a deletion in segment 6 and an insertion in segment 5. These insertions/deletions are variant and can cause established tests to fail. The recommendation is to test for segment 8 which, however, cannot distinguish pathogenic from non-pathogenic forms of ISAV which is not ideal for a notifieable virus and the legal dilemma triggered by notification. Recent work additionally appears to show that the same fish population can simultaneously harbour non-pathogenic, pathogenic and transition forms of the virus (Cardenas *et al.*, 2014). Interestingly, this study used a high-resolution melting curve analysis to distinguish the various ISAV types. It remains to be seen if the variation of these peaks would stand up to diagnostic rigor, if it would make any sense to use

Table 3.3 Commercially available real time PCR kits for virus detection in farmed aquatic species

Virus	Gene-reach[1]	Mylab[2]	Thermo[3] Fisher	Speedy[4] assay	Profound[5] Kestrel	Techne[6]	Bioin Gentech[7]	Primer design[8]	Aqua-culture species	Production in million tonnes*
IPNV			+			+		+		1.8 M (MC Europe)
ISAV			+			+		+		
SAV							+		Salmonids	
PMCV										
PRV								+		
OMV							+			
VNNV	+						+	+	Serranids	3.3 M (MC Asia)
SVCV	+		+			+				40.3 M (IL Asia) 0.4 M
VHSV			+			+			Cyprinids	
IHNV			+			+		+		
KHV	+		+				+	+		(IL Europe)
WSSV	+	+	+	+	+					3.5 M (MC Asia)
YHV	+	+	+	+	+					
TSV	+		+	+	+					
IMNV	+		+	+					Paneid shrimp	
IHHNV	+		+	+	+			+		
PmNV				+						
HPV				+						

[1]http://www.iq2000kit.com/products_1.php?bgid=2,
[2]http://mylablifesolutions.com/mylab/wssv/,
[3]https://www.thermofisher.com/nuk/en/home/industrial/animal-health/aquaculture-fish.html,
[4]http://www.speedyassay.com,
[5] http://profoundkestrel.com/index.php?page=shrimp-viral-detection-2
[6] http://www.techne.com/product.asp?dsl=7085
[7] http://realtimepcrkit.com/index.php/cPath/48_9/osCsid/3j2k38ap9e9uencihf0gslmim0
[8]http://www.genesig.com/products
MC: marine and costal aquaculture, IL: inland aquaculture.
*Numbers FAO. 2016. *The State of World Fisheries and Aquaculture 2016. Contributing to food security and nutrition for all.* Rome. 200 pp.

this type of assay for diagnostics (Sepulveda *et al.*, 2012). Clearly, there is a need to better understand the molecular epidemiology of ISAV in order to design bespoke EQA panels with prevalent non-pathogenic and pathogenic ISAV types. These recent relevations also make a case for defining a clinical threshold for the presence of pathogenic ISAV in water and in diseased fish.

Despite some progress on VHSV (He *et al.*, 2014; Kahns *et al.*, 2012; Sandlund *et al.*, 2014), ISAV (Godoy *et al.*, 2013, 2014; Kibenge *et al.*, 2009; Lyngstad *et al.*, 2012) and SAV (Hjortaas *et al.*, 2016; Jansen *et al.*, 2010, 2016; Kahns *et al.*, 2012; Karlsen *et al.*, 2014), concise molecular epidemiology describing the variety of virus strains and their sequences of many viruses affecting aquaculture species still needs more effort, especially by using NGS methods to obtain more complete genome sequences (see Table 3.2).

There are few reports on the development of internal positive controls (IPC) using mimic-IPCs (Pierce *et al.*, 2013; Snow *et al.*, 2009). An irritating feature of viruses affecting fish is that they are very promiscuous; for example, IPNV has been detected in more than 50 fish species. If a particular virus affects a certain fish family, it may also affect several farmed species such as salmon and trout. One group addressed this by developing a detection assay for ELF1-alpha as a trans-species IPC present in all three salmonid species cultured in Chile (Sepulveda *et al.*, 2013).

A few multiplex real-time assays have been reported for the detection of rhabdoviruses infecting finfish (Liu *et al.*, 2008a; Vazquez *et al.*, 2016), and for several virus combinations affecting penaeid shrimp (Panichareon *et al.*, 2010, 2011; Xie *et al.*, 2008). Virus infections in shrimp usually emerge in the grow-out phase. Therefore, the combinations WSSV/IHHNV/TSV (China) (Xie *et al.*, 2008) and WSSV/YHV/HPV (Thailand) (Panichareon *et al.*, 2011) appear to reflect the economic impact inflicted by these viruses in different countries. For commercialization, this means that multiplex assays need to be tailored for certain geographic needs. Commercial kits would also need to contain an IPC, which is not the case in all the published assays and multiplex SYBR Green assays would not be the ideal choice because of the less acceptable melting curve analysis specificity control (Panichareon *et al.*, 2011). In general, the rationale for the development of a multiplex assay can be the differential analysis of a syndrome allowing for husbandry and management decisions or to cover the biggest threats and the implicated legal reporting requirements.

Another important issue is the matter of representative sample size. As aquaculture diagnostics focus on populations of hosts and less on the individual animal, it needs to derive the necessary information from a representative sample to decide if the presence of an infectious agent actually also means the presence of disease or the potential for an outbreak of disease. Sample size requirements published in the 1980s emphasized the need to take into account the relative efficiency of the detection method used (Simon and Schill, 1984). Therefore, field testing and assessment of sensitivity and specificity are absolutely necessary. Pooling of samples is widely accepted and supported by the OIE but statistical approaches on the reliability of using pooled samples are not available. Recently, an approach to testing the reliability of an assay for pooled samples was described in which estimates of the probability of the positivity of individuals in a positive pool and the real number of positive individuals in the pool were correlated through logistic regression. The comparison of results for RT-PCR assays and virus isolation for ISAV and SAV suggests that only highly sensitive assays should be used for testing of pools (Hall *et al.*, 2013, 2014).

Traditionally, pathologists have been instrumental in describing fish diseases. The approach to testing for antigens in the affected tissues has therefore been transferred straight to molecular diagnostics and therefore fish tissues (head, kidney, heart, liver, muscle, etc.) are the prominent sample types. In recent years, however, evidence has accumulated indicating that viruses infecting fish replicate in the blood. Betanodavirus replication was demonstrated by PCR in the serum of wild meagre (*Argyrosomus regius*) (Lopez-Jimena *et al.*, 2010). VHSV and IHNV were detected in the blood of experimentally infected wrasse (*Ctenolobus pipesterus*) (Matejusova, 2014) and zebrafish (*Danio rerio*) respectively (Ludwig *et al.*, 2011). ENV infects pacific herring (*Clupea pallasii*) and salmonids (Meyers, 2007), and can be detected in blood and experimentally passed between live fish via blood (Glenn *et al.*, 2012). ISAV was initially thought to enter only vascular endothelial cells but was later shown to attach, enter and replicate in leucocytes (Moneke *et al.*, 2005) and erythrocytes (Workenhe *et al.*, 2007). Most recently, the elusive ISAV HRP0 type from which the virulent ISAV evolves was finally isolated (Marshall, 2014) by using a trout blood-derived monocyte cell line RTS11 (Ganassin and Bols, 1998) after several unsuccessful attempts using other cell types. The strongest case for viruses infecting salmon is a recent publication describing PRV replication in the blood of live salmon. In a detailed analysis, the major PRV load was detected in erythrocytes (Finstad *et al.*, 2014).

Therefore, using blood as a sample material may allow for non-lethal sampling procedures and more simple nucleic acid extraction for molecular diagnostics in the future.

Crustaceans and molluscs do not produce antibodies. Detection of antibodies such as IgM, IgD and mucosal IgT in finfish is very unreliable. In many fish, IgM is the most prevalent immunoglobulin; IgM concentrations vary between individual fish and can range from 1 mg/mL to 12 mg/mL in different fish species (human total Ig 13 mg/mL) (Hordvik, 2015).

Little is known about the proliferation of antibodies, such as the time windows of titre development and therefore the diagnostic window for antibodies induced by individual fish viruses. It has been observed that antibody titre development also depends on temperature. Neutralizing antibodies are not common and only induced by some viruses in some aquaculture species (see Table 3.1).

Fish antibodies tend to be of low avidity in comparison to their mammalian counterparts. This is reflected in low sensitivity and specificity of ELISA assays developed for the detection of antibodies (Jaramilla *et al.*, 2016). These are therefore mostly use as screening tools, such as for screening vaccinated populations.

In general, there is a high variation in immune response among individual fish. Therefore, immune response has to be assessed as a function of a representative sample with a sufficient number of individual fish to allow linking an antibody immune response to absence or presence of an infection in a population of fish (Ronald, 2012).

Serological assays for virus detection in finfish, crustaceans and molluscs usually have antigen detection formats (IFAT, antigen capture ELISA, antigen detection in fixed or lysed infected cells, tissue stamps, dot blots) with comparable sensitivities to molecular detection methods (Adams and Thompson, 2008). Commercial antibodies to build antigen detection formats are available for only a few viruses and commercial kits are very rare indeed (Table 3.4). In recent years, there has been pronounced activity to develop monoclonal antibodies against rhabdoviruses affecting cyprinids (Chen *et al.*, 2008; Li *et al.*, 2015; Liu *et al.*, 2014; Luo *et al.*, 2014; Xu *et al.*, 2014).

Out of the nine or so isothermal methods that have emerged in the last 15 years, loop-mediated amplification (LAMP) and recombinase polymerase amplification (RPA) are the two that have been applied to virus detection in aquaculture. These methods allow amplification at one temperature, thus reducing the complexity of the amplification and

Table 3.4 Commercial antibodies

Virus	Antibody registry [1]	Aquatic diagnostics [2]	IFAT kit[3]	NT kit [3]	ELISA kit [4]	LFD kit[2,5]	Aquaculture species
IPNV	4	1	1	1			
ISAV	46	1				1	
SAV							Salmonids
PMCV							
PRV							
OMV							
VNNV		1					Serranids
SVCV							
VHSV	2						Cyprinids
IHNV	2						
KHV		1			3		
WSSV	1	1				1	
YHV							
TSV	3						Penaeid shrimp
IMNV							
IHHNV							
PmNV							
HPV							

[1] http://antibodyregistry.org
[2] www.aquaticdiagnostics.com
[3] www.ango.co/aquaculture-diagnostic-kits/
[4]www.kovax.co.il/products/kv3-elisa-kit/, www.vetmed.ucdavis.edu/vmth/lab_services/clinical_labs/Featured_tests/koi_herp_virus.cfm, www.absolute-koi.com/article7.html
[5] www.fkkasei.co.jp/english/product/medical/reagent/01.html
ELISA, enzyme-linked immunosorbent assay; IFAT, indirect fluorescent antibody test; LFD, lateral flow assay; NT, neutralization test.

detection device. They are considered as choice point-of-care tests (POCT) to allow on-site testing by non-specialized staff in order to reduce time to result. For RPA, there are dried reagents (pellets) available and various companies are working on pellets for LAMP (personal communication). RPA has been shown to work effectively in a diagnostic suitcase laboratory in field conditions (Faye *et al.*, 2015). Especially in Asia, there has been intense development of LAMP assays mainly for viruses infecting shrimp (Table 3.5). However, commercial kits have hardly emerged. The company GeneReach has recently started marketing a whole panel of isolated isothermal PCR (iiPCR) assays for shrimp and finfish viruses (www.iipcr.com/products.php). This PCR system uses the convection flow of the reaction volume in a temperature gradient generated in a capillary for the cyclic PCR reaction (Tsai *et al.*, 2014). With a detector (Pockit: www.iipcr.com/products.php) similar in size to the ones used for LAMP (Genie II: Pro-Lab Diagnostics) and RPA (Tubescanner: www.qiagen.com/gb/about-

Table 3.5 Overview of published isothermal methods for the detection of viruses infecting aquaculture species

Virus	LAMP	LAMP-LFD	RPA	RPA-LFD	Commercial kits	Aquaculture species
ISKNV		1				
IHMV	1					
IPNV	4					
KHV	6				2	
NNV	5					
SVCV	2					
CMNV	1					
HPV		1				
IHHNV	2	1	2	1		
IMNV	1	2				
LSNV	1	1				
MrNV	1	2				
PmNV	1	1				
PvNV	1					
TSV	2	3			1	
WSSV	4	1	1			
YHV	3				1	

Finfish viruses: ISKN (Suebsing *et al.*, 2016), IHMV (Gunimaladevi *et al.*, 2005), KHV (Cheng *et al.*, 2011; Gunimaladevi *et al.*, 2004; Liang *et al.*, 2014; Soliman and El-Matbouli, 2005, 2009; Yoshino *et al.*, 2009), NNV (Hwang *et al.*, 2016; Mekata *et al.*, 2014; Suebsing *et al.*, 2012; Sung and Lu, 2009; Xu *et al.*, 2010), SVCV (Liu *et al.*, 2008b; Shivappa *et al.*, 2008), IPNV (Soliman *et al.*, 2009; Suebsing *et al.*, 2011a,2011b, 2016), IPNV VSHV, IHNV (Suebsing *et al.*, 2011c). **Shrimp viruses**: CMNV (Zhang *et al.*, 2015), HPV (Nimitphak *et al.*, 2008), IHHNV (Arunrut *et al.*, 2011a; He *et al.*, 2010; Jaroenram and Owens, 2014a,2014b; Sudhakaran *et al.*, 2008; Sun *et al.*, 2006; Xia *et al.*, 2015), IMNV (Andrade and Lightner, 2009; Puthawibool *et al.*, 2009), LSNV (Arunrut *et al.*, 2011b, 2014), MrNV (Lin *et al.*, 2014; Pillai *et al.*, 2006; Puthawibool *et al.*, 2010), PmNV (Chaivisuthangkura *et al.*, 2009; Nimitphak *et al.*, 2010), PvNV (Suebsing *et al.*, 2013), TSV (Kiatpathomchai *et al.*, 2007, 2008; Sappat *et al.*, 2011; Teng *et al.*, 2007), WSSV (Caipang *et al.*, 2012; Chou *et al.*, 2011; Jaroenram *et al.*, 2009; Kono *et al.*, 2004; Mekata *et al.*, 2009a; Seetang-Nu *et al.*, 2013; Waiwijit *et al.*, 2015; Xia *et al.*, 2014), YHV (Jaroenram *et al.*, 2012; Khunthong *et al.*, 2013; Mekata *et al.*, 2006, 2009b; Yang *et al.*, 2016) . **Commercial kits**: http://loopamp.eiken.co.jp/e/products/primer/, http://www.technology-x.net/CN43/201310019401.html, www.biotec.or.th/biogallery/index.php/food-and-agriculture/shrimp-disease
LAMP, loop-mediated amplification; LFD, lateral flow assay; RPA, recombinase polymerase amplification.

us/contact/oem-services/ese-instruments/esequant-ts2/), this system may compete with real isothermal amplification assays. It remains to be seen which type of assay convinces in field trials. All these systems will, however, have to address the question of POC extraction and extraction throughput (sample size).

Especially in Asia, several attempts have been made to combine microfluidic platforms with fluorescent PCR (Kuo *et al.*, 2012; Lee *et al.*, 2007; Lien *et al.*, 2009), or LAMP (Chang *et al.*, 2013; Wang *et al.*, 2011), or direct detection through hybridization (Su *et al.*, 2015). At least one study actually tested the platform in the field. It is to be expected that miniaturized systems of this type will become available for multiplex monitoring of viral and bacterial agents in the future. But as with any kind of multiplexing, the cost-benefit analysis will only be positive if system developers conceptually include veterinary experiences so that they are able to design systems which will help to answer relevant questions.

References

Adams, A. and Thompson, K.D. (2008) Recent applications of biotechnology to novel diagnostics for aquatic animals. *Revue Scientifique et Technique*, **27**, 197–209.

Andrade, T.P. and Lightner, D.V. (2009) Development of a method for the detection of infectious myonecrosis virus by reverse-transcription loop-mediated isothermal amplification and nucleic acid lateral flow hybrid assay. *Journal of Fish Diseases*, **32**, 911–924.

Arunrut, N., Prombun, P., Saksmerprome, V., Flegel, T.W. and Kiatpathomchai, W. (2011a) Rapid and sensitive detection of infectious hypodermal and hematopoietic necrosis virus by loop-mediated isothermal amplification combined with a lateral flow dipstick. *Journal of Virological Methods*, **171**, 21–25.

Arunrut, N., Seetang-Nun, Y., Phromjai, J., Panphut, W. and Kiatpathomchai, W. (2011b) Rapid and sensitive detection of Laem-Singh virus by reverse transcription loop-mediated isothermal amplification combined with a lateral flow dipstick. *Journal of Virological Methods*, **177**, 71–74.

Arunrut, N., Suebsing, R., Withyachumnarnkul, B. and Kiatpathomchai, W. (2014) Demonstration of a very inexpensive, turbidimetric, real-time, RT-LAMP detection platform using shrimp Laem-Singh virus (LSNV) as a model. *PloS One*, **9**, e108047.

Caipang, C.M.A., Sibonga, M.F.J., Geduspan, J.S. and Amar, M.J.A. (2012) An optimized loop-mediated isothermal amplification (LAMP) assay for the detection of white spot syndrome virus (WSSV) among cultured shrimps in The Philippines. *Journal of Animal and Plant Sciences*, **22**, 927–932.

Cardenas, C., Carmona, M., Gallardo, A., Labra, A. and Marshall, S.H. (2014) Coexistence in field samples of two variants of the infectious salmon anemia virus: a putative shift to pathogenicity. *PloS One*, **9**, e87832.

Carman, B. (2001) Molecular techniques should now replace cell culture in diagnostic virology laboratories. *Reviews in Medical Virology*, **11**, 347–349.

Chaivisuthangkura, P. *et al.* (2009) Rapid and sensitive detection of *Penaeus monodon* nucleopolyhedrovirus by loop-mediated isothermal amplification. *Journal of Virological Methods*, **162**, 188–193.

Chang, W.H., Yang, S.Y., Wang, C.H., *et al.* (2013) Rapid isolation and detection of aquaculture pathogens in an integrated microfluidic system using loop-mediated isothermal amplification. *Sensors and Actuators B - Chemical*, **180**, 96–106.

Chen, Z.Y., Liu, H., Li, Z.Q. and Zhang, Q.Y. (2008) Development and characterization of monoclonal antibodies to spring viraemia of carp virus. *Veterinary Immunology and Immunopathology*, **123**, 266–276.

Cheng, L., Chen, C. Y., Tsai, M.A., *et al.* (2011) Koi herpesvirus epizootic in cultured carp and koi, Cyprinus carpio L., in Taiwan. *Journal of Fish Diseases*, **34**, 547–554.

Chou, P.H., Lin, Y.C., Teng, P.H., Chen, C.L. and Lee, P.Y. (2011) Real-time target-specific detection of loop-mediated isothermal amplification for white spot syndrome virus using fluorescence energy transfer-based probes. *Journal of Virological Methods*, **173**, 67–74.

Faye, O., Faye, O., Soropogui, B., *et al.* (2015) Development and deployment of a rapid recombinase polymerase amplification Ebola virus detection assay in Guinea in 2015. *Euro Surveillance*, **20**(44). DOI: 10.2807/1560-7917.ES.2015.20.44.30053.

Finstad, O.W., Dahle, M.K., Lindholm, T.H., *et al.* Piscine orthoreovirus (PRV) infects Atlantic salmon erythrocytes. *Veterinary Research*, **45**, 35.

Ganassin, R.C. and Bols, N.C. (1998) Development of a monocyte/macrophage-like cell line, RTS11, from rainbow trout spleen. *Fish and Shellfish Immunology*, **8**, 457–476.

Gardner, I.A., Burnley, T. and Caraguel, C. (2014) Improvements are needed in reporting of accuracy studies for diagnostic tests used for detection of finfish pathogens. *Journal of Aquatic Animal Health*, **26**, 203–209.

Glenn, J.A., Emmenegger, E.J., Grady, C.A., *et al.* (2012) Kinetics of viral load and erythrocytic inclusion body formation in Pacific herring artificially infected with erythrocytic necrosis virus. *Journal of Aquatic Animal Health*, **24**, 195–200.

Godoy, M.G., Kibenge, M.J., Suarez, R., *et al.* (2013) Infectious salmon anaemia virus (ISAV) in Chilean Atlantic salmon (*Salmo salar*) aquaculture: emergence of low pathogenic ISAV-HPR0 and re-emergence of virulent ISAV-HPR: HPR3 and HPR14. *Virology Journal*, **10**, 344.

Godoy, M.G., Suarez, R., Lazo, E.S., *et al.* (2014) Genetic analysis and comparative virulence of infectious salmon anemia virus (ISAV) types HPR7a and HPR7b from recent field outbreaks in Chile. *Virology Journal*, **11**, 204.

Gunimaladevi, I., Kono, T., Venugopal, M.N. and Sakai, M. (2004) Detection of koi herpesvirus in common carp, *Cyprinus carpio* L., by loop-mediated isothermal amplification. *Journal of Fish Diseases*, **27**, 583–589.

Gunimaladevi, I., Kono, T., Lapatra, S.E. and Sakai, M. (2005) A loop mediated isothermal amplification (LAMP) method for detection of infectious hematopoietic necrosis virus (IHNV) in rainbow trout (*Oncorhynchus mykiss*). *Archives of Virology*, **150**, 899–909.

Hall, L.M., Wallace, I. and Munro, L. (2013) Reliability of individual and pooled test procedures for detecting the pathogenic agent for clinical infectious salmon anaemia. *Journal of Fish Diseases*, **36**, 741–74.

Hall, L.M., Munro, L. and Wallace, I. (2014) An approach to evaluating the reliability of diagnostic tests on pooled groups of infected individuals. *Preventive Veterinary Medicine*, **116**, 305–312.

He, L., Xu, H.S., Wang, M.Z. and Rong, H.N. (2010) [Development of rapid detection of infectious hypodermal and hematopoietic necrosis virus by loop-mediated isothermal amplification.] *Bing Du Xue Bao*, **26**, 490–495.

He, M., Yan, X.C., Liang, Y., Sun, X.W. and Teng, C.B. (2014) Evolution of the viral hemorrhagic septicemia virus: divergence, selection and origin. *Molecular Phylogenetics and Evolution*, **77**, 34–40.

Hjortaas, M.J., Bang Jensen, B., Taksdal, T., *et al.* (2016) Genetic characterization of salmonid alphavirus in Norway. *Journal of Fish Diseases*, **39**, 249–257.

Hordvik, I. (2015) Immunoglobulin isotypes in Atlantic salmon, *Salmo salar*. *Biomolecules*, **5**, 166–177.

Hwang, J., Suh, S.S., Park, M., *et al.* (2016) Detection of coat protein gene of nervous necrosis virus using loop-mediated isothermal amplification. *Asian Pacific Journal of Tropical Medicine*, **9**, 235–240.

Jansen, M.D., Gjerset, B., Modahl, I. and Bohlin, J. (2010) Molecular epidemiology of salmonid alphavirus (SAV) subtype 3 in Norway. *Virology Journal*, **7**, 188.

Jansen, M.D., Bang Jensen, B., McLoughlin, M., *et al.* (2016) The epidemiology of pancreas disease in salmonid aquaculture: a summary of the current state of knowledge. *Journal of Fish Diseases*, DOI:10.1111/jfd.12478.

Jaramillo, D., Durr, S., Hick, P. and Whittington, R. (2016) Bayesian estimation of diagnostic sensitivity and specificity of a nervous necrosis virus antibody ELISA. *Preventive Veterinary Medicine*, **123**, 138–142.

Jaroenram, W. and Owens, L. (2014a) Separation of endogenous viral elements from infectious *Penaeus stylirostris* densovirus using recombinase polymerase amplification. *Molecular and Cellular Probes*, **28**, 284–287.

Jaroenram, W. and Owens, L. (2014b) Recombinase polymerase amplification combined with a lateral flow dipstick for discriminating between infectious *Penaeus stylirostris* densovirus and virus-related sequences in shrimp genome. *Journal of Virological Methods*, **208**, 144–151.

Jaroenram, W., Kiatpathomchai, W. and Flegel, T.W. (2009) Rapid and sensitive detection of white spot syndrome virus by loop-mediated isothermal amplification combined with a lateral flow dipstick. *Molecular and Cellular Probes*, **23**, 65–70.

Jaroenram, W., Arunrut, N. and Kiatpathomchai, W. (2012) Rapid and sensitive detection of shrimp yellow head virus using loop-mediated isothermal amplification and a colorogenic nanogold hybridization probe. *Journal of Virological Methods*, **186**, 36–42.

Kahns, S., Skall, H.F., Kaas, R.S., *et al.* (2012) European freshwater VHSV genotype Ia isolates divide into two distinct subpopulations. *Diseases of Aquatic Organisms*, **99**, 23–35.

Karlsen, M., Gjerset, B., Hansen, T. and Rambaut, A. (2014) Multiple introductions of salmonid alphavirus from a wild reservoir have caused independent and self-sustainable epizootics in aquaculture. *Journal of General Virology*, **95**, 52–59.

Khunthong, S., Jaroenram, W., Arunrut, N., *et al.* (2013) Rapid and sensitive detection of shrimp yellow head virus by loop-mediated isothermal amplification combined with a lateral flow dipstick. *Journal of Virological Methods*, **188**, 51–56.

Kiatpathomchai, W., Jareonram, W., Jitrapakdee, S. and Flegel, T.W. (2007) Rapid and sensitive detection of Taura syndrome virus by reverse transcription loop-mediated isothermal amplification. *Journal of Virological Methods*, **146**, 125–128.

Kiatpathomchai, W., Jaroenram, W., Arunrut, N., Jitrapakdee, S. and Flegel, T.W. (2008) Shrimp Taura syndrome virus detection by reverse transcription loop-mediated isothermal amplification combined with a lateral flow dipstick. *Journal of Virological Methods*, **153**, 214–217.

Kibenge, F.S., Godoy, M.G., Wang, Y., *et al.* (2009) Infectious salmon anaemia virus (ISAV) isolated from the ISA disease outbreaks in Chile diverged from ISAV isolates from Norway around 1996 and was disseminated around 2005, based on surface glycoprotein gene sequences. *Virology Journal*, **6**, 88.

Kilburn, R., Murray, A.G., Hall, M., *et al.* (2012) Analysis of a company's production data to describe the epidemiology and persistence of pancreas disease in Atlantic salmon (*Salmo salar* L.) farms off Western Scotland. *Aquaculture*, **368**, 89–94.

Knusel, R., Bergmann, S. M., Einer-Jensen, K., *et al.* (2007) Virus isolation vs RT-PCR: which method is more successful in detecting VHSV and IHNV in fish tissue sampled under field conditions? *Journal of Fish Diseases*, **30**, 559–568.

Kono, T., Savan, R., Sakai, M. and Itami, T. (2004) Detection of white spot syndrome virus in shrimp by loop-mediated isothermal amplification. *Journal of Virological Methods*, **115**, 59–65.

Kuo, H.C., Wang, T.Y., Hsu, H.H., *et al.* (2012) An automated microfluidic chip system for detection of piscine nodavirus and characterization of its potential carrier in grouper farms. *PLoS One*, 7(8), e42203.

Lee, S.H., Ou, M.C., Chen, T.Y., *et al.* (2007) Integrated microfluidic chip for fast diagnosis of piscine nodavirus. 14th International Conference on Solid-State Sensors, Actuators and Microsystems, Lyon, France, June 10–14. Available at: http://ieeexplore.ieee.org/document/4300287/ (accessed 13 December 2016).

Li, Z., Zhang, Q., Luo, P., *et al.* (2015) Monoclonal antibody against M protein of spring viremia of carp virus. *Monoclonal Antibodies in Immunodiagnosis and Immunotherapy*, **34**, 122–125.

Liang, L.G., Xie, J. and Luo, D. (2014) Development of a rapid cyprinid herpesvirus 2 detection method by loop-mediated isothermal amplification. *Letters in Applied Microbiology*, **59**, 432–437.

Lien, K.Y., Lee, S.H., Tsai, T.J., *et al.* (2009) A microfluidic-based system using reverse transcription polymerase chain reactions for rapid detection of aquaculture diseases. *Microfluidics and Nanofluidics*, 7(6), 795–806.

Lin, F., Liu, L., Hao, G.J., *et al.* (2014) [Rapid detection of *Macrobrachium rosenbergii* nodavirus isolated in China by a reverse-transcription loop-mediated isothermal amplification assay combined with a lateral flow dipstick method.] *Bing Du Xue Bao*, **30**, 502–507.

Liu, H., Zheng, X., Shi, X., *et al.* (2014) Selection and characterization of single-chain recombinant antibodies against infectious haematopoietic necrosis virus from mouse phage display library. *Journal of Virological Methods*, **205**, 61–67.

Liu, Z.X., Teng, Y., Liu, H., *et al.* (2008a) Simultaneous detection of three fish rhabdoviruses using multiplex real-time quantitative RT-PCR assay. *Journal of Virological Methods*, **149**, 103–109.

Liu, Z., Teng, Y., Xie, X., *et al.* (2008b) Development and evaluation of a one-step loop-mediated isothermal amplification for detection of spring viraemia of carp virus. *Journal of Applied Microbiology*, **105**, 1220–1226.

Lopez-Jimena, B., Cherif, N., Garcia-Rosado, E., *et al.* (2010) A combined RT-PCR and dot-blot hybridization method reveals the coexistence of SJNNV and RGNNV betanodavirus genotypes in wild meagre (*Argyrosomus regius*). *Journal of Applied Microbiology*, **109**, 1361–1369.

Ludwig, M., Palha, N., Torhy, C., *et al.* (2011) Whole-body analysis of a viral infection: vascular endothelium is a primary target of infectious hematopoietic necrosis virus in zebrafish larvae. *Plos Pathogens*, 7, e1001269.

Luo, P., Ruan, X., Zhang, Q., *et al.* (2014) Monoclonal antibodies against G protein of spring viremia of carp virus. *Monoclonal Antibodies in Immunodiagnosis and Immunotherapy*, **33**, 340–343.

Lyngstad, T.M., Kristoffersen, A.B., Hjortaas, M.J., *et al.* (2012) Low virulent infectious salmon anaemia virus (ISAV-HPR0) is prevalent and geographically structured in Norwegian salmon farming. *Diseases of Aquatic Organisms*, **101**, 197–206.

Marshall, S.M. (2014) Molecular signatures supporting ongoing evolution of infectious salmon anemia virus in Chile. Paper presented at the 9th International Symposium on Viruses of Lower Vertebrates, Malaga, 2014.

Matejusova, I. (2014) Susceptibility of goldsinny Wrasse (*Ctenolabrus rupestris*) to viral haemorrhgaic septicaemia virus (VHSV). Paper presented at the 9th International Symposium on Viruses of Lower Vertebrates, Malaga, 2014.

Mekata, T., Kono, T., Savan, R., *et al.* (2006) Detection of yellow head virus in shrimp by loop-mediated isothermal amplification (LAMP). *Journal of Virological Methods*, **135**, 151–156.

Mekata, T., Sudhakaran, R., Kono, T., *et al.* (2009a) Real-time quantitative loop-mediated isothermal amplification as a simple method for detecting white spot syndrome virus. *Letters in Applied Microbiology*, **48**, 25–32.

Mekata, T., Sudhakaran, R., Kono, T., *et al.* (2009b) Real-time reverse transcription loop-mediated isothermal amplification for rapid detection of yellow head virus in shrimp. *Journal of Virological Methods*, **162**, 81–87.

Mekata, T., Satoh, J., Inada, M., *et al.* (2014) Development of simple, rapid and sensitive detection assay for grouper nervous necrosis virus using real-time loop-mediated isothermal amplification. *Journal of Fish Diseases*, DOI:10.1111/jfd.12297.

Meyers, T.R. (2007) First report of erythrocytic inclusion body syndrome (EIBS) in chinook salmon *Oncorhynchus tshawytscha* in Alaska, USA. *Diseases of Aquatic Organisms*, **76**, 169–172.

Moneke, E., Ikede, B.O. and Kibenge, F.S.B. (2005) Viremia during infectious salmon anemia virus infection of Atlantic salmon is associated with replicating virus in leucocytes. *Diseases of Aquatic Organisms*, **66**, 153–157.

Nimitphak, T., Kiatpathomchai, W. and Flegel, T.W. (2008) Shrimp hepatopancreatic parvovirus detection by combining loop-mediated isothermal amplification with a lateral flow dipstick. *Journal of Virological Methods*, **154**, 56–60.

Nimitphak, T., Meemetta, W., Arunrut, N., Senapin, S. and Kiatpathomchai, W. (2010) Rapid and sensitive detection of *Penaeus monodon* nucleopolyhedrovirus (PemoNPV) by loop-mediated isothermal amplification combined with a lateral-flow dipstick. *Molecular and Cellular Probes*, **24**, 1–5.

Panichareon, B., Khawsak, P., Deesukon, W. and Sukhumsirichart, W. (2010) Development of multiplex real-time PCR and high-resolution melt analysis for detection of three viruses in penaeid shrimp. *Journal of Biotechnology*, **150**, S127.

Panichareon, B., Khawsak, P., Deesukon, W. and Sukhumsirichart, W. (2011) Multiplex real-time PCR and high-resolution melting analysis for detection of white spot syndrome virus, yellow-head virus, and *Penaeus monodon* densovirus in penaeid shrimp. *Journal of Virological Methods*, **178**, 16–21.

Pierce, L.R., Willey, J.C., Crawford, E.L., *et al.* (2013) A new StaRT-PCR approach to detect and quantify fish Viral Hemorrhagic Septicemia virus (VHSv): enhanced quality control with internal standards. *Journal of Virological Methods*, **189**, 129–142.

Pillai, D., Bonami, J.R. and Sri Widada, J. (2006) Rapid detection of *Macrobrachium rosenbergii* nodavirus (MrNV) and extra small virus (XSV), the pathogenic agents of white tail disease of *Macrobrachium rosenbergii* (De Man), by loop-mediated isothermal amplification. *Journal of Fish Diseases*, **29**, 275–283.

Puthawibool, T., Senapin, S., Kiatpathomchai, W. and Flegel, T.W. (2009) Detection of shrimp infectious myonecrosis virus by reverse transcription loop-mediated isothermal amplification combined with a lateral flow dipstick. *Journal of Virological Methods*, **156**, 27–31.

Puthawibool, T., Senapin, S., Flegel, T.W. and Kiatpathomchai, W. (2010) Rapid and sensitive detection of *Macrobrachium rosenbergii* nodavirus in giant freshwater prawns by reverse transcription loop-mediated isothermal amplification combined with a lateral flow dipstick. *Molecular and Cellular Probes* **24**, 244–249.

Ronald, J.R. (2012) The virology of teleosts, in *Fish Pathology*, Blackwell, Oxford, pp.186–291.

Sandlund, N., Gjerset, B., Bergh, O., *et al.* (2014) Screening for viral hemorrhagic septicemia virus in marine fish along the Norwegian coastal line. *PloS One*, **9**, e108529.

Sappat, A., Jaroenram, W., Puthawibool, T., *et al.* (2011) Detection of shrimp Taura syndrome virus by loop-mediated isothermal amplification using a designed portable multi-channel turbidimeter. *Journal of Virological Methods*, **175**, 141–148.

Seetang-Nun, Y., Jaroenram, W., Sriurairatana, S., Suebsing, R. and Kiatpathomchai, W. (2013) Visual detection of white spot syndrome virus using DNA-functionalized gold nanoparticles as probes combined with loop-mediated isothermal amplification. *Molecular and Cellular Probes*, **27**, 71–79.

Sepulveda, D., Cardenas, C., Carmona, M. and Marshall, S.H. (2012) Novel strategy to evaluate infectious salmon anemia virus variants by high resolution melting. *PloS One*, **7**(6), e37265.

Sepulveda, D., Bohle, H., Labra, A., Grothusen, H. and Marshall, S.H. (2013) Design and evaluation of a unique RT-qPCR assay for diagnostic quality control assessment that is applicable to pathogen detection in three species of salmonid fish. *BMC Veterinary Research*, **9**, 183.

Shivappa, R.B., Savan, R., Kono, T., *et al.* (2008) Detection of spring viraemia of carp virus (SVCV) by loop-mediated isothermal amplification (LAMP) in koi carp, *Cyprinus carpio* L. *Journal of Fish Diseases*, **31**, 249–258.

Simon, R.C. and Schill, W.B. (1984) Tables of sample-size requirements for detection of fish infected by pathogens – 3 confidence levels for different infection prevalence and various population sizes. *Journal of Fish Diseases*, **7**, 515–520.

Snow, M., McKay, P. and Matejusova, I. (2009) Development of a widely applicable positive control strategy to support detection of infectious salmon anaemia virus (ISAV) using Taqman real-time PCR. *Journal of Fish Diseases*, **32**, 151–156.

Soliman, H. and El-Matbouli, M. (2005) An inexpensive and rapid diagnostic method of Koi Herpesvirus (KHV) infection by loop-mediated isothermal amplification. *Virology Journal*, **2**, 83.

Soliman, H. and El-Matbouli, M. (2009) Immunocapture and direct binding loop mediated isothermal amplification simplify molecular diagnosis of Cyprinid herpesvirus-3. *Journal of Virological Methods*, **162**, 91–95.

Soliman, H., Midtlyng, P.J. and El-Matbouli, M. (2009) Sensitive and rapid detection of infectious pancreatic necrosis virus by reverse transcription loop mediated isothermal amplification. *Journal of Virological Methods*, **158**, 77–83.

Su, Y.C., Wang, C.H, Chang, W.H., *et al.* (2015) Rapid and amplification-free detection of fish pathogens by utilizing a molecular beacon-based microfluidic system. *Biosensors and Bioelectronics*, **63**, 196–203.

Sudhakaran, R., Mekata, T., Kono, T., *et al.* (2008) Rapid detection and quantification of infectious hypodermal and hematopoietic necrosis virus in whiteleg shrimp *Penaeus vannamei* using real-time loop-mediated isothermal amplification. *Fish Pathology*, **43**, 170–173.

Suebsing, R., Jeon, C.H., Oh, M.J. and Kim, J.H. (2011a) Reverse transcriptase loop-mediated isothermal amplification assay for infectious hematopoietic necrosis virus in *Oncorhynchus keta*. *Diseases of Aquatic Organisms*, **94**, 1–8.

Suebsing, R., Oh, M.J. and Kim, J.H. (2011b) Evaluation of rapid and sensitive reverse transcription loop-mediated isothermal amplification method for detecting infectious pancreatic necrosis virus in chum salmon (*Oncorhynchus keta*). *Journal of Veterinary Diagnostic Investigation*, **23**, 704–709.

Suebsing, R., Kim, J.H., Kim, S.R., Park, M.A. and Oh, M.J. (2011c) Detection of viruses in farmed rainbow trout (*Oncorhynchus mykiss*) in Korea by RT-LAMP assay. *Journal of Microbiology*, **49**, 741–746.

Suebsing, R., Oh, M.J. and Kim, J.H. (2012) Development of a reverse transcription loop-mediated isothermal amplification assay for detecting nervous necrosis virus in olive flounder *Paralichthys olivaceus*. *Journal of Microbiology and Biotechnology*, **22**, 1021–1028.

Suebsing, R., Prombun, P. and Kiatpathomchai, W. (2013) *Reverse transcription loop-mediated* isothermal amplification (RT-LAMP) combined with colorimetric gold nanoparticle (AuNP) probe assay for visual detection of *Penaeus vannamei* nodavirus (PvNV). *Letters in Applied Microbiology*, **56**, 428–435.

Suebsing, R., Pradeep, P.J., Jitrakorn, S., *et al.* (2016) Detection of natural infection of infectious spleen and kidney necrosis virus in farmed tilapia by hydroxynapthol blue-loop-mediated isothermal amplification assay. *Journal of Applied Microbiology*, **121**, 55–67.

Sun, Z.F., Hu, C.Q., Ren, C.H. and Shen, Q. (2006) Sensitive and rapid detection of infectious hypodermal and hematopoietic necrosis virus (IHHNV) in shrimps by loop-mediated isothermal amplification. *Journal of Virological Methods*, **131**, 41–46.

Sung, C.H. and Lu, J.K. (2009) Reverse transcription loop-mediated isothermal amplification for rapid and sensitive detection of nervous necrosis virus in groupers. *Journal of Virological Methods*, **159**, 206–210.

Teng, P.H., Chen, C.L., Sung, P.F., *et al.* (2007) Specific detection of reverse transcription-loop-mediated isothermal amplification amplicons for Taura syndrome virus by colorimetric dot-blot hybridization. *Journal of Virological Methods*, **146**, 317–326.

Tsai, Y.L., Wang, H., Lo, C., *et al.* (2014) Validation of a commercial insulated isothermal PCR-based POCKIT test for rapid and easy detection of white spot syndrome virus infection in Litopenaeus vannamei. *PloS One*, **9**(3), e90545.

Vazquez, D., Lopez-Vazquez, C., Skall, H.F., *et al.* (2016) A novel multiplex RT-qPCR method based on dual-labelled probes suitable for typing all known genotypes of viral haemorrhagic septicaemia virus. *Journal of Fish Diseases*, **39**, 467–482.

Vendramin, N., Zrncic, S., Padros, F., *et al.* (2016) Fish health in Mediterranean aquaculture, past mistakes and future challenges. *Bulletin of the European Association of Fish Pathologists*, **36**, 38–45.

Waiwijit, U., Phokaratkul, D., Kampeera, J. *et al.* (2015) Graphene oxide based fluorescence resonance energy transfer and loop-mediated isothermal amplification for white spot syndrome virus detection. *Journal of Biotechnology*, **212**, 44–49.

Wallace, P.S. and MacKay, W.G. (2013) Quality in the molecular microbiology laboratory. *Methods in Molecular Biology*, **43**, 49–79.

Wang, C.H., Lien, K.Y., Wang, T.Y., *et al.* (2011) An integrated microfluidic loop-mediated-isothermal-amplification system for rapid sample pre-treatment and detection of viruses. *Biosensors and Bioelectronics*, **26**(5), 2045–2052.

Workenhe, S.T., Wadowska, D.W., Wright, G.M., Kibenge, M.J.T. and Kibenge, F.S.B. (2007) Demonstration of infectious salmon anaemia virus (ISAV) endocytosis in erythrocytes of Atlantic salmon. *Virology Journal*, **4**, 3.

Xia, X., Yu, Y., Weidmann, M., *et al.* (2014) Rapid detection of shrimp white spot syndrome virus by real time, isothermal recombinase polymerase amplification assay. *PloS One*, **9**, e104667.

Xia, X., Yu, Y., Hu, L., *et al.* (2015) Rapid detection of infectious hypodermal and hematopoietic necrosis virus (IHHNV) by real-time, isothermal recombinase polymerase amplification assay. *Archives of Virology*, **160**, 987–994.

Xie, Z.X., Xie, L.J., Pang, Y.S., *et al.* (2008) Development of a real-time multiplex PCR assay for detection of viral pathogens of penaeid shrimp. *Archives of Virology*, **153**, 2245–2251.

Xu, H.D., Feng, J., Guo, Z.X., Ou, Y.J. and Wang, J.Y. (2010) Detection of red-spotted grouper nervous necrosis virus by loop-mediated isothermal amplification. *Journal of Virological Methods*, **163**, 123–128.

Xu, L.M., Liu, M., Zhao, J.Z., *et al.* (2014) Epitope mapping of the infectious hematopoietic necrosis virus glycoprotein by flow cytometry. *Biotechnology Letters*, **36**, 2109–2116.

Yang, H.L., Qiu, L., Liu, Q., *et al.* (2016) A novel method of real-time reverse-transcription loop-mediated isothermal amplification developed for rapid and quantitative detection of a new genotype (YHV-8) of Yellow head virus. *Letters in Applied Microbiology*, **63**(2), 103–110.

Yoshino, M., Watari, H., Kojima, T., Ikedo, M. and Kurita, J. (2009) Rapid, sensitive and simple detection method for koi herpesvirus using loop-mediated isothermal amplification. *Microbiology and Immunology*, **53**, 375–383.

Zhang, Q., Liu, S., Yang, H., *et al.* (2015) Reverse transcription loop-mediated isothermal amplification for rapid and quantitative assay of covert mortality nodavirus in shrimp. *Journal of Invertebrate Pathology*, DOI:10.1016/j.jip.2015.09.001.

4

Parasitic Diseases in Aquaculture: Their Biology, Diagnosis and Control

Giuseppe Paladini[1], Matt Longshaw[2], Andrea Gustinelli[3] and Andrew P. Shinn[2,4]

[1] *Institute of Aquaculture, University of Stirling, Stirling, Scotland, UK*
[2] *Benchmark Animal Health Ltd, Edinburgh Technopole, Milton Bridge, Scotland, UK*
[3] *Department of Veterinary Medical Sciences, Alma Mater Studiorum, University of Bologna, Bologna, Italy*
[4] *Fish Vet Group Asia Ltd, Chonburi, Thailand*

Introduction

It is an immutable fact that a significant proportion of organisms on Earth are parasitic for part or all of their life. The use of emerging technologies such as environmental DNA (eDNA) has increased the identification of potential new parasites severalfold, even if they have not yet been formally described (Bass *et al.*, 2015). If one considers the number of other associations such as symbiosis, commensalism and mutualism, then the proportion of organisms in this category markedly increases. Additionally, it is highly probable that every species plays host to at least one parasitic species during its lifetime and it is rare to find any aquaculture species that is not troubled by at least one problematic parasite during the farming process. Even closed, recirculation systems, often seen as the panacea to minimize disease issues through good biosecurity, can be subject to parasite infections (Gratzek *et al.*, 1983; Jørgensen *et al.*, 2009; Moestrup *et al.*, 2014; Noble, 1996; Noble *et al.*, 1997). Parasite infections on farms can be devastating with serious socioeconomic, ecological and welfare consequences (Shinn *et al.*, 2015a). Financial losses on a farm can be direct through mortality of the stock, increased costs of removing or checking for mortalities, reduced growth and feed conversion ratios, incurred veterinary costs, and rejection or downgrading of product during processing. Indirectly, concerns over welfare of the farmed stock, increased susceptibility to other infections and the potential legislative burdens, as well as the inability to move infected stock to other sites, means that it is imperative that any infection is either pre-emptively or rapidly (and correctly) identified and appropriate control measures are put in place.

Parasites with direct life-cycles, or those with simple life-cycles with a water-borne infectious stage, tend to dominate within aquaculture. This is exemplified by infections with protistans, monogeneans and parasitic crustaceans. Parasites with water-borne stages also include the Myxozoa and Digenea and these can reach epidemic proportions in a farm, even with good biosecurity. In spite of changes in farming practices and the use of intervention and control strategies described in the current chapter, expected changes in climate and the need to increase food production to account for increased human populations mean that it is highly probable that parasitic diseases will continue to be problematic (Callaway *et al.*, 2012).

Diagnosis and Control of Diseases of Fish and Shellfish, First Edition. Edited by Brian Austin and Aweeda Newaj-Fyzul.

Current aquatic farming practices and the species that are grown worldwide are extraordinarily varied and reflect the diversity of habitats, ecological niches and biological diversity of the vertebrates and invertebrates cultured. No single review chapter could hope to provide comprehensive cover of all parasite species impacting on aquaculture-based activities, the mode of diagnosis or the methods to control those infections and therefore this chapter represents an attempt to provide general principles and the underlying rationale for decision making, while providing global and local examples where possible. The chapter covers the major parasite groups of concern in both vertebrate and invertebrate farmed hosts and signposts the reader to the most important publications for those groups. There are, however, several other minor parasite and/or commensal groups, outwith the purpose of this chapter, which rarely cause issues on farms. These include, but are not limited to, the Aspidogastrea, Diptera, Hirudinea, Oligochaeta, Ostracoda, Temnocephala and Turbellaria, among others. The chapter also covers a diagnostic summary with some considerations and approaches regarding treatment strategies, prophylaxis methods and farm management practices. There is, however, some variability on the length of the different sections presented below, which reflects the importance of certain parasite groups and the risk that they pose to the aquaculture industry.

Protista

Biology and Taxonomy

Protistans (Figure 4.1) are a large paraphyletic group of organisms that parasitize most, if not all, animal (and plant) groups. Typical groups found in or on aquatic animals include representatives of the flagellates (e.g. *Amyloodinium, Cryptobia, Gymnodinium, Hexamita, Ichthyobodo, Piscinoodinium, Spironucleus, Trypanosoma, Trypanoplasma*), amoebae or rhizopodes (e.g. *Vermamoeba* [=*Hartmannella*], *Paramoeba, Thecamoeba*), alveolates (e.g. *Perkinsus*), apicomplexans (e.g. *Aggregata, Eimeria, Goussia, Haemogregarina, Margolisiella* [=*Pseudoklossia*]), cercozoans (e.g. *Bonamia, Haplosporidium, Marteilia, Paramarteilia*) and ciliates (e.g. *Anophryoides, Apiosoma, Capriniana, Chilodonella, Cryptocaryon, Epistylis, Ichthyophthirius, Tetrahymena, Trichodina, Uronema*).

Life-Cycle

Generally, protistans have simple life-cycles, reproducing by binary fission, with transmission between and within hosts through contact. In addition, some protistans utilize vectors and/or intermediate hosts in transmission. This includes leeches in the life-cycle of trypanosomes, crustaceans and oligochaetes in coccidian life-cycles, and fomites/substrate in the life-cycle of *Ichthyophthirius multifiliis, Cryptocaryon irritans* and *Amyloodinium ocellatum*.

Public Health

The vast majority of protistans, while problematic for aquatic animals, are not generally considered to be of zoonotic concern. Although the zoonotic *Cryptosporidium parvum* has been identified in several fish species, the risk of fish-to-human transmission has not been unequivocally demonstrated (Koinari *et al.*, 2013; Reid *et al.*, 2010). Additionally, shellfish are known to carry the zoonotic parasites *Giardia duodenalis* and *C. parvum* (see Giangaspero *et al.*, 2014;

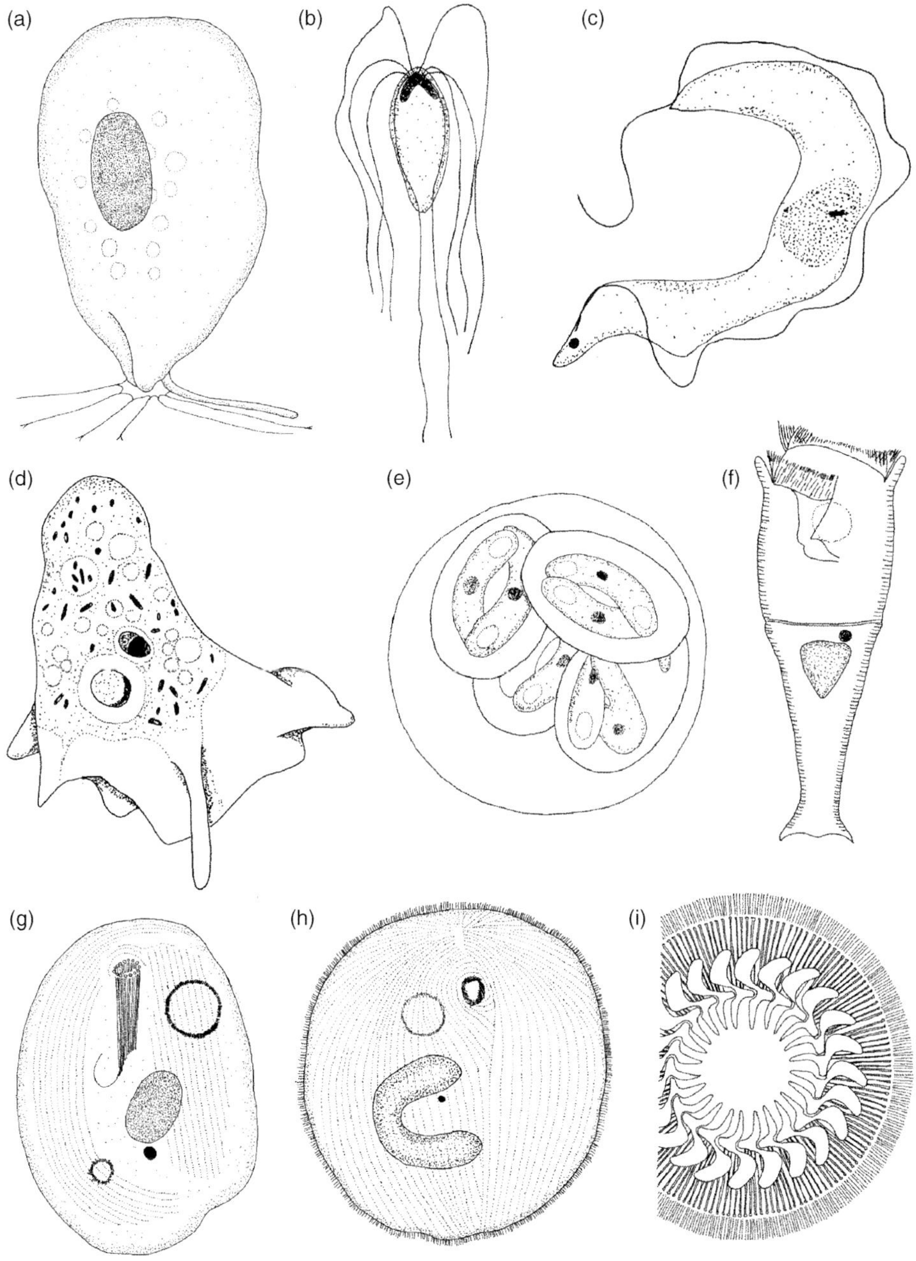

Figure 4.1 Representative drawings of protistans typically found associated with farmed aquatic animals. (a) Trophont of *Amyloodinium* sp. (flagellate); (b) *Spironucleus* sp. (flagellate); (c) *Trypanosoma* sp. (flagellate); (d) *Paramoeba* sp. (rhizopod); (e) *Goussia* sp. (coccidian); (f) *Apiosoma* sp. (ciliate); (g) *Chilodonella* sp. (ciliate); (h) Trophont of *Ichthyophthirius multifiliis* (ciliate); (i) *Trichodina* sp. (ciliate). Figures b, c, e–i after Lom and Dykova (1992), Figure a original, Figure d modified from Page (1970).

Willis *et al.*, 2013), which they probably acquire through the process of filter feeding followed by subsequent sequestration into their tissues. It is probable that shellfish are a more likely route of infection to humans compared with fish.

Significant Pathogens within the Group

The majority of problems associated with protistans in aquaculture are mainly due to their ability to transmit without the need for an intermediate host. In many instances, outbreaks on farms are a result of increased stress in the host animal or decreased water quality and, thus, environmental manipulation to reduce these may help to mitigate the lethal outcome of infection. The marine dinoflagellate *Amyloodinium ocellatum* and the freshwater flagellate *Ichthyobodo necator*, occurring on the external surfaces of their hosts, have been implicated in the loss of farmed, wild and aquarium fish in a number of regions around the world (Isaksen *et al.*, 2011). Blood-borne *Trypanosoma* spp. and *Trypanoplasma* spp. occur in marine and freshwater fish, with several species considered of economic importance. These include *Trypanosoma carassii* and *Trypanoplasma borreli* in freshwater carps, *Trypanoplasma salmositica* in salmonids and *T. bullocki* in a range of marine fish. Infected fish are anaemic and often exhibit exophthalmia and ascites (Scholz, 1999a). A major issue in marine salmon farming is caused by the free-living, facultative amoeba *Paramoeba* [=*Neoparamoeba*] *perurans*, the causative agent of amoebic gill disease (AGD) which leads to gill damage and death of infected fish (Mitchell and Rodger, 2011). The freshwater counterparts, such as *Acanthamoeba*, *Naegleria*, *Protacanthamoeba*, *Rhogostoma*, *Vannella* and *Vermamoeba*, have been associated with high mortalities in rainbow trout, *Oncorhynchus mykiss*, in the Czech Republic, Germany and Italy (Dyková and Tyml, 2016; Dyková *et al.*, 2010; Quaglio *et al.*, 2016). Also of concern are the ciliates which have led to mortalities in a number of wild and farmed vertebrate and invertebrate hosts. While they often occur as harmless ectocommensals, under poor environmental conditions or stress, some ciliates such as *Trichodina* spp., *Uronema* spp. and *Epistylis* spp. can rapidly increase in number, leading to morbidity and mortality. Additionally, the freshwater ciliate *Ichthyophthirius multifiliis* and the marine *Cryptocaryon irritans* are devastating to farmed and wild fish, causing the parasitic white spot disease.

Shellfish diseases of concern include the alveolate *Perkinsus marinus*, the causative agent of Dermo disease which leads to mortalities in bivalve molluscs held at high temperature and relatively low salinities. Another important group of shellfish protistans are the cercozoans which include *Bonamia ostreae* and *Bonamia exitiosa*; both infect the haemocytes of their ostreid hosts, with the antipodean *B. exitiosa* being invasive in Europe (Longshaw *et al.*, 2013). Additionally, *Marteilia* spp., normally found in the digestive glands of their hosts, have been implicated in mass mortalities of bivalve molluscs in Europe. These shellfish diseases are all included in the list of notifiable diseases by the World Organization for Animal Health (OIE, 2016). Parasites of cephalopods and crustaceans include several species of the apicomplexan *Aggregata*, an intracellular coccidian infecting the digestive tracts of cephalopods as definitive hosts (e.g. cuttlefish, *Sepia officinalis*; flying squid, *Todarodes sagittatus*; common octopus, *Octopus vulgaris*) and crustaceans as intermediate hosts (e.g. blue-leg swimming crab, *Liocarcinus* [=*Macropipus*] *depurator*) (see Castellanos-Martínez *et al.*, 2013; Gestal *et al.*, 2002; Hochberg, 1990; Levine, 1985; Mladineo and Jozić, 2005).

Reviews

General and specific reviews of protistans include books by Bauer (1984), Paperna (1991), Lom and Dyková (1992), Bower *et al.* (1994), Scholz (1999a), Lee *et al.* (2000), Gaevskaya

(2004), Woo (2006), Dyková and Lom (2007) and Eiras *et al.* (2012a). Reviews and important articles on the biology and taxonomy of the flagellates include Cone and Wiles (1984), Urawa *et al.* (1998), Todal *et al.* (2004), Poynton *et al.* (2004), Jørgensen and Sterud (2006, 2007), Lynn (2011) and Isaksen *et al.* (2012). Publications on amoebic infections include those by Johnson (1977), Leiro *et al.* (1998), Dyková and Lom (2004), Young *et al.* (2007), Santos *et al.* (2010), Kudryavtsev *et al.* (2011), Crosbie *et al.* (2012) and Feehan *et al.* (2013). Important publications on apicomplexans and alveolates include Goggin and Lester (1995), Desser and Bower (1997), Davies and Johnston (2000), Tenter *et al.* (2002), Villalba *et al.* (2004), Duszynski *et al.* (2007), Ghimire (2010) and Ogedengbe *et al.* (2011). Publications on cercozoans include those by Burreson and Ford (2004), Berthe *et al.* (2004), Stentiford (2008), Feist *et al.* (2009), Hine *et al.* (2009), Murray *et al.* (2012), Longshaw *et al.* (2013), Engelsma *et al.* (2014), Carnegie *et al.* (2014) and Arzul and Carnegie (2015). Important articles on ciliates include those by Colorni (1985), van As and Basson (1989), Morado and Small (1995), Colorni and Burgess (1997), Gaze and Wootten (1998), Matthews (2005), and Mitchell and Rodger (2011).

Identification

The taxonomy and identification of protistans are based on the morphology of the various life stages. It is clear, however, that there is a great deal of plasticity in these features and as such, there has been a move towards use of molecular tools to discriminate species and genera within the Protista. Flagellates typically have one or more flagellum, generally a single nucleus and body shape is pleomorphic. Parasite size, the organ it infects in its host and the species of host have all been used to discriminate species. Amoebae are also pleomorphic and while traditionally described on the basis of size, shape and other characteristics, there is an increasing reliance on molecular tools to help discriminate species. For apicomplexans, the structure and the arrangement of the oocyst and sporocyst are of paramount importance in discriminating species and genera. Ciliates, as the name suggests, possess cilia during one or more of their life stages. The arrangement and position of the cilia are of taxonomic importance. Cercozoans are discriminated on the basis of the number, arrangement and size of cells, as well as spore morphology for spore-forming types.

Diagnostic Methods

As described above, protistans are primarily identified using morphological characteristics and the majority of species have been described on this basis. Techniques utilized include light microscopy methods like phase contrast, bright-field and differential interference contrast microscopy. Stained, fixed and permanent preparations of blood and tissue smears and imprints can be made to assist with diagnosis. For some protistans, such as *Uronema* and *Tetrahymena*, the silver nitrate impregnation method (Foissner, 2014; Klein, 1943) to show the ciliary meridians is fundamental. Histology and stains such as Giemsa have been extensively utilized to localize infections and to describe any associated pathology. Refinements to light microscopy methods include the use of *in situ* hybridization (ISH), monoclonal and polyclonal antibodies and lectins to facilitate the visualization of protistans in histological sections. Transmission electron microscopy has been used extensively to diagnose protistans as internal cellular structures are important in discriminating species and genera. Finally, molecular tools are paramount and of increasing importance in the description of new species – their application in the identification of protistans cannot be overestimated.

Myxozoa

Biology and Taxonomy

Myxozoans (Figure 4.2) are highly specialized cnidarian parasites comprising two classes – the Myxosporea and the Malacosporea. Around 64 genera, with approximately 2000–2500 species, have been described in hosts from tropical, temperate and polar regions (Atkinson *et al.*, 2015).

Life-Cycle

The life-cycle of most myxozoans is still unknown but, for those in which the life-cycle has been demonstrated, they alternate between a vertebrate and an invertebrate host, with a small number apparently able to transmit without the need for a second host (Estensoro *et al.*, 2010). Development within a host typically proceeds via cell-within-cell division (pluricellularity), leading to the formation of infectious spores. Invertebrate hosts (where sexual reproduction takes place) include Monogenea (where they are hyperparasitic), oligochaetes (the typical invertebrate host), polychaetes and bryozoans. Vertebrate hosts include fish, amphibians, terrestrial shrews and waterfowl (Canning and Okamura, 2003). The majority of myxozoans have been described from fish in marine, estuarine and freshwater across all continents, except Antarctica.

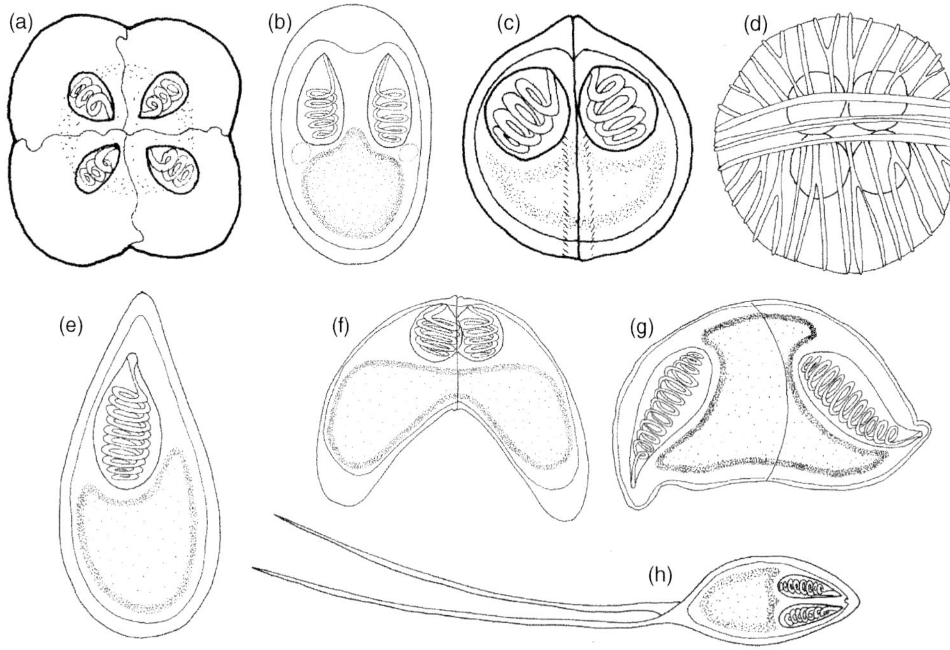

Figure 4.2 Representative drawings of myxozoans reported in farmed fish. (a) *Kudoa* sp.; (b) *Myxobolus* sp.; (c) *Sphaerospora* sp.; (d) *Chloromyxum* sp.; (e) *Thelohanellus* sp.; (f) *Ceratonova* sp.; (g) *Enteromyxum* sp.; (h) *Henneguya* sp. Figures a-e and h, original drawings, Figure f modified from Atkinson *et al.* (2014), Figure g modified from Palenzuela *et al.* (2002).

Public Health

Although not normally of concern for human health, there have been incidental findings of non-viable myxozoans in stool samples (Boreham *et al.*, 1998; McClelland *et al.*, 1997) and more recently, reports of food poisoning in Japan due to *Kudoa septempunctata* through the consumption of raw olive flounder, *Paralichthys olivaceus* (see Iwashita *et al.*, 2013) and allergic reactions associated with the consumption of fish infected with a *Kudoa* sp. (see Martínez de Velasco *et al.*, 2008).

Significant Pathogens within the Group

Genera and species reported as deleterious to farmed (and wild) fish include *Tetracapsuloides bryosalmonae* (causative agent of proliferative kidney disease – PKD), *Myxobolus cerebralis* (causative agent of whirling disease – WD), *Ceratonova* [=*Ceratomyxa*] *shasta*, *Kudoa* spp. and *Parvicapsula* spp. in salmonids and other fish species; *Enteromyxum* spp., *Sphaerospora* [=*Polysporoplasma*] *sparis* and *Sphaerospora* [=*Leptotheca*] *sparidarum* in sparids; *Sphaerospora dicentrarchi* and *S. testicularis* in European seabass, *Dicentrarchus labrax* and *Myxobolus lentisuturalis* in goldfish; *Carassius auratus* (see Kent *et al.*, 2001) and *Chloromyxum* spp. in several fish species (Eiras *et al.*, 2012b); *Thelohanellus hovorkai* in carp (Yokoyama *et al.*, 1998) and *Henneguya* spp. in several hosts, including ornamental fish species and salmonids (Li *et al.*, 2015; Tossavi *et al.*, 2015; Yokoyama *et al.*, 2012).

Reviews

Major reviews of the group, selected genera or geographical distribution include Jaysari and Hoffman (1982), Dyková and Lom (1988), Gioia and Silva Cordeiro (1996), Moran *et al.* (1999), Kent *et al.* (2001), Eiras and Adriano (2012), and Eiras *et al.* (2012, 2014).

Identification

Traditionally, myxozoans have been classified using morphological criteria of the spores, such as their overall shape and size, and the number and arrangement of polar capsules and of spore walls (Lom and Arthur, 1989; Lom and Dyková, 2006; Lom *et al.*, 1997). However, spore morphology can be variable between tissues in the same host and between different hosts, leading to possible misidentifications (Urawa *et al.*, 2009, 2011). Furthermore, in the absence of supporting data, it remains possible that cryptic speciation in myxozoans occurs. Tissue tropism does have some utility in diagnosis, helping to further define the species under investigation (Molnár, 2002a,b, 2007; Molnár and Székely, 2014). Often, histozoic species (those residing within tissues) form cysts of various colours (usually white or yellow), sizes and shapes (branched, oval, round). Gross signs of infection are extremely varied but, in many cases, clinical signs can be pathognomonic for the disease in question, such as reno- and splenomegaly associated with PKD, blackened tail associated with WD and myoliquefaction associated with *Kudoa* spp. Host specificity can be used in preliminary identification but caution should be exercised as this can vary between parasite species (Longshaw *et al.*, 2003, 2005).

Diagnostic Methods

Diagnostic methods for identification include the use of phase contrast or differential interference microscopy for fixed or fresh spores. Blood and tissue smears or imprints stained with

May–Grünwald–Giemsa, Giemsa or silver nitrate are useful for observing both spores and extrasporogonic stages (Lom *et al.*, 1983; Longshaw *et al.*, 2003; Parker and Warner, 1970; Reed *et al.*, 2002). Scanning electron microscopy (SEM) can be useful for elucidating detail of surface morphology (e.g. *Chloromyxum*) (Ali, 2009; Lom and Dyková, 1993); ultrastructural studies using transmission electron microscopy (TEM) have limited value as a diagnostic tool but can provide valuable data on cellular development. Histology should be used as a frontline tool to elucidate tissue specificity as well as determining any pathology caused by a myxozoan infection; specific identity of myxozoans by histology is, however, not always possible. Furthermore, low-level infections and early development stages can be difficult to detect in histological sections. To an extent, this problem can be overcome by applying a number of specialist tools such as lectins (Marin de Mateo *et al.*, 1993; Muñoz *et al.*, 1999), monoclonal and polyclonal antibodies (Hedrick *et al.*, 2004; Morris *et al.*, 1997) and *in situ* hybridization to sectioned material to assist with visualization and parasite identity (Baxa *et al.*, 2002).

Recent advances in molecular-based tools are important for discriminating species as well as providing data on phylogeny of the group (Bartošová *et al.*, 2009; Bartošová-Sojková *et al.*, 2015; Fiala, 2006; Fiala and Bartosová, 2010; Jirků *et al.*, 2011; Salim and Desser, 2000). Molecular methods include, but are not limited to, restriction fragment length polymorphism (RFLP) (Eszterbauer, 2002; Eszterbauer *et al.*, 2001), small and large subunit (SSU/LSU) amplification and sequencing (Li *et al.*, 2013; Rosser *et al.*, 2015) and loop-mediated isothermal amplification (LAMP) assays (Biswas and Sakai, 2014; El-Matbouli and Soliman, 2005; Sarker *et al.*, 2015). Finally, attempts have been made to culture a number of myxozoans of concern (Morris, 2012; Redondo *et al.*, 2003; Wolf and Markiw, 1976). While they have limited utility currently as a diagnostic tool, it may be possible that with further refinement, *in vitro* cultivation could be used to amplify various myxozoan stages to provide additional material for testing. Alternatively, if species-specific *in vitro* culture conditions are found to exist, then these could be refined as a useful diagnostic tool.

Mesomycetozoea, Fungi and Fungal-Like Organisms

Biology and Taxonomy

This section covers a wide range of species, genera and taxa that loosely fit together under the fungi and fungal-like organisms or have previously been included in the fungi. This includes the phyla Oomycota (or slime molds), Ascomycota, Chytridiomycota and Microsporidia (Figure 4.3). The Microsporidia have previously been considered as Protista, but recent molecular evidence suggests they are basal fungi (Gill and Fast, 2006; Hirt *et al.*, 1999; Lee *et al.*, 2008). Furthermore, the Mesomycetozoea (or DRIPs clade, an acronym for the first protistan taxa allocated to this clade) are included in this section as some members of this group were traditionally included in the fungi.

Life-Cycle

Fungi and fungal-like organisms have direct life-cycles and in some cases may have resting stages outside their host. While fungi and fungal-like organisms show some level of host specificity, this varies according to species; tissue specificity can also be variable and all tissues and organs are equally susceptible to infections by this group.

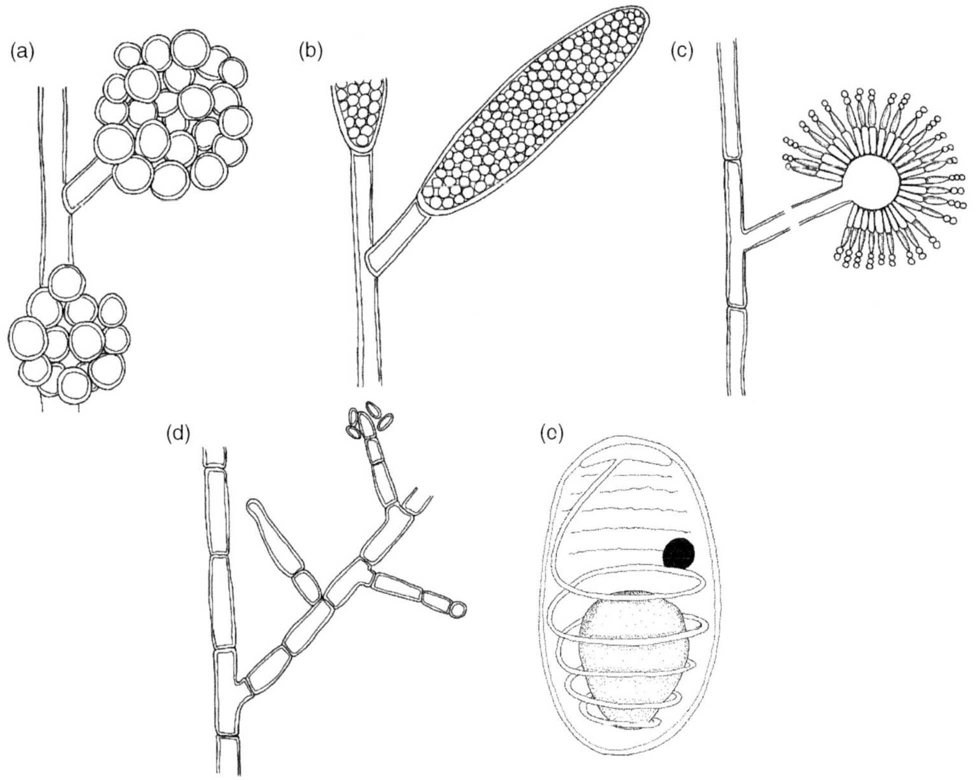

Figure 4.3 Representative drawings of fungi and fungal-like organisms reported from aquatic animals. (a) Primary zoospores of *Aphanomyces* sp., an oomycete associated with crayfish plague and with epizootic ulcerative syndrome in fish (b) Asexual zoosporangium of *Saprolegnia* sp.; (c) Conidia of *Aspergillus* sp.; (d) Conidia of *Exophiala* sp.; (e) drawing of a typical microsporidian, showing main features including polar filament coiled within main body. All images original.

Public Health

Fungi and fungal-like organisms have been reported in all major animal groups as well as plants and humans, but those infecting aquacultured species are not normally considered as harmful to human health. Early reports of AIDS patients infected by fish-infecting opportunistic microsporidians do not appear to be substantiated (Mathis *et al.*, 2005).

Significant Pathogens within the Group

Important genera and species reported as deleterious to farmed and wild aquatic hosts include *Aphanomyces astaci* (Phylum Oomycota; agent of crayfish plague in freshwater crayfish), *Aphanomyces invadans* (Phylum Oomycota; causative agent of epizootic ulcerative syndrome (EUS) in teleosts), *Saprolegnia* spp. (Phylum Oomycota; in freshwater fish, fish eggs and shellfish species), *Aspergillus* spp., *Exophiala* spp., *Fusarium* spp. and *Phoma* spp. (Phylum Ascomycota; in various fish and shellfish hosts), *Batrachochytrium dendrobatidis* (Phylum Chytridimycota; the agent of chytrid disease principally in amphibians), *Dermocystidium* spp., *Sphaerothecum destruens* (Rosette agent), *Ichthyophonus* spp. (Phylum Mesomycetozoea; in various fish and shellfish species), and the microsporidians *Enterospora* spp., *Loma* spp., *Pseudoloma* spp., *Pleistophora* spp., *Enterocytozoon hepatopenaei*, *Kabatana* [=*Kabataia*] spp., *Nosema* spp. and *Thelohania* spp. in various fish and shellfish species.

Reviews

Reviews of the major groups of fungi and fungal-like organisms include those by Mendoza *et al.* (2002), Arkush *et al.* (2003), Lom and Nilsen (2003), Mazzoni *et al.* (2003), Diéguez-Uribeondo *et al.* (2009), Corradi and Slamovits (2011), Glockling *et al.* (2013), Rowley *et al.* (2013), Gozlan *et al.* (2014), McLaughlin and Spatafora (2014) and Brannelly *et al.* (2015).

Identification

Classification criteria for the different groups vary but have previously been based mainly on established morphological characters. Additionally, biochemical methods such as determining the presence or absence of pigments, or structure of the cell wall, have been used. While these methods have utility in the initial placement of an organism in the wider group, the use of molecular tools has gained traction in the last few years to assist with the identification of fungi and fungal-like organisms.

Diagnostic Methods

Diagnostic methods include light microscopy (including phase contrast and differential interference microscopy) and histology. The latter is useful for assessing pathology and tissue localization, particularly when coupled with specialist stains such as Luna stain (Peterson *et al.*, 2011), periodic acid-Schiff (PAS), Gomori methenamine silver (GMS), Fontana-Masson (FM), mucicarmine (MC), or when used in conjunction with molecular methods such as *in situ* hybridization. Direct stains include potassium hydroxide (KOH) and Chicago sky blue (CSB), both used in human medicine to dissolve keratin which allows the hyphae to be visible (Fonseka *et al.*, 2011); chlorazol black E, a chitin-specific blue and black stain; and calcofluor white, used under fluorescent microscope to highlight cellulose and chitin in the cell walls (Jain, 2012; Thomas *et al.*, 2008). As with other major parasite groups, molecular tools have been used to provide insights into phylogeny of the group and as specific diagnostic tools (Arkush *et al.*, 2003; Diéguez-Uribeondo *et al.*, 2009; Freeman *et al.*, 2003; Glockling *et al.*, 2013; Kozubíková-Balcarová *et al.*, 2013; McClymont *et al.*, 2005; Ragan *et al.*, 1996; Vrålstad *et al.*, 2014; Winters *et al.*, 2016). It is likely that molecular methods for identification will become essential for diagnosing infections in aquatic hosts.

Monogenea

Biology and Taxonomy

Monogeneans (Figure 4.4) are parasitic flatworms in the Class Monogenea [=Monogenoidea] (Phylum Platyhelminthes) and the two subclasses, the Monopisthocotylea [=Polyonchoinea] and the Polyopisthocotylea [=Oligonchoinea], with over 5500 species allocated to 750+ monogenean genera. They are commonly found on the skin and gills/buccal cavity of fish and within the urogenital system of anurans and chelonians. Species are also recorded, to a lesser extent, from the nares (e.g. *Nasicola* in *Thunnus* spp.), stomach (e.g. *Enterogyrus* in

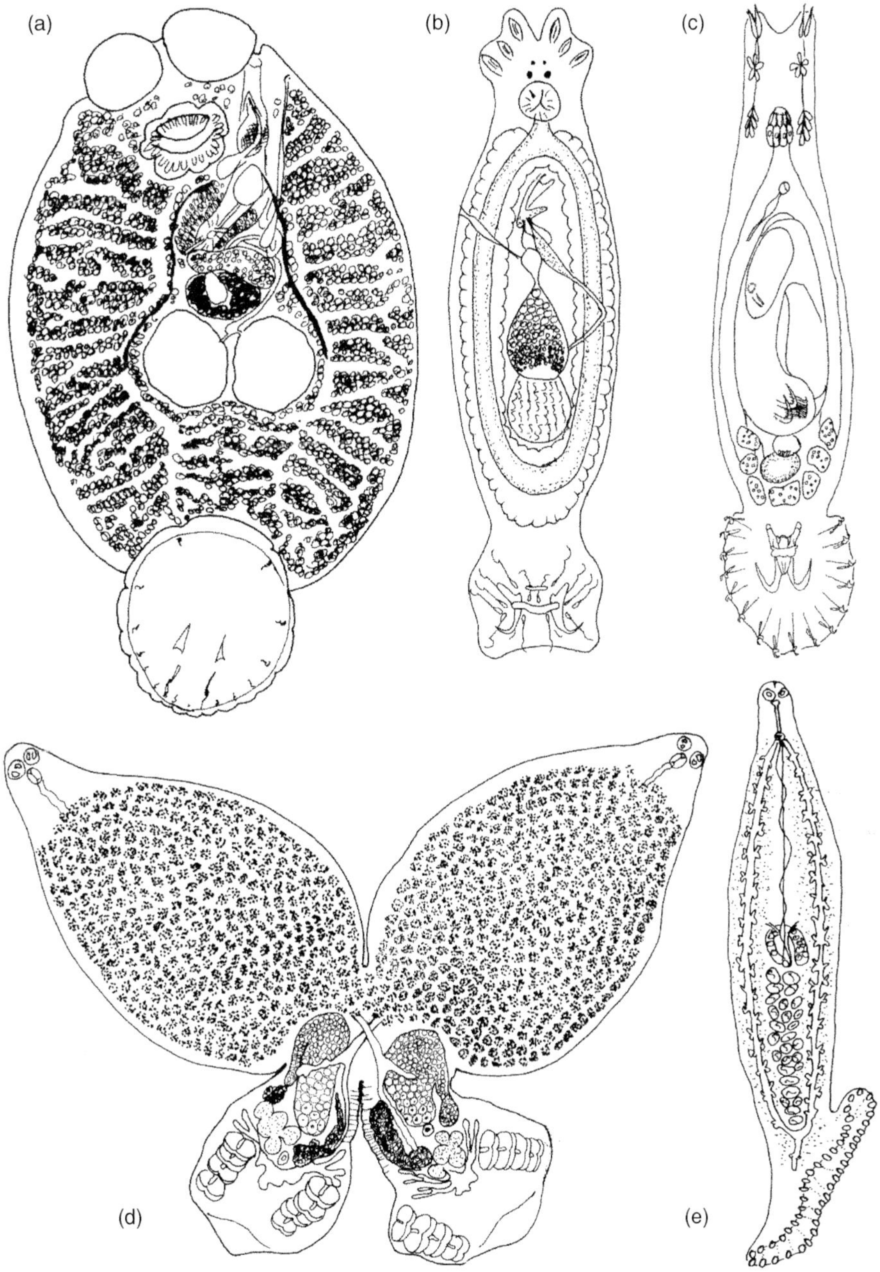

Figure 4.4 Representative drawings of monogeneans reported on the skin and gills of farmed fish, including the monopisthocotyleans (a) *Benedenia* sp. (after Ogawa *et al.*, 1995); (b) *Dactylogyrus* sp. (after Beverley-Burton, 1984); and (c) *Gyrodactylus* sp. (after Pugachev *et al.*, 2009); and the polyopisthocotyleans (d) *Diplozoon* sp. presented as a single twin-worm formed from the fusion of two individuals (after Khotenovsky, 1985); and (e) *Microcotyle* sp. (after Beverley-Burton, 1984).

tilapias), coelom and urogenital system (e.g. *Monocotyle* in rays), heart and circulatory system of fish (e.g. *Amphibdella* in *Torpedo*), from the mantle of cephalopods (e.g. *Isancistrum* in *Alloteuthis*), as hyperparasites of copepods (e.g. *Udonella* on *Lepeophtheirus*), and even from the eyes of hippopotami (e.g. *Oculotrema*).

Monogeneans vary in size from *ca.* 200 micrometres up to 4 cm long (typically 0.3–20 mm); display a high degree of host specificity; can be viviparous or oviparous; are hermaphrodite, commonly protandrous; attach to their host by means of a specialized muscular posterior attachment organ or opisthaptor which houses a variable array of sclerotized hooks, connecting bars, clamps or epidermal structures (i.e. tegumental spines or squamodisc sclerites), the number, shape and configuration of which are key to the identification and separation of species; the copulatory organs may also contain sclerotized elements and armature contributing to their identification. Monopisthocotyleans typically inhabit the skin and gills of their hosts; are epidermal grazers although there are some exceptions to this, most notably *Dactylogyrus* which is a blood feeder commonly found on the gills of cyprinids; may or may not possess eye spots (0–4); most are mobile, moving in a leech-like manner over their host, securing attachment through an opisthaptor bearing hooks and adhesive secretions of the prohaptor (anterior part of the body); typically possess a true vagina but lack a genital-intestinal canal. Polyopisthocotyleans, by comparison, typically occupy the gills of their hosts; are less motile; are blood feeders; the larvae possess eye spots but these disappear in the adult; typically possess a single pair of anchors but their marginal hooks are replaced by clamps which may vary in number from 0 to >200 pairs; they possess a genital-intestinal canal.

Life-Cycle

Monogeneans have a single definitive host in their life-cycles; however, the immature stages of two species of monogenean, *Gotocotyla acanthura* and *Pricea multae*, may use optional intermediate hosts which are predated upon by their final host. Most monogeneans produce eggs, apart from some genera within the Gyrodactylidae, which are viviparous. The eggs vary greatly in their morphology and may be operculated or non-operculated; bear one or two polar processes or filaments; may be hooked terminally, bear spines or sticky droplets; may be laid singly, in chains or deposited as egg masses which may be neutrally buoyant, sinking or are anchored to the substrate by adhesive or become immediately lodged within their host's gill apparatus or become entangled in cage netting (Kearn, 1986). Within each egg, a single oncomiracidium develops, the speed of which is temperature dependent (e.g. 4–5 days for *Dactylogyrus extensus* at 25 °C; 54 days for *Entobdella hippoglossi* at 5 °C). Egg hatching may be stimulated by a variety of environmental cues or chemical cues from potential hosts in close proximity. The larva or oncomiracidium emerging from an egg is typically 250–300 micrometres in length, ciliated and eyed. The oncomiracidium then swims off in search of a host, using a combination of active swimming (1–5 mm/s^{-1}) and passive sinking as it is borne along by the water current, with increases in its turn rate in response to host-generated chemical cues. On attachment, the ciliated cells are lost as are eyes in polyopisthocotylean species as the parasite matures.

Public Health

No monogenean species pose a risk to human health.

Significant Pathogens within the Group

Infections on captive reared aquaculture stocks can cause serious economic impacts (Shinn *et al.*, 2015a, 2015b; Thoney and Hargis, 1991). Significant monogenean parasites of captive reared stocks include *Benedenia seriolae, Cichlidogyrus* spp., *Dactylogyrus* spp., *Diplectanum aequans, Diplozoon* spp., *Gyrodactylus* spp., *Lamellodiscus* spp., *Microcotyle* spp., *Neobenedenia melleni, Sparicotyle chrysophrii,* and *Zeuxapta seriolae,* among others.

Reviews

Major reviews on monogenean taxonomy and phylogenetics can be found in Bychowsky (1957), Yamaguti (1963a), Beverley-Burton (1984), Gusev (1985), Lebedev (1988), Boeger and Kritsky (1993, 1997, 2001), Hoffman (1999), Baohua and Suo (2000), Littlewood and Bray (2001), Olson and Littlewood (2002), Pandey and Agrawal (2008) and Pugachev *et al.* (2009), with additional overviews on the Class Monogenea in Kearn (1998, 2005) and Rohde (2005). Further reviews on aspects of monogenean biology are available in the following: eggs (Kearn, 1986), larvae/oncomiracidia (Whittington *et al.*, 2000), infections in aquaculture and public aquaria (Shinn *et al.*, 2015a, 2015b; Thoney and Hargis, 1991), treatment of certain problematic species (Schelkle *et al.*, 2009, 2011; Shinn and Bron, 2012); economic losses in aquaculture (Shinn *et al.*, 2015a, 2015b).

Identification

The shape and configuration of the sclerotized elements of the opisthaptor and the copulatory apparatus are key to the morphological discrimination and identification of species. Most monopisthocotyleans possess an array of proteinaceous sclerotized elements housed within their opisthaptor which typically comprises one or two pairs of centrally positioned anchors or 'hamuli' connected by one or two bars and, commonly, 14–16 smaller marginal hooks distributed around the periphery of the opisthaptor. Polyopisthocotyleans possess sclerotized clamps, the skeletal arrangement of which is a key feature in their classification. The clamps may be 'simple' open structures that may or may not bear a central spine that effect attachment to their host by suction, or they may be articulated and independently able to grasp the lamellae of their host's gills.

Diagnostic Methods

Monogeneans may move or fall off dead hosts and so hosts should be examined immediately following euthanasia. Many small monogeneans will be destroyed by freeze-thawing and so the examination of hosts that were sampled and subsequently frozen is ill-advised.

Monogenean anatomy can be determined in a variety of ways; the method applied depends on which structures are under investigation. Large, whole parasites can be flattened and examined alive using a live-box or compressorium, or fixed compressed between two glass slides before routine staining as whole mounts with haematoxylin or carmine-based stains to visualize internal anatomy (Justine, 2005). The armature of the attachment organ and those of the reproductive organs can be examined directly, with the loss of internal anatomy, by:

- mounting live specimens on glass slides and then fixing, staining and clearing specimens *in situ* with ammonium picrate glycerine (Malmberg, 1957, 1970)
- proteolytic digestion (Fannes *et al.*, 2015; Paladini *et al.*, 2009a, 2009b, 2011; Shinn *et al.*, 1993) or by lactophenol-based methods (Justine, 2005) to remove enclosing tissue

- using chromotrope 2R-based or fluorescent dyes to visualize the sulfur-rich hooks of monopisthocotyleans and the clamp proteins of polyopisthocotyleans (García-Vásquez *et al.*, 2012; Kritsky *et al.*, 1978; Milne and Avenant-Oldewage, 2006).

The specimens prepared for light microscopy are typically viewed using phase contrast or differential interference contrast (DIC or Normarski) microscopy. In histological sections, monogeneans commonly inhabit the skin or gills of fish, while the presence of eggs *in utero*, or skeletal elements of the attachment or copulatory apparatus, which appear bright under phase contrast microscopy, can also facilitate their identification. Molecular methods include amplification and sequencing of informative regions of the parasites genome (Boeger and Kritsky, 1993, 1997, 2001; Littlewood and Bray, 2001; Mendoza-Palmero *et al.*, 2015; Messu Mandeng *et al.*, 2015; Olson and Littlewood, 2002; Pouyaud *et al.*, 2006).

Digenea

Biology and Taxonomy

Digeneans (Figure 4.5) are endoparasitic flatworms also known as 'flukes' or 'digenetic trematodes', principally infecting the alimentary canal or associated organs. There is, however, some controversy as to whether the Digenea should be considered a separate class or a subclass of the Trematoda. The current systematic classifications place the Digenea under the Class Trematoda, which also includes the Aspidogastrea, and, together with the Monogenea and Cestoda, forms the subphylum Neodermata under the Phylum Platyhelminthes (Cribb *et al.*, 2003; Gibson *et al.*, 2002; Olson *et al.*, 2003). More than 6000 species have been described from terrestrial (ca. 2000 digenean species) and aquatic hosts (ca. 4000 digenean species); however, there are a number of species (>200) that are infectious to humans, including species of *Schistosoma* which affect over 200 million people worldwide (King, 2011; Sturrock, 2001).

The principal developmental stages of digeneans are called miracidium, sporocyst, redia, cercaria, metacercaria, transitory migrating larva (e.g. 'diplostomule', 'schistomule', depending on the parasite genus) and adult. Egg morphology varies greatly and can be oval, operculated or non-operculated, usually unembryonated, occasionally possessing spines or filaments. The miracidium is generally ovoid and possesses cilia covering the body that allow the parasite to swim and search for the first intermediate host, which usually is represented by a snail.

The larval cercarial stages were initially subdivided into 13 groups based on gross morphology and then subsequently rearranged (Dawes, 1968; Galaktionov and Dobrovolskij, 2003; Roberts and Janovy, 2009; Smyth, 1994). Of these, the Furcocercariae (forked tail cercariae) and Xiphidiocercariae (anterior stylet-bearing cercariae) represent the two major groups of cercariae. The Furcocercariae possess a bifurcate caudal stem which is a feature of all taxa within the Order Strigeidida, which includes members from the families Aporocotylidae, Cyathocotylidae, Diplostomidae, Gymnophallidae, Sanguinicolidae, Schistosomatidae and Strigeidae (Galaktionov and Dobrovolskij, 2003). The Xiphidiocercariae possess a long unforked tail and are characterized by the presence of a stylet in the anterior margin of the oral sucker (Olsen, 1974); this includes all taxa belonging to the Order Plagiorchiida, which includes members of the families Allocreadiidae, Bunoderidae, Dicrocoeliidae, Lecithodendriidae, Microphallidae, Plagiorchiidae, Ochetosomatidae, Pleurogenidae, Renicolidae, etc. (Galaktionov and Dobrovolskij, 2003). Cercarial locomotion is effected through periods of

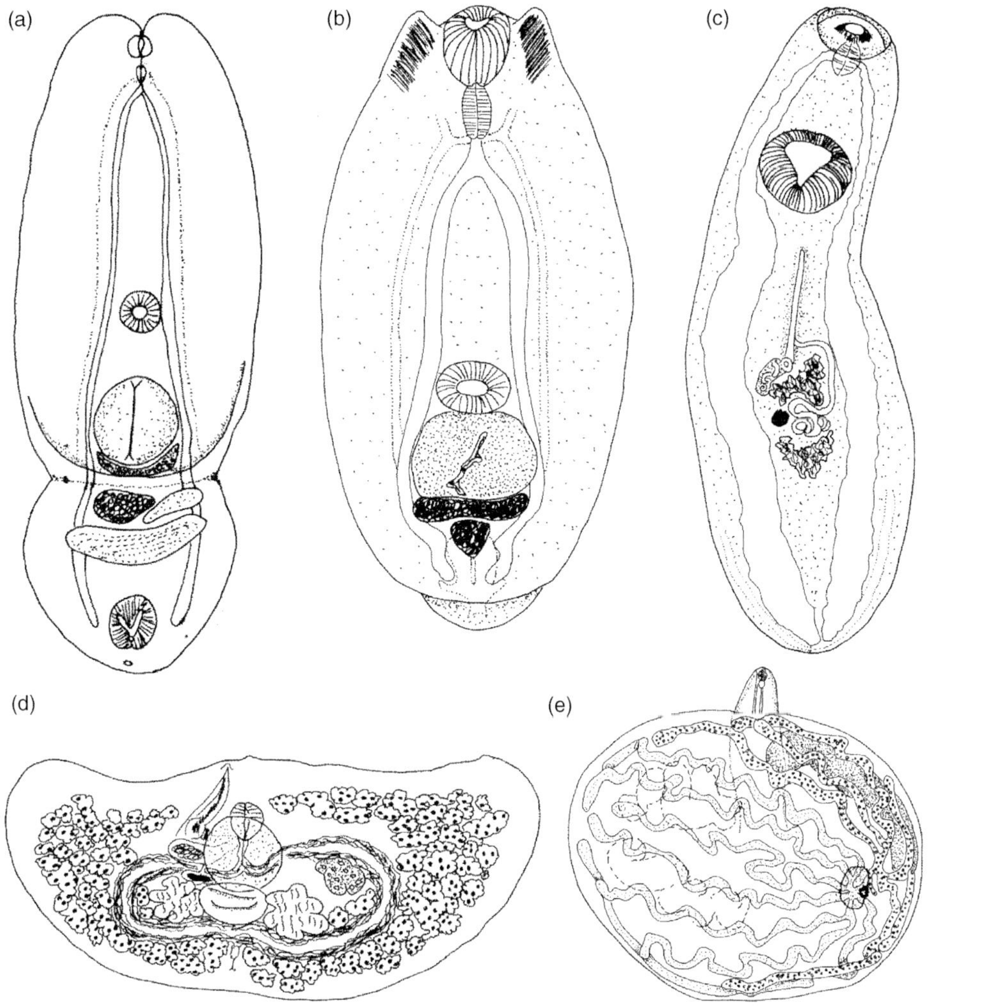

Figure 4.5 Representative drawings of digeneans reported from fish. (a) Metacercaria of *Posthodiplostomum* sp. (after Gibson, 1996); (b) Metacercaria of *Diplostomum* sp. (after Niewiadomska, 1986); (c) Metacercaria of *Clinostomum* sp. (after Caffara *et al.*, 2011); (d) Adult *Transversotrema* sp. (after Gibson *et al.*, 2002); (e) Adult *Didymocystis* sp. (after Kohn and Justo, 2008).

active swimming and passive floating (Galaktionov and Dobrovolskij, 2003). The morphology of the metacercarial stage varies slightly; they are typically ovoid with a thick tegument for protection while encysted. Exceptions include the metacercariae of *Diplostomum* which are free (non-encysted) and continue to feed within the brain, lens and humour of the eye (Cavaleiro *et al.*, 2012; Dezfuli *et al.*, 2007). The adults are usually flattened dorsoventrally, although round and filamentous forms occur, and typically possess two muscular suckers – an anteriorly positioned oral sucker and a medially positioned ventral sucker or acetabulum. The tegument is generally smooth, but in certain genera can have varying degrees of spined armature (Gibson *et al.*, 2002).

Life-Cycle

Digeneans have a complex and indirect life-cycle involving 2–4 hosts; fish can represent the intermediate or the definitive host, depending on the species and the availability of hosts. If fish are definitive hosts, the adult digeneans are usually localized in the gastroenteric apparatus (some exceptions to this include aporocotylids which are commonly located in the vascular system and didymozoids found in the gills and muscle). If fish are intermediate hosts, the metacercarial stages can infect several organs including the eyes, gills, skin, musculature, heart and kidney. Fish can also serve as second intermediate hosts, such as is the case with *Opisthorchis* spp., which represent important fish-borne disease agents. When eggs are laid in water, the operculum opens and a free-swimming, ciliated miracidium emerges. The miracidium penetrates the first intermediate host, typically a mollusc, after which it loses its cilia and develops into a sporocyst which contains embryonic cells. These cells further develop into rediae or 'daughter sporocysts' which subsequently produce hundreds of cercariae. The cercariae possess a tail, a digestive tract and primitive suckers; once released, these then seek out a second intermediate host, which in the aquatic environment is generally represented by a fish. Once the cercariae locate and penetrate their host, they migrate to their body organ of preference and subsequently encyst as metacercariae; in some taxa this migrating larval form is referred to as a diplostomule, schistostomule, etc., according to the genus name.

Many digeneans can cause changes in their host's behaviour to facilitate completion of the parasite's life-cycle. Such changes include modifications to the typical predator escape response; obstructing cryptic colouration ability; reducing shoaling ability (in fish), generally making them more susceptible to predation by the next host; and, by altering their depth preference towards the surface, increasing their likelihood of being predated by facilitating aerial attacks by birds (Gopko *et al.*, 2015; Levri and Lively, 1996; Mikheev *et al.*, 2010; Poulin, 2010; Seppälä *et al.*, 2012). Following transmission to the final host, the metacercariae excyst and develop into an adult, commonly within the final host's intestinal tract.

Public Health

There are over 200 digenean species of major concern to human health. Among these, *Schistosoma* spp., responsible for the water-borne disease called 'snail fever', is perhaps the most significant. This digenean affects over 200 million people, with infection and consequential medical complications resulting in >5500 deaths per year, and poses a major health risk to a further 600 million people working in and around aquatic environments (King, 2011; Sturrock, 2001). Humans become infected by free-swimming cercaria, liberated from snails, penetrating the skin assisted by the release of proteolytic enzymes (Basch, 1991; Hansell *et al.*, 2008; Knudsen *et al.*, 2005; McKerrow and Salter, 2002). Metacercarial stages encysted within the musculature of fish, notably species belonging to the Opisthorchiidae, Heterophyidae and Plagiorchiidae, also pose a risk to human health when improperly cooked aquatic products are consumed (Lima dos Santos and Howgate, 2011). Within the Opisthorchiidae, several species deserve particular attention, most notably *Clonorchis sinensis*, *Opisthorchis viverrini* and *Opisthorchis felineus* which can infect humans following the consumption of raw, improperly cooked or underprocessed infected fish (Tran *et al.*, 2009). Recently, *C. sinensis* and *O. viverrini*, because of the consequential effects of infection, have been classified as carcinogens by the International Agency for Research on Cancer (Lima dos Santos and Howgate, 2011). Likewise, *Paragonimus* spp., belonging to the Plagiorchiidae, poses a risk to those eating infected freshwater crustaceans (Liu *et al.*, 2008). Collectively, around 975 million people are estimated to be at risk of infection with *Opisthorchis*, *Clonorchis* and *Paragonimus* species (Keiser and Utzinger, 2005). Amongst the family Heterophyidae, public health issues have been reported for the genera *Ascocotyle*, *Centrocestus*, *Haplorchis*, *Heterophyes* and *Metagonimus* (Chai, 2007; Chai *et al.*, 2009; Fried *et al.*, 2004; Toledo *et al.*, 2006; Yu and Mott, 1994). A human case of *Clinostomum complanatum* infection has also been reported from a Korean patient following consumption of raw perch, *Lateolabrax japonicus* (see Park *et al.*, 2009).

Other aquatic food-borne zoonoses are associated with species from the Echinostomatidae in bivalves (clams), crustaceans and fish (Bandyopadhyay and Nandy, 1986); the Gastrodiscidae in squid and crayfish (Fried *et al.*, 2004); the Gymnophallidae in oysters (Lee *et al.*, 1993); the Microphallidae in crabs and shrimp (Schell, 1985); and the Nanophyetidae in salmonids (Schell, 1985).

Significant Pathogens within the Group

There are a number of digenean species that pose problems for captive reared aquatic species. Groupers are reported to be infected by several species, including *Prosorhynchus epinepheli*, *Prosorhynchus pacificus*, *Helicometra fasciata*, *Erilepturus hamate* and *Transversotrema patialense* in Vietnam, for which some of them resulted in market downgrades and subsequent losses (Vo *et al.*, 2008, 2011). Members of the Didymozoidae, such as *Didymocystis* spp., have been reported to infect the gills of Atlantic bluefin tuna and other related species (Mladineo, 2006; Mladineo and Block, 2010; Mladineo and Tudor, 2004); *Unitubulotestis sardae* from Atlantic bonito, *Sarda sarda* (see Marino *et al.*, 2003); *Didymocylindrus simplex* from skipjack tuna, *Katsuwonus pelamis* (see Nascimento Justo *et al.*, 2013); and unidentified didymozoids have also been reported from groupers (Vo *et al.*, 2008, 2011). Other commonly encountered digenean infections in mariculture include *Galactosomum* spp. in Japanese amberjack (*Seriola quinqueradiata*), Japanese pufferfish (*Takifugu rubripes*), striped beakfish (*Oplegnathus fasciatus*) (see Kimura and Endo, 1979; Yasunaga *et al.*, 1981); *Stephanostomum tenue* in *O. mykiss* (see McGladdery *et al.*, 1990); *Cardicola* spp. in gilthead bream, *Sparus aurata* (see Holzer *et al.*, 2008) and various species of *Thunnus* spp. (Aiken *et al.*, 2006, 2008; Cribb *et al.*, 2000, 2011; Hardy-Smith *et al.*, 2012; Kirchhoff *et al.*, 2011; Shirakashi *et al.*, 2012a, 2012b; Sugihara *et al.*, 2014); *Paradeontacylix* spp. from greater amberjack, *Seriola dumerili* (see Crespo *et al.*, 1992; Ogawa and Fukudome, 1994; Ogawa *et al.*, 1989, 1993; Repullés-Albelda *et al.*, 2008); *Psettarium* spp. in *T. rubripes* (see Yoshinaga *et al.*, 2009).

In freshwater aquaculture, there are a number of species that are reported to be pathogenic, including *Bolbophorus damnificus* which results in morbidity and mortality of channel catfish, *Ictalurus punctatus*, in the USA (Levy *et al.*, 2006; Overstreet *et al.*, 2002; Yost *et al.*, 2005). Infections of the eye fluke species *Diplostomum spathaceum* and *Tylodelphys* spp. can cause cataract and blindness in a range of fish species (Dwyer and Smith, 1989; Karvonen *et al.*, 2003; Whyte *et al.*, 1991); 'black spot disease' has been associated with the presence of *Posthodiplostomum cuticola* and the marine host-infecting digenean *Cryptocotyle lingua*, which encyst within the epidermis of fish skin with the resultant surrounding accumulation of melanophores, and infections reduce the marketability of harvested stock (Kristoffersen, 1992; Ondracková *et al.*, 2004); *Centrocestus formosanus* infecting the gills of cultured tropical fish (Pinto and Melo, 2012), and recently reported from tilapia in Brazil (Pinto *et al.*, 2014) where associated losses were estimated at US$3.5 M to pisciculture in the USA (Mitchell *et al.*, 2005); *Clinostomum complanatum*, the causative agent of the 'yellow grub disease', and other *Clinostomum* species are reported from several freshwater species (Aohagl *et al.*, 1992), including tilapia in Brazil (Schafer da Silva *et al.*, 2008) resulting in the rejection of product with resultant economic loss (Lane and Morris, 2000).

Although snails typically serve as the first intermediate host, infections in other molluscs such as scallops are also common. Examples include *Proctoeces* spp., *Himasthla* spp. and *Stephanostomum* spp. causing black spots, while various sanguinicolid species are reported to result in parasitic castration in *Argopecten* spp. (Linton, 1915; Karlsson, 1991; Pérez-Urbiola and Martínez-Diaz, 2001; Stunkard, 1938). Similarly, *Bucephalus*-like digeneans can cause castration in *Pecten* spp. by displacement of the gonad (Heasman *et al.*, 1996; Sanders and Lester, 1981), while *Microphallus* spp. infecting various crustaceans also results in parasitic castration of their hosts (Overstreet *et al.*, 1992a; Pina *et al.*, 2011).

Reviews

Comprehensive reviews of the Digenea, which encompass keys to identification, systematics, geographical distribution and their biology, are detailed within Yamaguti (1958), Smyth (1994), Bray and Cribb (1998), Gibson *et al.* (2002), Galaktionov and Dobrovolskij (2003), Olson *et al.* (2003), Cribb *et al.* (2003), Jones *et al.* (2005), Bray *et al.* (2008), Roberts and Janovy (2009), Lima dos Santos and Howgate (2011), Shimazu (2013), Bray and Justine (2014) and Ogawa (2015).

Identification

General body features of both the cercariae and adult digeneans can facilitate their identification, notably the size and configuration of the suckers and other body organs. Some of the older terminology (e.g. '*stoma*' in Greek meaning 'mouth', not 'sucker') is used to characterize such body features, such as 'monostome' with a single, orally positioned sucker; 'amphistome' with one oral sucker and a posterior *acetabulum*; and 'distome' with two suckers, one oral and one ventral (Roberts and Janovy, 2009). Subsequent identification nomenclature includes additional terms to describe body forms, such as 'holostome' (e.g. *Diplostomum*) 'schistosome' (e.g. *Schistosoma*) and echinostome (e.g. *Echinostoma*). When using cercariae to identify species, the shape of the body and the tail, the number of flame cells, body spination and the presence or absence of a stylet are all important diagnostic features. Metacercariae, however, are more challenging to identify, although a presumptive diagnosis can be made using the nature and site of infection of the encysted parasite, such as *Diplostomum* in the lens.

Diagnostic Methods

Ideally, digeneans are best examined alive following collection from their hosts. When the examination of fresh samples is not possible then specimens can be fixed in 70–95% ethanol for subsequent morphological and molecular analyses. Several staining methods can be used to visualize their internal anatomy, including iron acetocarmine (Georgiev *et al.*, 1986; Kostadinova *et al.*, 2003), Semichon's acetocarmine or Ehrlich's haematoxylin (Choudhury and Nelson, 2000), and van Cleave's haematoxylin (Overstreet, 1976), among others. Following staining and differentiation, specimens can be dehydrated through graded alcohols, cleared in an appropriate medium (e.g. clove oil) and then flattened and permanently mounted in Canada balsam. Specimens for histological examination can either be fixed in formalin (Cribb and Bray, 2010) or in aqueous Bouin's fixative for 24 hours, then rinsed in 70% ethanol and subsequently stored in 70% ethanol (Dezfuli *et al.*, 2013; Humason, 1979).

Although material fixed in 10% neutral buffered formalin can be used for molecular studies, it is more problematic and it is advised that, where possible, additional specimens specifically for molecular analysis are fixed in 95% molecular grade ethanol.

As already mentioned, the diagnosis of metacercariae is difficult and usually is only presumptive, based on information relating to the type of cyst (e.g. shape, presence of a single or double wall) and the site of infection; sequencing of taxonomically informative parts of the genome can lead to precise identifications (Dzikowski *et al.*, 2004). Experimental infection of a suitable definitive host (usually a piscivorous bird) may provide adult worms; however, in the interests of reducing the number of animals used in scientific studies, this sort of investigative approach should be the final resort and should be limited to studies of strategic importance. Metacercariae encysted within the musculature of fish can be released either by mechanical pressure using a needle to rupture cysts and release the parasite within or by using proteolytic digestion (e.g. pepsin, HCl, trypsin and/or sodium taurocholate-based solutions) (Bass and LeFlore, 1984). Eye fluke infections, such as *Diplostomum* spp., can be diagnosed by the naked eye looking at the pathognomonic symptoms of the cataract formed on the surface of the fish eye; frequently, live metacercariae can be seen within the eye. Alternatively, the fish can be euthanized and the eye dissected to collect the unencysted metacercariae within. ELISA can also be used for determining plasma antibody levels to a particular digenean species as an indication of potential infection not evident from gross examination and dissection of body organs (Höglund and Thuvander, 1990; Whyte *et al.*, 1987). Molecular diagnostic methods for the identification include the use of internal transcribed spacers (ITS) (Born-Torrijos *et al.*, 2012), the complete small subunit ribosomal RNA gene (SSU) and regions D1–D3 of the large subunit ribosomal RNA gene (LSU) (Olson *et al.*, 2003).

Cestoda

Biology and Taxonomy

Tapeworms (Figure 4.6) are cosmopolitan endoparasites. Adult cestodes have a flattened body composed of an adhesive apical part called the 'scolex', a germinative short segment referred to as the 'neck' and the strobilum with a variable number of hermaphroditic proglottids. Cestodes feed through a metabolically active tegument consisting of microtriches and filtering tissue. The Class Cestoda includes 13 Orders and approximately 5000 species, among which the Bothriocephalidea, Caryophyllidea, Diphyllobothriidea, Lecanicephalidea, Proteocephalidea, Pseudophyllidea, Tetraphyllidea and Trypanorhyncha are of particular ichthyoparasitological interest.

Life-Cycle

Cestode life-cycles are always heteroxenous, requiring a definitive host and at least one or, more frequently, two intermediate hosts. Fish can act either as an intermediate host to different parasite larval stages, such as procercoid and plerocercoid, or as a definitive host. When fish play the role of second intermediate host, the larval stages of several tapeworm species can have different tissue tropisms, while when the fish act as definitive host, cestodes that reach the adult phase and sexual maturity usually produce eggs in the gut. First intermediate hosts are invertebrate organisms belonging to different taxa, mainly aquatic crustaceans. Given the

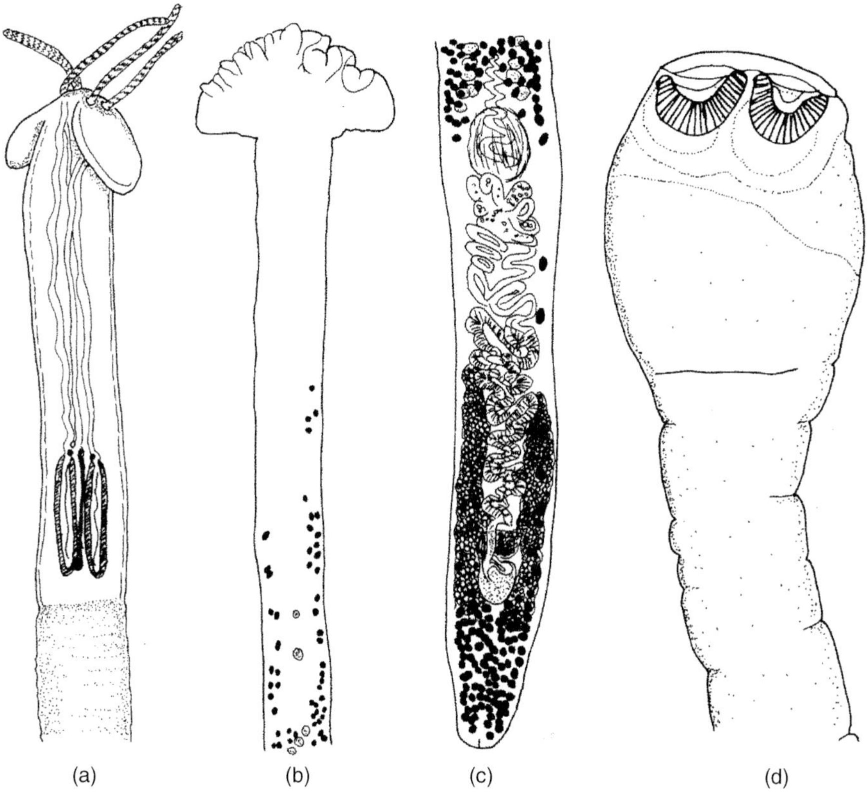

Figure 4.6 Representative drawings of cestodes reported in fish. (a) *Gilguinia* sp. (after Khalil *et al.* 1994); (b) Anterior portion, including scolex, of *Khawia* sp. (adapted from Scholz *et al.*, 1970); (c) Posterior portion of *Khawia* sp. (adapted from Scholz *et al.*, 1970); (d) Scolex of *Proteocephalus* sp. (adapted from Scholz and Hanzelová, 1970).

complex nature of cestode life-cycles, conditions leading to infection in aquaculture environments are rather limited; consequentially, only a few species are of concern in farmed animals. In marked contrast to this, wild fish are commonly infected with cestodes and they therefore pose a potential risk to farmed aquatic hosts through indirect transmission via feeding on these infected hosts. Cestodes, similar to digeneans, can also change their host's behaviour to allow the parasite's life-cycle to be completed, for example by increasing their susceptibility to predation; by affecting the foraging and shoaling behaviour of the infected fish; and by suppressing the satiation response (e.g. in sticklebacks infected with *Schistocephalus*) to ensure that both parasite and host gain sufficient nutrition (Barber and Huntingford, 1995; Barber *et al.*, 1995, 2008).

Public Health

Several species of aquatic (and terrestrial) cestode have public health implications, and humans, being at the apex of the food chain, can be involved as the definitive host for those species of tapeworm linked to the aquatic environment. Among these, the most important zoonotic fish-borne cestodes belong to the Diphyllobothriidae, which are aetiological agents of around 20 million human cases of diphyllobothriasis worldwide (Scholz *et al.*, 2009). The most common species are the freshwater *Diphyllobothrium latum* and *D. dendriticum* and the marine species *Adenocephalus* [=*Diphyllobothrium*] *pacificum*. Human infections are invariably linked to the ingestion of plerocercoid larvae through the consumption of raw or undercooked fish products.

Significant Pathogens within the Group

Significant pathogens include *D. dendriticum*, *D. latum*, *Eubothrium crassum*, *E. salvelini* and *Gilquinia squali* in farmed salmonids, *Monobothrium wageneri* in tench, *Tinca tinca* (see Dezfuli *et al.*, 2011), *Triaenophorus crassus* in coregonids, *Schyzocotyle* [=*Bothriocephalus*] *acheilognathi* in cyprinids, *Hepatoxylon trichiuri* in Atlantic bluefin tuna, *Thunnus thynnus*, and *Tylocephalum* metacestodes in pearl oysters. Species of *Proteocephalus* infecting several fish species in the Palearctic region, including salmonids, cyprinids and percids, in addition to species of *Khawia* infecting cyprinids, are also worthy of note. The impact of the adult and larval stages of tapeworms on fish health can vary, even within the same species, and in general, their pathogenic effect is dependent on parasitic burden. Usually the survival strategy of adult cestodes in the intestine of suitable fish species is not to kill their host; instead, the sublethal impact of the parasite on its host can include nutrient depletion, mechanical damage to the intestinal mucosa by the cestode's attachment apparatus (i.e. adhesive organs of the scolex, such as suckers, bothria, bothrids, hooks) and alterations to the immune status/profile of their host (Alvarez-Pellitero, 2008). For the larval stages, pathogenicity is strongly connected to intensity and localization within target organs; for example, the functionality of vital visceral organs can be threatened by high numbers of larvae; high burdens of infection within the musculature can reduce host fitness, predisposing them to increased likelihood of predation by the definitive host. Heavy cestode burdens can reduce the food conversion ratios of aquaculture reared stock and their evident presence can negatively affect the marketability of stocks.

Reviews

General and specific reviews on the systematics of cestodes can be found within Yamaguti (1959), Mackiewicz (1972), Schmidt (1986), Khalil *et al.* (1994), Hoffman (1999), Scholz (1999b), Palm (2004), Kuchta *et al.* (2008) and Scholz *et al.* (2011), among others.

Identification

The identification of cestode species is based on the 'classic' analysis of the main morphological features: the scolex and its characteristic structures (number and shape of suckers, hooks, spines, bothria and bothriids, etc.); morphology of the proglottids and anatomy of the sexual organs in gravid proglottids (number and position of testes, shape and position of the cirrus, ovary and uterus, etc.), egg morphometry. Species identification, especially for the larval stages which cannot be readily discriminated by morphology, is made, for example, by the dual application of molecular techniques based on DNA/RNA amplification and sequencing, and DNA barcoding.

Diagnostic Methods

Diagnosis by morphological analysis is conducted using a combination of different techniques. Cestodes should be isolated from the host, cleaned and rinsed in water, then fixed in hot formalin (usually not suitable for subsequent molecular analyses) or in 70–99% ethanol. At this stage, the cestodes can be kept preserved indefinitely. Clarification by Amman's lactophenol or glycerol and differential staining techniques (e.g. carmine-based stains, Malzacher's stain, among others), together with SEM and TEM, allow for features of taxonomic importance to be visualized. Histology of adult tapeworms is useful in determining the key anatomical features of proglottids, as well as gaining a better understanding of any pathology caused by the parasite in its host. Molecular techniques are becoming increasingly helpful in diagnostic support, but it is always judicious to combine these with morphology-based approaches since their application is dependent upon the availability of publicly accessible sequences.

Nematoda

Biology and Taxonomy

Nematodes (roundworms) are a widespread group of parasites infecting both wild and, to a lesser extent, farmed fish (Figure 4.7). Molluscs and crustaceans can act as intermediate hosts harbouring the larval stages of these parasites. Adult nematodes usually live (but not exclusively) within the intestinal lumen of their fish host; other notable species may reside within the gonads, for example, some species of *Philometra* (see Moravec *et al.*, 2016); the gall bladder and pyloric caeca, for example, *Hysterothylacium fabri* in migratory fish (Urquhart *et al.*, 2010); the swimbladder, for example, *Anguillicoloides crassus* in eels (Lefebvre *et al.*, 2012) and *Cystidicola farionis* in salmonids (Lankester and Smith, 1980). Larval stages of nematodes have a wide range of organ tropism. The body is typically cylindrical with an anterior cephalic extremity characterized by structures such as lips, teeth and/or papillae, a posterior tail, an elongated body which can be covered by spines and/or ridges, and have sensory structures called phasmids. A cuticle secreted by the syncytial epidermis covers the body. Internally, there are four longitudinal muscles and two longitudinal nerves running along the length of the parasite. The pseudocoelomatic cavity contains a digestive and an excretory system. Nematodes show sexual dimorphism and morphological features unique to adult males and females that are of taxonomical relevance.

Life-Cycle

Most nematodes infecting an aquatic host have a complex life-cycle that involves a fish as either an intermediate or definitive host. When the definitive host is a fish, typically there is only a single intermediate host. If the final host is not a fish, then there are typically two intermediate hosts, one of which is a fish. In some cases, when the transmission is linked to the trophic chain (e.g. as with anisakid nematodes), many fish species can also play a paratenic host role, in which the parasite does not undergo a biological developmental step but the strategy contributes to the spread of the parasite in the aquatic environment. In intensive aquaculture, where only a commercial pelleted feed is typically used, conditions leading to a possible contact between the different hosts are much more difficult to establish. Changes to husbandry practices (e.g. poor feed management, starvation) and environmental factors could result in altered feeding behaviour of the farmed fish, promoting the transmission of nematodes. In addition to those routes of infection, a few nematode species, such as *Capillaria* spp., can transmit directly by fish-to-fish contact and, as such, can represent a threat to ornamental fish kept in confined environments such as aquaria.

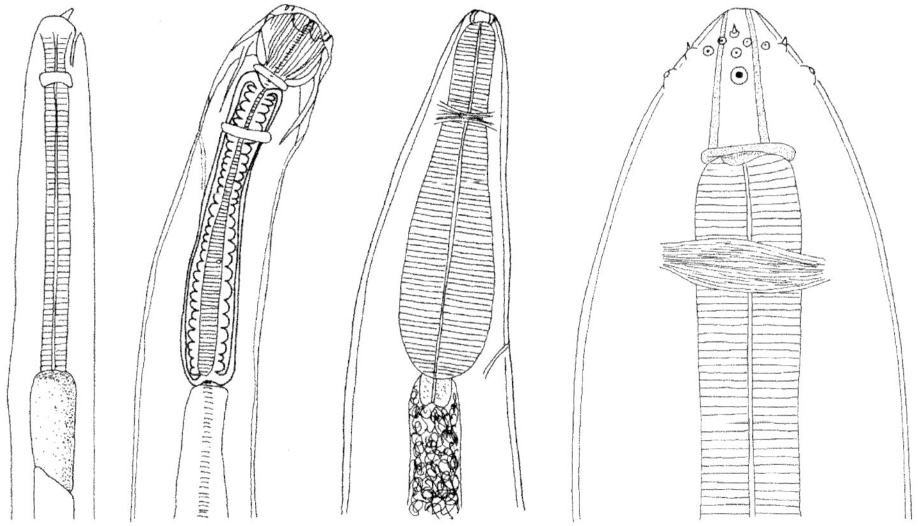

Figure 4.7 Representative drawings of nematodes found in farmed and/or wild fish. (a) Head of L3 larva of *Anisakis* sp. (original); (b) Head of a female fourth stage larva of *Camallanus* sp. (after Rigby *et al.*, 1997); (c) Adult *Anguillicoloides* sp. (after Moravec, 2002); (d) Cephalic end of a male fourth stage larva of *Eustrongylides* sp. (after Moravec and van As, 2015).

Public Health

Several species of aquatic nematodes are of public health concern. The most important zoonotic roundworms are the marine anisakid nematodes, in particular species belonging to the genera *Anisakis*, *Pseudoterranova* and, to a lesser extent, *Contracaecum*. Globally, thousands of human cases are reported each year, always linked to the traditional consumption of raw or undercooked fish products. There are typically over 2000 cases of gastrointestinal anisakiasis in Japan each year (Bucci *et al.*, 2013). Marine mammals, and birds for some species of *Contracaecum*, are the definitive hosts but man acts as an incidental or 'dead-end' host; human infections by anisakid larvae are usually self-limiting and lead to rapid death of the parasite but in some cases can result in invasive or allergic syndromes, and parasites can only be removed by surgical intervention. The consumption of certain raw or undercooked aquatic organisms from freshwater environments, notably in Asia and South America, can also lead to accidental human infections by the larval stages of *Gnathostoma* spp., with consequential gastrointestinal or more severe *larva migrans* syndromes (Diaz, 2015). Infection by *Capillaria philippinensis* resulting in intestinal capillariasis is widespread throughout South-East Asia as is, to a lesser extent, infection by the cosmopolitan, red nematode *Eustrongylides* spp. (see Cole, 1999). For both latter species, fish-eating birds are the most suitable definitive hosts. The consumption of raw infected fish products, though, can lead to human intestinal infections; female worms within the gut produce fertilized eggs and larvae, which are able to spread into the environment or reinfect the same host.

Significant Pathogens within the Group

The pathogenicity of adult worms is generally low in mild infections but can intensify with increases in parasitic burden. Pathological effects are usually linked to the haematophagous activity of the parasite (e.g. *Anguillicoloides crassus*) (see Molnár *et al.*, 1991) or to the mechanical damage to host tissue caused by penetration structures such as buccal capsules (e.g. *Camallanus* spp.) or cephalic teeth. Larval stages are usually hypobiotic, which means that the larval development is prolonged but temporarily arrested. Pathogenicity is correlated to parasite intensity and localization within the host – the functionality of vital visceral organs can be threatened by high numbers of larvae, whereas high burdens within the musculature can result in diminished fitness, predisposing the host to an increased probability of predation by the definitive host. Heavy nematode burdens may impact on the quality, aesthetic appeal and marketability of fish.

Reviews

General reviews on nematode systematics are detailed in Yamaguti (1962), Moravec (1994, 1998, 2001, 2002, 2004), Anderson (2000), Anderson *et al.* (2009) and Gibbons (2010).

Identification

The morphological identification of adult nematodes to the species level is usually made by studying specific anatomical features, such as cephalic structures, the number and distribution of anterior and posterior papillae, the position of excretory pores, the features pertaining to the digestive system, the morphometry of the reproductive organs, etc. The larval stages are not easily discriminated and morphological identification is usually limited to the genus level. Molecular taxonomy in combination with information derived from morphology, however, is regarded as the 'gold standard' approach through the sequencing of informative regions of the genome. Other methods used in the discrimination of species include multilocus enzyme electrophoresis (Mattiucci and Nascetti, 2008).

Diagnostic Methods

Diagnosis by morphology should follow isolation of parasites from the host, cleaning in an appropriate medium (e.g. physiological saline) and ethanol fixation. Thereafter, parasites can be kept preserved indefinitely. Nematodes should be cleared in either Amman's lactophenol or in glycerol, as differential staining and permanent mounting are of limited use since parasites should be mounted in a medium to allow for their rotation and orientation to assess all potential diagnostic features, such as excretory pores, papillae, phasmids, transversal and longitudinal ridges, etc. Although SEM cannot be used as a routine technique, it is a very useful tool for mapping and examining surface structures. The best diagnostic approach is a combination of morphology and molecular-based tools, by partitioning samples so that appropriate sections of each worm can be evaluated by both methods, that is, the anterior and posterior third of each worm being used for morphology, the middle section for DNA sequencing.

Acanthocephala

Biology and Taxonomy

Acanthocephalans, also known as 'thorny headed' or 'spiny headed' worms, are characterized by an eversible proboscis that is differentially armed with an array of hooks, the number and

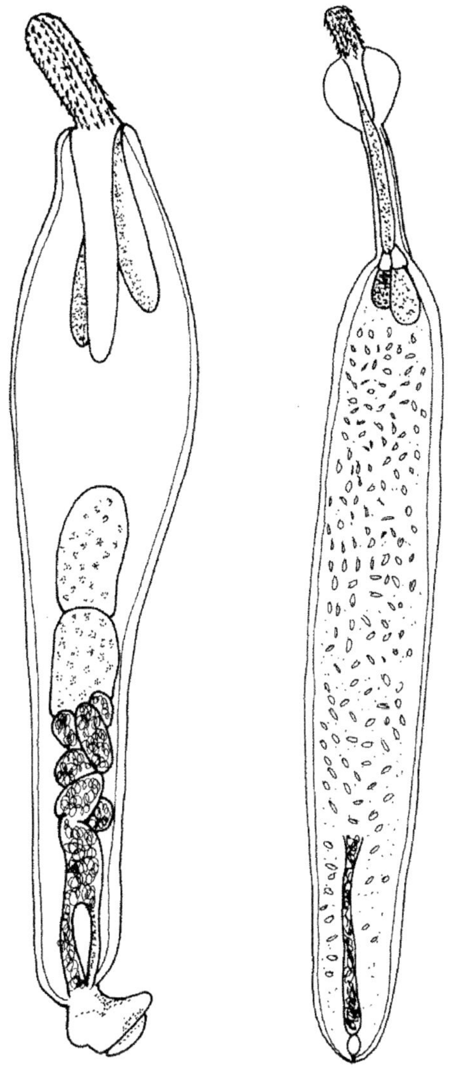

Figure 4.8 Representative drawings of acanthocephalans reported from fish. (a) Male individual of *Echinorhynchus* sp. (after Arai, 1989); (b) Female individual of *Pomphorhynchus* sp. (after Špakulová *et al.*, 2011).

pattern of which have taxonomical importance (Figure 4.8). The body is limited by a syncytial epidermis and acanthocephalans, which lack a digestive layer, feed by nutrient uptake through the cuticular layer. Acanthocephalans are sexually dimorphic: males possess, depending on the species, a variable number of testes, a copulatory bursa and 'cement glands' which are used to seal the female's vagina after reproduction (Kennedy, 2006).

Life-Cycle

Adult parasites typically live within the gut of their definitive host, where they reproduce sexually. Fertilized eggs develop inside the female to the acanthor stage at which point the eggs are then released within its host's faecal waste into the aquatic environment. When ingested by a suitable intermediate host, the embryonated eggs hatch into an acanthella stage which subsequently encysts in its host's tissues as a fully developed larval cystacanth until consumed, and released, by its definitive host. For some parasite species, such as *Acanthocephalus anguillae*, the fish can act as a paratenic host. Fish also play a role as definitive hosts to species such as *Pomphorhynchus laevis* in trout, *A. anguillae* in European eels, *Anguilla anguilla*, and *Acanthocephalus lucii* in northern pike, *Esox lucius* (see Schmidt and Nickol, 1985), while other piscine species can act as a postcyclic host, such as when adults occupying one host are ingested and able to survive within the predatory host (Kennedy, 1999). This reduction of the typical complex life-cycle suggests that infections could propagate between piscivorous aquaculture species who consume their congeners rather than the commercial feed.

Public Health

Acanthocephalans have been rarely reported in humans, and in cases where infections are known, these are typically as a result of accidental infection. *Acanthocephalus rauschi*, *Bolbosoma* spp. and *Corynosoma strumosum* are the only acanthocephalans reported in man following the ingestion of raw fish (Golvan, 1969; Schmidt, 1971; Tada *et al.*, 1983).

Significant Pathogens within the Group

Sanitary problems caused by acanthocephalans are strictly derived from the intensity of the adult parasitic infection, in terms of the mechanical damage inflicted on the mucosa during the process of parasite attachment (Dezfuli *et al.*, 2002; Wanstall *et al.*, 1986), and in the nutrient resources drawn from the host (Wanstall *et al.*, 1982; Woo, 2006). Significant pathogens within the group include *Acanthocephalus* spp., *Bolbosoma* spp., *Echinorhynchus* spp. and *Pomphorhynchus* spp., among others.

Reviews

Reviews dedicated to the taxonomy of the Acanthocephala include those by Yamaguti (1963b), Amin (1987, 2000, 2013) and Khatoon and Bilqees (2011); parasite–host interactions are covered by Taraschewski (2000) and population dynamics are reviewed by Kennedy (2006). Acanthocephalans also represent interesting species for biological modelling and act as bioindicators of pollution and environmental contamination (Jankovská *et al.*, 2011; Nachev and Sures, 2016; Nachev *et al.*, 2013; Sures, 2001).

Identification

The identification of acanthocephalans follows the traditional morphological approach based on the evaluation of taxonomically informative morphological features such as the presence/absence of spines on the trunk; the number, shape and distribution pattern of hooks on the proboscis; the number of cement glands in the male; the shape of the paired lemnisci and that of the proboscis receptacle, etc. There are several generic texts on the identification of Acanthocephala, including those of Yamaguti (1963b), Brown *et al.* (1986), Amin (1985, 1987, 2013) and Hoffman (1999). As with most parasite taxa, morphological analyses should be supported, where possible, with parallel investigations employing molecular taxonomy-based methods (i.e. DNA extraction, PCR-based amplification and sequencing), notably in facilitating the identification of larval stages recovered from intermediate hosts, whose morphological identification is not usually straightforward.

Diagnostic Methods

Adult acanthocephalans within their definitive host exhibit intestinal tropism and parasites are found securely attached to the intestinal wall by their armed proboscis; in some cases, parasite attachment results in gut perforation, with some parasites subsequently occupying the visceral cavity. Collected parasites typically have to be liberated from host tissue to which they are attached by using dissecting needles, ensuring that the proboscis remains intact. Once released from enclosing host tissue, the acanthocephalans can be fixed in 70–95% ethanol for subsequent morphological and molecular-based analyses. Brown *et al.* (1986) provide a detailed methodology for the collection, fixation, preservation and examination of acanthocephalan parasites. Alcohol-fixed specimens can be cleared using glycerol or can be stained using Mayer's acid carmine, to assist with the elucidation of the internal anatomy of these helminths. SEM can assist in mapping and studying the armature of the proboscis and body spination, while histology serves as an essential means to investigate host–parasite interactions and the pathogenicity of acanthocephalan infection.

Arthropoda

Biology and Taxonomy

Arthropods (Figure 4.9) are a highly diverse, species-rich phylum of organisms and their taxonomy is complex. The subphylum Crustacea, for example, includes 971 families, 9598 genera and around 64 663 extant species, of which an estimated 8000+ species have parasitic stages. This section will therefore comment on only a small number of important taxa within the subphylum Crustacea that contain noted parasite pathogens of aquaculture, namely species within the subclasses Copepoda and Branchiura and the Order Isopoda.

Life-Cycles

Parasitic Copepods

The life-cycle of a parasitic copepod is generally direct. Parasitic stages may be found mobile over the external surfaces of its host, attached by specialized attachment structures, partially embedded or completely embedded within its host's tissues. Parasitic copepods are dioecious, the adult male being much smaller than the female, for example *Chondracanthus* spp. where the female is around 15–20 times larger than the male. Females extrude their eggs into paired egg sacs or uniseriate egg strings; several batches may be produced by a female over her lifetime. Egg development is temperature dependent. Nauplii hatch from the eggs that are carried by the female. Parasitic copepods have two life phases: typically a free-living, dispersive, lecithotrophic naupliar phase within which there may be up to six naupliar stages, and a copepodid phase which is marked by a change in body morphology and a switch to a parasitic mode of life. The nauplii have an unsegmented body and three pairs of functional appendages, antennules, antennae and mandibles, while on transition to the copepodid stages, the parasite develops a segmented body, a full set of cephalic appendages and two pairs of swimming legs. There may be a maximum of five copepodid stages; the fifth copepodid moults into the definitive adult stage which, in some species, is marked by a profound metamorphosis and gross transformation of the body morphology, with the resultant loss of appendages and/or the development of specialized attachment structures. The males may guard preadult females

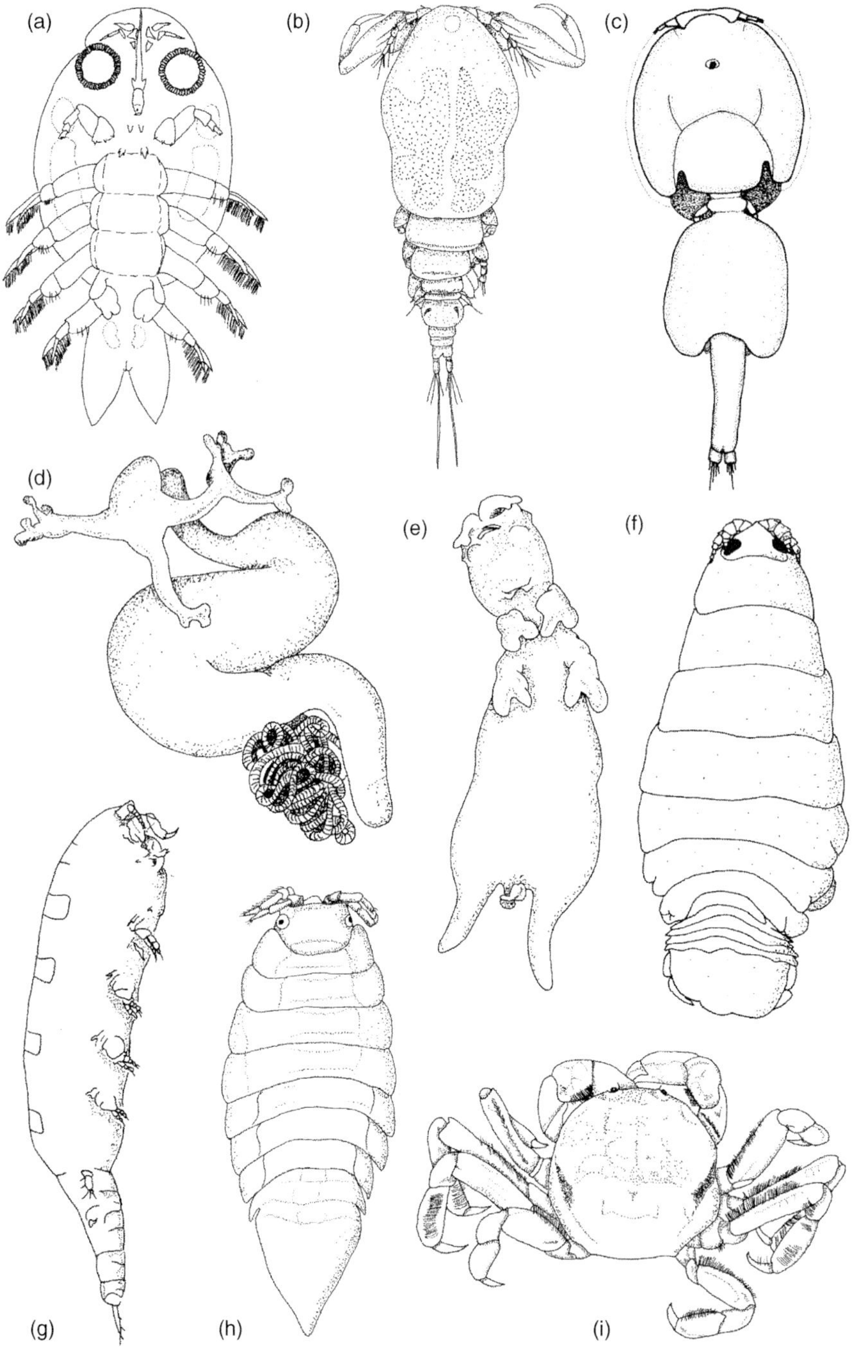

Figure 4.9 Representative drawings of parasitic Arthropoda reported as pathogens of farmed fish and/or shellfish. Examples of fish parasites include: (a) Female *Argulus* sp. (Branchiura); (b) *Ergasilus* sp. (Copepoda); (c) *Lepeophtheirus salmonis* (Copepoda); (d) *Lernaeocera branchialis* (Copepoda); (e) Female *Chondracanthus* sp. (Copepoda) with a single parasitic male on the posterior edge of the main body; and, (f) *Ceratothoa* sp. (Isopoda) occurring in the mouth of a number of marine fish hosts. Examples of farmed bivalve parasites include: (g) *Myicola ostreae* (Copepoda); (h) *Edotia* sp. (Isopoda); and (i) *Nepinnotheres novaezelandiae* (Decapoda). Figure a after Cressey (1978), Figures b, d and e after Kabata (1979), Figure c original, Figure f after Horton (2000), Figure g after Ho and Kim (1991), Figure h after Brandt (1990), Figure i after Page (1983).

and then mate, depositing spermatophores on the female once she has moulted. Adult copepods do not moult. The life-cycles of parasitic copepods are generally shorter than free-living copepods. Parasite activity in attaching, burrowing and/or feeding can result in damage to the host and mortality.

Isopods

Adult isopods are dorsoventrally flattened crustaceans that lack a carapace, have a head that is fused to the first thoracic somite, have sessile eyes and a thorax with seven somites, each with a pair of uniramous swimming legs. Isopods are dioecious but cymothoid isopods are protandrous hermaphrodites – the first male attaching to a fish changes into a female, which may then prevent the development of other males into females. Some species are obligate parasites (e.g. *Cymothoa*) and pose a serious threat to certain aquaculture stocks, while other species, such as *Cirolana borealis*, for example, are free-living scavengers, which have been reported as occasional parasites of farmed stocks. Gravid females release eggs into a brood pouch or marsupium within which the eggs embryonate, hatch and undergo two moults to form the manca or pullus II stages, which have only six pairs of legs, large compound eyes and heavily setose pleopods facilitating their rapid swimming performance. These juvenile stages are then released from the pouch, the parent then moults, feeds and subsequently produces the next batch of eggs. The manca are active, rapid swimmers for a short period but then switch to a parasitic mode of life, taking a blood meal within two days of their release from the parent; for obligate species such as *Ceratothoa*, the manca may move to their preferred site and remain attached. For species that exhibit temporary parasitism, they continue to move on and off their hosts to feed and to moult until they attain adulthood, marked by the appearance of a seventh pair of legs. For gnathiids (Gnathiidae, Cymothoida, Isopoda), however, only the larvae or praniza are normally parasitic on the gills and skin of fish (some exceptions include heavy infections of adult parasites on fish under aquarium conditions), where they feed on blood and within the gastral cavities of anemones and tunicates. The praniza moult after each blood meal; after the third moult the gnathiid transforms into an adult and then switches to a non-parasitic, sediment dwelling mode of life.

Branchiurans

Adult branchiurans such as *Argulus* are dioecious and highly mobile and temporary parasites, moving on, off and between their hosts to feed and lay eggs. In appearance, argulids are ovoid with a dorsoventrally flattened carapace, possess a modified pair of first maxillae which are evident as large suctorial organs, have compound eyes, a piercing preoral stylet, four pairs of swimming legs and a tubular mouth with denticulated mandibles. Branchiurans feed on tissue fluids and haemolymph of their hosts. Branchiuran eggs are not carried in egg strings, as is the case with parasitic copepods; instead, the females carry their eggs within a single ovary until they can be laid, in rows one layer thick, onto an appropriate substrate. Egg development is temperature dependent and cohorts of eggs may overwinter. The first-stage larvae, which in *Argulus* is a developmentally advanced metanauplius stage, must seek out and parasitize a host within 2–3 days of hatching or die. The parasite then passes through 11–12 moults until it reaches sexual maturity; branchiurans continue to moult in adulthood.

Public Health

No parasitic crustaceans pose a risk to human health.

Significant Pathogens within the Group

Infections on captive-reared aquaculture stocks commonly impose serious economic impacts. In fresh water, significant pathogens of aquaculture reared stocks include *Argulus foliaceus, Ergasilus sieboldi, Lernaea cyprinacea* and *Salmincola salmoneus.* Although the caligid copepod *Lepeophtheirus salmonis* is occasionally seen on Atlantic salmon (*Salmo salar*), in fresh water, this is a marine parasite that is carried into fresh water on its anadromous host. *Caligus elongatus, Caligus rogercresseyi* and *L. salmonis* on Atlantic salmon are the most significant metazoan parasites of marine aquaculture, reputedly costing the global salmon industry around US$584 million p.a. (Shinn *et al.*, 2015a, 2015b). Other caligid species are also reported as impacting on the health and welfare of captive stocks of, for example, black porgy, *Acanthopagrus schlegelii* (see Lin *et al.*, 1994); flathead grey mullet, *Mugil cephalus* (see Paperna and Lahav, 1974); Japanese amberjack (Ogawa *et al.*, 1993); milk fish, *Chanos chanos* (see Lin, 1989); rainbow trout (Urawa and Kato, 1991); European seabass, *Dicentrarchus labrax* (see Er and Kayiş, 2015); and southern bluefin tuna, *Thunnus maccoyii* (see Hayward *et al.*, 2008). Important scientific publications on other significant parasitic copepods include, among others, those on *Lernaeocera branchialis* on Atlantic cod, *Gadus morhua* (see Brooker *et al.*, 2007; Khan *et al.*, 1990), *Lernanthropus kroyeri* on European seabass, *Dicentrarchus labrax* (see Athanassopoulou *et al.*, 2001; Vagianou *et al.*, 2006), *Diergasilus kasahara* on milkfish (Lin and Ho, 1998), *Ergasilus lobus* on grouper species (Lin and Ho, 1998) and *Ergasilus lizae* on flathead grey mullet (Paperna, 1975).

A number of scavenging and parasitic species of isopod are reported as pathogens of farmed stocks of fish, including *Alitropus typus* on *C. chanos* (see Regidor and Arthur, 1986); *Ceratothoa gaudichaudii* on Chilean populations of *S. salar* (see Sievers *et al.*, 1996); *Ceratothoa oestroides* and *C. parallela* on gilthead seabream, *S. aurata*, and European seabass, *D. labrax* (see Horton and Okamura, 2003; Papapanagiotou and Trilles, 2001; Šarušic, 1999); *Cirolana fluviatilis* on barramundi, *Lates calcarifer* (see Sanil *et al.*, 2009); *Emetha audouini* and *Nerocila orbignyi* on European seabass (Bragoni *et al.*, 1984; Papapanagiotou *et al.*, 1999); and *Natatolana borealis* (see Johansen and Brattegard, 1998).

In mollusc aquaculture, notable copepod pathogens include *Modiolicola gracilicaudus, Myicola ostreae, Mytilicola intestinalis, Mytilicola orientalis, Ostrincola koe* and *Pectenophilus ornatus* (see Bower *et al.*, 1994; Elston, 1993; Ho and Zheng, 1994; Lauckner, 1983; Nagasawa and Nagata, 1992; Pogoda *et al.*, 2012; Robledo *et al.*, 1994; Villalba *et al.*, 1997). The isopod *Edotia doellojuradoi* damages the gills of farmed mussels (Valencia and George-Nascimento, 2013), while the parasitic pea crab *Nepinnotheres novaezelandiae* causes significant damage and economic loss to farmed New Zealand green-lipped mussel, *Perna canaliculi* (see Trottier *et al.*, 2012).

In shrimp culture, the bobyrid isopod *Orbione bonnieri* is a commonly encountered parasite of cultured *Metapenaeus* species (Printrakoon and Purivirojkul, 2012).

Reviews

Taxonomy and Systematics

For general reviews of the subphylum Crustacea, see, among others, the accounts of Yamaguti (1963c), Kabata (1970, 1979, 1981, 1984), Möller and Anders (1986), Grabda (1991), Martin and Davis (2001) and Lester and Hayward (2006). For reviews relating to the phylogenetics of parasitic Crustacea, see Ho (1990) and Bron *et al.* (2011).

For reviews of parasitic species within the **Amphipoda**, see Bousfield and Kabata (1988), Lützen (2005); for the **Asothoracida** see Grygier and Høeg (2005); for the **Branchiura** see Martin (1932), Meehan (1940), Yamaguti (1963c), Kabata (1988), Overstreet *et al.* (1992b), Boxshall (2005a); for **Cirripedia** see Høeg *et al.* (2005); for the **Copepoda** see Gurney (1934), Yamaguti (1963c), Hewitt (1963), Kabata (1981, 1988, 2003), Kazachenko (2001), Martin and Davis (2001), Ho and Lin (2004), Boxshall and Halsey (2004), Boxshall (2005b), Dojiri and Ho (2013); for **Isopoda** see Bruce (1987), Rafi (1988), Keable and Bruce (1997), Bunkley-Williams and Williams (1998), Lester (2005), Keable (2006); for **Rhizocephala** see Høeg *et al.* (2005); for the **Tantulocarida** see Boxshall (2005c); and for the **Thoracica** see Høeg *et al.* (2005).

For general taxonomic keys to regional communities of parasitic crustaceans within the following geographic zones, see: **Africa:** Barnard (1955), Fryer (1968), Kensley and Grindley (1973); **Asia and Australasia:** Heegaard (1962), Yin (1962), Hewitt (1963), Jones (1988), Ho and Lin (2004), Keable (2006); **Central and South America:** Boxshall and Montú (1997), Young (1998); **Europe:** Scott and Scott (1913), Gurney (1934), Fryer (1982), Boxshall (1974), Keable and Bruce (1997), Kabata (2003); and **North America:** Wilson (1905, 1915, 1917), Bousfield and Kabata (1988), Kabata (1988), Rafi (1988).

For pathology and impacts on hosts, see Kabata (1984), Roubal (1989), Jones *et al.* (1990), Bower *et al.* (1994), Dezfuli *et al.* (2003), Horton and Okamura (2003), Manera and Dezfuli (2003), Ferguson (2006), Lester and Hayward (2006), and Smith *et al.* (2007). For problematic species on farmed marine species, see Boxshall and Defaye (1993), Mladineo (2003), Johnson *et al.* (2004), Pike and Wadsworth (1999), Brooker *et al.* (2007), and Nagasawa (2015), among others. The economic costs of some of the main pathogens on, principally marine, aquaculture species are reviewed in Shinn *et al.* (2015a, 2015b).

For reviews on the collection, preparation and processing of parasitic arthropods, see Humes and Gooding (1964), Fryer (1982), Grutter (1995), and Boxshall *et al.* (2016).

Identification

Arthropods are dioecious and the morphology of both the adult male and female, which differs, is key to their taxonomy and identification. For parasitic copepods, their general body organization follows a podoplean body plan with the body divided into a prosome consisting of a cephalosome and four cephalic somites, of which one to four are leg bearing, and a urosome which has a fifth leg-bearing somite, a genital somite, four abdominal somites and a pair of caudal rami on the anal somite. The cephalosome bears seven pairs of segmented appendages (i.e. antennules, antennae, mandibules, maxillules, maxillae, maxillipeds and the first pair of swimming legs), the collective morphological information provided by each facilitating the discrimination of species within taxa. The genital somite and the first abdominal somite may fuse in adult females to form a genital double somite. Gravid females possess paired egg sacs/strings. Branchiurans are typified by a large dorsal carapace, compound eyes and a pair of modified maxillules which have developed as powerful suckers. They possess nine pairs of limbs – the body of a branchiurian is divided into a head with five limbs (antennules, antennae, mandibles within a tubular mouth, modified maxillules as suckers and maxillae), a thorax with four pairs of swimming legs and a short bilobed abdomen which differs between sexes. Argulids also possess a retractable preoral stylet. A typical isopod has a body that is divided into a head or cephalon (that bears sessile eyes, antennae, antennules, mandibles, two pairs of maxillae and maxillipeds), a thorax or peraeon with six or seven somites each with a pair of legs or peraeopods, and an abdomen or pleon which consists of five pleonites and a pleotelson which bears a pair of uropods, composed of an inner (endopod) and outer (exopod) ramus. Bopyrid isopods, which are parasites of crustaceans, have seven pairs of peraeopods and a marsupium or brood pouch formed from oostegites. Daijid isopods, which are typically parasites of prawns, possess five pairs of peraeopods and a brood pouch formed from oostegites, while entoniscid isopods, which are internal parasites of decapods, have lost most signs of their peraeopods and oostegites.

Diagnostic Methods

When screening hosts for parasitic arthropods, it is important to remember that in addition to the evident presence of certain species attached to the external surface of its host, other attached species may occupy less visible microhabitats, for example the nares or between the epithelial folds of the pharyngeal cavity. Parasites may also be partially embedded in host tissue as a result of active penetration or the consequential host reaction that subsequently encloses them. Copepod examples of this include species belonging to the families Chondracanthidae, for example *Chondracanthus* spp. (Tang *et al.*, 2007); Lernaeidae, for example *Lernaea polymorpha* (see Shariff and Roberts, 1989), *Lernaea cyprinacea* (see Piasecki *et al.*, 2004); and Pennellidae, for example *Lernaeocera branchialis* (see Brooker *et al.*, 2007), *Lernaeolophus sultanus* (see Grabda, 1991). The rhizocephalan cirripede *Sacculina carcini* which infects the shore crab, *Carcinus maenas*, is another good example (Høeg *et al.*, 2005). The parasite may also become completely internal, for example the isopod *Natatolana borealis* within the abdominal cavity of various fish species (Johansen and Brattegard, 1998); *Ichthyotaces pteroisicola* and other species belonging to the Philichthyidae which inhabit the lateral line sensory canals (Shiino, 1932) or skull bones (Quignard, 1968) of their hosts; *Sarcotaces pacificus* from galls on their host (Izawa, 1973); or species belonging to the Monstrilloida which have endoparasitic naupliar stages within their polychaete/molluscan host (Boxshall, 2005b).

As the life-cycles and host associations exhibited by parasitic arthropods are highly varied, it is also important to consider that there are free-living stages, and stages that may move on and off their hosts to feed (e.g. *Argulus* spp.). Appropriate sampling methods should therefore be employed in evaluating the potential impact or risk posed by parasites to aquaculture stocks. Such methods might include plankton sampling as well as the post-mortem evaluation of stock as part of a rigorous health surveillance programme. For methods for the collection and processing of free-living copepod stages, see Kilburn *et al.* (2010) and Boxshall *et al.* (2016). The sorting of copepods in the collected filtrate can be assisted by the use of neutral red as a vital stain (1:67 000 w/v solution). For parasite stages attached to their hosts, they can either be carefully picked off using fine tweezers or dissected out of their hosts tissues at post-mortem. If the parasite stages are mobile, they can be dislodged from live hosts using either an appropriate anaesthetic (e.g. 1: 4000 formalin solution, 5% MS222 or 0.4% chloretone prepared in filtered seawater) or narcotizing agent (e.g. carbonated water or ENO-salt™ (sodium bicarbonate Ph. Eur. (*Pharmacopoeia Europaea*) 46.4 g, citric acid Ph. Eur. 43.6 g, anhydrous sodium carbonate Ph. Eur. 10 g)) and then recovering them by either siphoning or filtering the treatment water. For dead or euthanized hosts, some parasites can be dislodged by using fresh water (for marine hosts) or by placing the host in a bag with 70% ethanol and then shaking for a few seconds. Parasites can then be harvested and either fixed directly in 95% ethanol, RNAlater® or frozen for molecular studies, or transferred to an ethanol, formalin and glycerol mixture (7:2:1) as a general preservative. The use of formalin, however, is best avoided for any studies involving a molecular basis. Boxshall *et al.* (2016) provide a discussion on which fixatives to use but conclude that the use of DESS, a dimethylsulfoxide, EDTA and saturated NaCl solution, allows for the long-term, effective storage of specimens which can be subsequently used for either morphological or molecular-based analyses. Mucus and host tissue adhering to specimens that cannot be removed using mounted needles or a fine paint brush can be removed by tumbling specimens in 16% glycerol for six hours before rinsing them and returning them to their fixative.

For morphology-based studies, the dissection of specimens is facilitated by transferring them to lactic acid which makes the cuticle supple; the dissected parts can then, depending on preference, be stained by adding a few drops of a 1% w/v solution of either chlorazol black E, lignin pink or methylene blue, made up in distilled water or 70% ethanol. Permanent mounts can be made by fixing specimens in AFA (85% ethanol: formalin: glacial acetic acid; 85:10:5), stain with eosin and orange-G, then destain, dehydrate and clear by passing the specimen through phenol, stop the destaining process by transferring specimens into methyl salicylate and then mount in Canada balsam (Thatcher, 1987). Drawings of the dissected parts can then be made using a *camera lucida* attached to a compound microscope. Brooker *et al.* (2012), however, discuss the rapid production of taxonomic drawings and digital e-types by using laser scanning confocal microscopy as a tool. Specimens can be prepared for SEM either by (1) dehydrating them through graded ethanol to 96%, then immersing in hexamethyldisilazane (HMDS) for two hours and then allowing to air dry before critical-point drying and sputter coating with gold or (2) washing specimens in 0.1 M phosphate buffer solution at pH 7.3, then fixing in 0.5% osmium tetroxide before passing through a graded alcohol series to 100%, critical-point drying and sputter coating with gold.

The use of molecular tools serves a critical role in the rapid identification of species and their placement (i.e. DNA barcoding) and should be used in parallel with morphology-based methods. There is a rich literature regarding the utility of various genomic regions (e.g. 18S, 28S, COI) for this purpose and these are reviewed, for example, in the works of Bucklin *et al.* (2011), and Blanco-Bercial *et al.* (2014).

Treatment, Prophylaxis and Farm Management Practices

Chemical Approaches

It is normal practice that initial attempts to control parasitic infection in aquaculture tend to use pesticides or insecticides. Many of the compounds currently utilized in aquaculture have derived from historical use in agriculture or from mammalian veterinary applications. Rarely, if ever, are compounds developed for exclusive use in aquaculture without first being developed for use elsewhere. The major investment in drug development for aquaculture has been in chemicals for use against parasitic Copepoda and against Monogenea. This is in part explained by the fact that these two groups tend to have direct life-cycles leading to rapid build-up of numbers on a farm, partly due to the wide range of potential targets compared with other groups and partly due to the economic cost of infections versus the cost of development and subsequent sale of any successful compounds. This is a reflection of the need for commercial companies to have a financial return on any investment. Given the high cost of developing new drugs and the relatively low returns from chemotherapeutants in aquaculture compared with mammalian and human health, it explains why most drugs utilized in aquaculture are derived from other spheres. It should be noted, however, that investment in research and development by pharmaceutical companies and by private and public funding bodies continues, with new and novel compounds being marketed. This is evidenced by the large number of publications produced annually and by patent applications detailing new and novel compounds trialled against parasites of concern.

With the range of compounds in use, in development or in the pipeline, it was felt that the best approach for this section was to highlight relevant publications signposting the reader to current and historical treatments, and to provide an overview of the main targets of interest. It is expected that future developments will seek to refine the approach to drug discovery through the use of *in silico* methods and continued use of bioassays. The increasing sophistication of molecular and omics technologies means that previously unknown or underutilized targets will probably be found and used to control infections. Application of any new compounds will need to consider the risks posed to the environment as well as trying to minimize the possibility of developing resistance in the target population.

The route to market for any antiparasiticide is relatively formulaic, with a similar path being followed for each compound; minor variations are to be expected between countries and can be dependent on the final formulation, the route of application and the label claims being made. In essence, once a target parasite and potential compounds have been identified either *in silico* or through prior knowledge, a bioassay should be conducted. This minimizes the use of animals and helps to refine dose ranges as well as confirming the ability of the compound to kill the target parasite, albeit through an *in vitro* route. Those compounds showing promise are then further tested *in vivo*. Additional tests and information include the need to refine the dose or dose range; determination of efficacy of the compound at that dose; assessment of the pharmacokinetics of the compound for the host species under consideration which would include the absorption, distribution, metabolism and excretion (ADME) of the compound; possibly determination of duration of protection; assessment of nature of residues and time taken to metabolize the compound which would allow for an application for a maximum residue limit (MRL) for food fish; and determination of the safety of the compound at increased dosing regimens (typically 1×, 3× and 5× overdose, and 3× duration for bath exposure routes).

Additional work may be required to find the best route of application (usually bath or in-feed, rarely via injection); data may be required on environmental impact and on non-target organism safety (including environmental, as well as human/mammalian toxicology) and field efficacy data should be collected. Further data will need to be obtained on packaging type and labelling, as well as a number of other minor but important facets of final product before the relevant authorities can consider allowing sale of the successful candidate molecule to the industry. Needless to say, such data collection and collation can take many years which will need to follow advisory and regulatory guidelines; there will be a concomitant cost associated with this. Some compounds will fail to progress to final authorization but that is the nature and risk of pharmaceutical development.

Reviews

Major texts concerned with aquatic medicines and their use in control include those by Herwig (1979), Stoskopf (1993), Treves-Brown (2000), Noga (2010) and Lewbart (2011). In addition, general books covering insect and pest control should be considered to gain a broader understanding of potential and actual targets for control. Major published reviews and primary data papers include Herman (1970); Schmahl and Taraschewski (1987); Mehlhorn *et al.* (1988); Schmahl (1991, 1993); Baticados and Paclibare (1992); Brown (1993); Roth (2000); Rae (2002); Iglesias *et al.* (2002); Shinn *et al.* (2003); Direkbusarakom (2004); Poléo *et al.* (2004); Athanassopoulou *et al.* (2009); Schelkle *et al.* (2009); Reimschuessel *et al.* (2011); Shinn and Bron (2012); Picón-Camacho *et al.* (2012b); Igboeli *et al.* (2013); Reverter *et al.* (2014); Ali *et al.*, (2016).

Parasiticide Mode of Action

Parasiticides can be classified according to their chemical structure and include carbamates, insect growth regulators, neonicotinoids, organophosphates and pyrethroids. An alternative way of classifying the different parasiticides is through the mode of action, many of which are shared across the various compound classes. This approach is taken by the Insecticide Resistance Action Committee (IRAC) which considers that the classification is the definitive list of target sites of insecticides and which should be used as a tool to maximize the development of insecticide resistance management strategies (IRAC, 2016); clearly this approach applies equally well to parasiticides. IRAC lists 28 broad categories based on the physiological function affected and including impacts on nerve and muscles, on growth, on respiration, on midgut function and those of unknown or non-specific action. Those affecting nerve and muscle function which have been used as parasiticides in aquaculture are further subdivided into specific groups, including:

- acetylcholinesterase (AChE) inhibitors that include carbamates and organophosphates (e.g. azamethiphos, triclorfon) that have been used extensively
- sodium channel modulators, such as pyrethroids and pyrethrins (e.g. cypermethrin)
- glutamate-gated chloride channel (GluCl) allosteric modulators (e.g. emamectin benzoate).

Additional groups that act on nerves and muscles that have not been fully developed as antiparasitics but have been tested by, for example, Brooker *et al.* (2011), Aaen and Horsberg (2016) and Aaen *et al.* (2016) include:

- nicotinic acetylcholine receptor (NAChR) competitive modulators such as neonicotinoids, NAChR allosteric modulators (e.g. active ingredient Spinosad) and NAChR channel blockers
- GABA-gated chloride channel blockers such as cyclodiene organochlorides and phenylpyrazoles
- octopamine receptor agonists
- voltage-dependent sodium channel blockers
- ryanodine receptor modulators
- chordotonal organ modulators which include pyridine azomethine derivatives.

The second group of compounds classified according to mode of action are those that affect growth and development. Only one group of compounds, the one acting as chitin synthesis inhibitors, has been extensively developed for use in aquaculture. The others in the group of compounds affecting growth include:

- juvenile hormone mimics
- mite growth inhibitors
- moulting disruptors
- ecdysone receptor agonists
- inhibitors of acetyl CoA carboxylase.

None of these have been exploited as antiparasitics in aquaculture but have been tested for potential efficacy through bioassays (Aaen and Horsberg, 2016; Aaen *et al.*, 2016).

The third group of compounds categorized by IRAC on the basis of mode of action includes molecules affecting respiration:

- inhibitors of mitochondrial ATP synthase
- uncouplers of oxidative phosphorylation via disruption of the proton gradient, which have been tested *in vitro* (Aaen and Horsberg, 2016; Aaen *et al.*, 2016)
- mitochondrial complex I, II, III and IV electron transport inhibitors (e.g. cyanide and rotenone).

Microbial disruptors of insect midgut membranes, such as *Bacillus* spp. have not been utilized in aquaculture, possibly due to their specificity of action against terrestrial pathogens.

The final group proposed by IRAC includes compounds that are either non-specific or multisite inhibitors. While this is a somewhat large box to place the rest of the compounds in, it serves to demonstrate that many compounds in use are developed because they have an effect (*i.e.* usually death of the parasite); however, their mode of action is unknown. In addition, more widely, there will be subtleties in mode of action for a range of other compounds.

Non-Chemical Approaches in Parasite Control

Although the use of chemical-based antiparasitics is invariably the first choice for the management and control of parasite infections, there are a series of non-chemical approaches that can be implemented as part of an integrated pest management strategy to either minimize the probability of infections establishing or to control established infections. The rigour of strategies, however, is grounded in having a comprehensive understanding of the potential parasite threats, their probable routes of entry and their life-cycles. These approaches include the design and position of the aquaculture production site, the source and movement of water through the system, the stock, the feed, husbandry practices, the implementation of a veterinary health plan, adherence to biosecurity codes of practice, and the use of physical, biological and mechanical interventions, where appropriate.

Biosecurity

Biosecurity should be regarded as an overall management system and should look at the entire production pipeline including the brood stock, the source and quality of juveniles, stocking densities, feed and feeding regimes, hatchery disinfection and management, water system preparation and monitoring of quality, disease surveillance, training and record keeping. On-site biosecurity measures should address the potential risks of parasite entry, establishment and spread, and should include restricting access to the site and prohibiting entry with the use of physical barriers (e.g. personnel and vehicles having recently visited sites with disease, drive-through disinfection troughs); the use of zoning to minimize cross-contamination between different sections, for example separating hatchery/nursery areas from grow-out; the use of quarantining and disease testing using a combination of histology and molecular testing to verify that stock are free of general and specific pathogens; regular health assessments to monitor the health of hatchery and farm stock and to control the on-site sanitary status.

Farm Infrastructure

Site design and location are critical factors in determining the general health risk of an aquaculture facility. Important considerations include the relevant biosecurity risks of siting a production unit in open water, in a protected bay, in a river, a pond or as a land-based facility. The position of each will be dictated by the year-round availability of a ready, good-quality water source. For marine salmonid sites, understanding the local hydrodynamics, flush rates and patterns of dispersion may provide insights as to whether the site will have, for example, a high probability of lice infections. Likewise, the surrounding terrain, the local microclimate and potential sources of freshwater input will have an impact on water salinity – low-saline sites have a reduced likelihood of amoebic gill disease (AGD) caused by *Paramoeba perurans*. For freshwater sites, while borehole water may be a more biosecure option, the water path through a farm site is critical; each fish-holding facility should have an independent water supply, that is, flow-through from one tank or pond to another should be avoided. For both freshwater and marine sites, the sharing of common water sources and the relative proximity of one site to other culture sites will have a bearing on the probability and frequency of parasite-based disease events (Jansen *et al.*, 2012; Kristoffersen *et al.*, 2013).

Husbandry-Based Practices

Many routine husbandry practices can be considered within a portfolio of non-chemical control strategies. These can include the effective brushing and cleaning of tank systems to either prevent the growth of biofilms and organic loading, which may facilitate the proliferation of certain parasites, or to dislodge stages attached to the culture enclosure, for example the cysts of *Ichthyophthirius multifiliis*. Maintenance of the culture environment also includes regular net cleaning and changing which can be facilitated through the use of various net crawlers and cleaning rigs (AKVA Group, 2015; Yanmar, 2016). Good husbandry practice and highly trained staff can ensure that stress and damage to stock are minimized during handling and transport, optimal stocking densities are used, and regular grading and health assessments are conducted with the ability to recognize the early signs of disease as the frontline in disease management. Robust record keeping of stock numbers, movements, mortalities and disease events, therefore, can serve to build a disease calendar forewarning of high-risk periods and therefore allowing for advance planning in managing potential infections.

The use of dedicated protective clothing is advised and site visitors should use materials (e.g. boots, overalls, lifejackets, safety helmets, gloves) provided by the farm. Ideally, sites should use colour-coded footwear only to be worn in designated zones. Each culture unit should have its own dedicated equipment (i.e. nets, buckets) and by the same token, materials brought onto aquaculture sites should be kept to an absolute minimum and equipment should not be moved between sites.

Aquaculture enterprises should also be cognisant of potential parasite threats, windows of infection and/or high-risk periods and co-ordinate farm activities, stock movements and transfers during periods of low risk. Such practices may include transferring fully developed juvenile fish (e.g. transfer of young trout after their bones have ossified and are not subject to infection by *Myxobolus cerebralis*) or larger sized stock (e.g. larger Atlantic salmon smolts are less likely to consume cestode-infected copepods) so that they are less susceptible to infection. Stocking practices including monoculture, single year class, fallowing and 'all in, all out' harvesting can minimize the perpetuation of parasitic infection within aquaculture sites (Bron *et al.*, 1993).

For the safe disposal of aquatic products, it is advised that approved on-site incinerators are used or that carcasses and waste are stored in robust containers until collected and disposed of by waste specialists in accordance with national regulations. The integrity of the containers should be such that wild and domestic animals cannot get access to the mort bins, as many mammals serve as hosts for a wide array of aquatic parasites. Animal waste must not be buried and products must not be allowed to seep into water systems or ground water. The culling, on-site processing and/or storage of stock should also strictly adhere to national regulations to ensure that waste products, including parasite stages, do not contaminate local water sources.

Diet

Proper feed management can minimize the likelihood of parasite establishment and propagation. By monitoring feed requirements and intake, aggression, biting and stress in captive-reared populations can be minimized, as can the organic loading and amount of waste feed. Stress, low immunity and open wounds may allow various opportunistic oomycete, bacterial, viral and protistan pathogens to gain access. The quality of the feed given to stock, therefore, is important – there should be no feeding of trash fish and the food must be properly stored so it is free of fungal-like agents.

New diet formulations aim to accelerate growth rate, improve upon existing food conversion ratios (FCRs) and where possible to boost the stock animals' immunity and/or resistance to disease agents. Quicker growth to the target weight means a shorter time spent in the culture facility, which may mean a reduced probability of pathogen encounter and a disease event (e.g. *Enterocytozoon hepatopenaei* infections in whiteleg shrimp, *Penaeus* [=*Litopenaeus*] *vannamei* ponds).

Whether the addition of dietary supplements, herbal extracts and natural immunostimulants to the diet is regarded as non-chemical or not, their strategic use has proven effective in the control of certain parasitic agents (Harikrishnan *et al.*, 2011; Lauridsen and Buchmann, 2010; Sommerville, 2012). The new generation of diets also includes, for example, host-masking compounds that are used to disrupt the settlement of salmon lice (Ewos, 2016). Submerged feeding and lighting are also being used to draw fish away from zones where infective copepodids of *L. salmonis* may accumulate in the water column (Frenzl *et al.*, 2014a).

Biological Interventions

The use of biological agents has also proven effective in the management and control of certain parasite species. For example, ducks and/or selected fish species are used to control vegetation and snail populations in ponds. Cleaner fish, for example various wrasse species (Leclercq *et al.*, 2014; Sayer *et al.*, 1996), lumpsuckers, *Cyclopterus lumpus* (see Imsland *et al.*, 2014) and the cunner, *Tautogolabrus adspersus*, among other species, are used for the control of *L. salmonis* infections on farmed marine salmon, while the co-habitation of leopard plecos, *Glyptoperichthys gibbiceps*, with blue tilapia (*Oreochromis aureus*) by grazing on parasite cysts served to keep *I. multifiliis* infections under control (Picón-Camacho *et al.*, 2012a).

As certain parasites have complex life-cycles involving more than one host, understanding their biology can allow for the strategic implementation of efficacious prophylactic and/or control measures to break the life-cycle. Such interventions can include the elimination or 'management' of intermediate hosts, for example, the use of molluscicides to control snails, the removal of vegetation to remove habitat and feed sources for snails, or preventing the access to culture sites of birds which might otherwise close a parasite life-cycle through the release of parasite eggs during feeding forays.

Genetic Breeding Programmes

The importance of genetic breeding programmes for the selection of traits/populations resistant against specific parasites cannot be overstated and these programmes have a critical role in animal welfare, production and parasite management. Although these are not reviewed in detail in the current chapter, there is a substantial body of research relating to this and the reader is referred to a variety of works including, for example, those of Ford *et al.* (1990); Jones (2001); Villalba *et al.* (2004); Kolstad *et al.* (2005); Nell and Perkins (2006); Frenzl *et al.* (2014a); and Gharbi *et al.* (2015).

Physical Measures

A series of physical defences can be installed to serve as control points or to minimize the likelihood of alien species entering pond/farm sites. Defences can include fencing around sites to prevent unauthorized entry, the use of gating, the use of defence/predator nets round cage and pond sites and water reservoirs to prevent access by species that may serve as intermediate hosts for many pathogens, such as non-target crustacean and fish species. Likewise, the maintenance of dykes and banks around pond sites to withstand flood events helps to minimize the likelihood of stock loss, mixing or the introduction of undesirable species. Although arguably considered a chemical method, the use of footbaths and drive-through troughs for vehicles is important as part of a rigorous biosecurity programme. Other physical control measures include the use of removable substrates onto which parasites, such as *Argulus*, can lay their eggs which are then periodically removed, cleaned and then redeployed (Bauer, 1970; Gault *et al.*, 2002; Hoffman, 1977). Dinoflagellate blooms and other harmful swarms can be controlled through the use of bubble curtains to protect stock (Rodger *et al.*, 2011). Alternatively, strategies to protect stocks from harmful blooms include submerging cages (Dempster *et al.*, 2009), the use of deep water pumps, towing cages away from high-risk areas and/or the use of protective pen enclosures (Rodger *et al.*, 2011).

Mechanical Measures

A diverse array of mechanical systems is employed to divert either the entry or establishment of parasitic agents in culture sites. Commonly used systems include:

- deterrents – bird scarers and nets to prevent access to pond sites and the likelihood of defaecation and the deposition of parasite stages in culture systems
- methods of water filtration, for example for the removal of *Diplostomum spathaceum* cercariae from the inbound water current (Heinecke and Buchmann, 2009; Larsen *et al.*, 2005) or the use of biofilters in recirculation/static systems
- devices to improve the quality of the culture environment, for example, suction devices to remove the attached cyst stages of *I. multifiliis* (see Shinn *et al.*, 2009); rotary tank cleaners (McRobbie and Shinn, 2011); replaceable/disposable tank mats for the management of *Cryptocaryon irritans* infections (Jiang *et al.*, 2016); net crawlers/cleaners to reduce biofouling and to facilitate the passage of water through cage sites but also to remove attached parasite stages, eggs, etc.
- topical applicants, for example cement sealers to reduce the surface area that would otherwise retain organic detritus, parasite stages (Shinn *et al.*, 2009) or paints containing biocides to deter the colonization of biofouling species or organisms that serve as intermediate hosts
- lures, traps – which admittedly have a chemical basis (Buchmann and Nielsen, 1999; Ingvarsdóttir *et al.*, 2002)
- systems for the physical dislodgement of attached parasite stages, such as the use of the Silkstream system to remove salmon lice, *L. salmonis* and *Caligus elongatus* (see Anonymous, 1996)
- UV sterilization of the water which, while expensive, is appropriate for smaller sized aquaria (Summerfelt, 2003)
- electrified grids to destroy cercariae (Schäperclaus, 1992)
- black plastic to cover inlet channels feeding trout farms, to deter the growth of vegetation and, therefore, a habitat for snails. This must, however, be used with caution and monitored as the plastic may serve as a suitable substrate for the colonization of other potential

parasite hosts, for example the freshwater bryozoan *Plumatella repens* which serves as a host for *Tetracapsuloides bryosalmonae*, a myxozoan responsible for proliferative kidney disease (PKD) in rainbow trout. Rubber butyl liners are also used, for example, in shrimp pond culture as a general contribution towards maintaining pond health through the removal of organic matter, thereby preventing the accumulation of bacterial pathogens and microsporideans such as *E. hepatopenaei*.

The impact that salmon lice have on the industry has been the impetus for a new generation of state-of-the-art salmon pen/farms that include 'the Egg' (Hauge Aqua, 2016), the 'Ocean farm' (Blank, 2015) and the use of net snorkels and skirts (Stien *et al.*, 2012, 2016) to completely enclose culture units. Modern technologies also include the use of lasers to detect and remove salmon lice (Stingray Marine Solutions AS, 2016) and 20 kHz ultrasound transmitters to control the juvenile stages of *Caligus rogercresseyi* (see Anonymous, 2014).

Conclusion

It is critical that any diagnostics conducted are underpinned by good science and unequivocal taxonomy. Incorrect diagnosis of a disease agent can have unintended economic, ecological and welfare consequences for wild and farmed animals as well as impacting detrimentally on national and international trade. The inability to diagnose certain disease conditions as a result of poor or non-existent diagnostic tools (Gaughan, 2002) may lead to the unintentional translocation of disease agents across borders. The subsequent financial cost to eradicate or control such diseases may exceed several million dollars (Lafferty *et al.*, 2015; Morant *et al.*, 2013; Stebbing *et al.*, 2014). While this chapter seeks to signpost the reader to a range of specialist taxonomy papers, it should be noted that a number of more general texts have been written over the past century and readers are encouraged to seek these as a starting point for any assessment of the parasite fauna of their chosen hosts. It is, however, incumbent on researchers and diagnosticians to ensure that the most up-to-date literature is also referenced and reviewed to ensure accurate disease diagnosis.

Correct identification of the various organs and tissues of the host is equally important, particularly for those parasites that have very narrow tissue specificity. For example, the complexity of the eye structure is often overlooked when describing an ocular pathogen and yet it is such complexity that can assist in parasite identity; initial discrimination of the eye flukes *Diplostomum* and *Tylodelphys* can be achieved by determining if the parasite occurs in the lens or in the vitreous humour. Similarly, certain myxozoans are known to be strictly cell specific, for example *Myxobolus corneus* in corneas of bluegills (Cone *et al.*, 1990) and *Henneguya episclera* in the sclera of pumpkinseed fish (Minchew and Sleight, 1977). Recommended texts that provide detail on tissue and organs of various aquatic hosts as well as descriptions of dissection methodology include Willemse (1979), Gupta and Mullins (2010), and De Iuliis and Pulerá (2011).

It is recognized that study-specific tissues might be examined by diagnosticians but this does not preclude the examination and collection of other tissues as part of an integrated approach to diagnostics. This is particularly important where the hosts are either new to science or from new geographical areas or where mortality or morbidity due to parasitism is suspected. Failure to examine all available tissues may lead inevitably to a misdiagnosis. As a rule, it is strongly recommended that all tissues are examined and where time, resources and space allow, tissues are appropriately stored for additional studies. This includes, but is not limited to, material for bacterial and viral analyses, material for histology and electron microscopy, tissue imprints and smears (e.g. blood, bile, urine), tissues for molecular identification of host and pathogen as well as, for example, gut contents to understand diet choices. In addition, it is imperative to collect morphometric and morphological host data, age, sex, as well as contemporaneous environmental data to assist with further understanding of the potential underlying causes of observed mortalities. Such data can be shared with specialists in order to more widely understand the drivers of individual and population health.

A laboratory information management system (LIMS) to assist with the effective management of samples and data is an important addition to any diagnostic laboratory and should be implemented at the earliest opportunity. An understanding of the level of detail gleaned from the different approaches is critical before any final decision is made on the validity of the results. In particular, there is a clear distinction between a presumptive result based on a limited number of criteria and a confirmatory result based on a gold standard diagnostic test.

Finally, it is important to stress the need for standardization and demonstration of competence. Standards such as ISO17025 are useful to demonstrate competence of diagnostics labs, with chartered status of individual diagnosticians being recognized through postnominal qualifications such as chartered veterinarians or diagnosticians. Accessing the skills and knowledge of government, intergovernmental and learned societies and their respective websites which include, but are not limited to, global disease reference laboratories and the OIE is recommended for up-to-date data on parasite distribution, legislative information and standardized, validated diagnostics methods.

References

Aaen, S.M. and Horsberg, T.E. (2016) A screening of multiple classes of pharmaceutical compounds for effect on preadult salmon lice *Lepeophtheirus salmonis*. *Journal of Fish Diseases*, **39**, 1213–1223.

Aaen, S.M., Hamre, L.A. and Horsberg, T.E. (2016) A screening of medicinal compounds for their effect on egg strings and nauplii of the salmon louse *Lepeophtheirus salmonis* (Krøyer). *Journal of Fish Diseases*, **39**, 1201–1212.

Aiken, H.M., Hayward, C.J. and Nowak, B.F. (2006) An epizootic and its decline of a blood fluke, *Cardicola forsteri*, in farmed southern bluefin tuna, *Thunnus maccoyii*. *Aquaculture*, **254**, 40–45.

Aiken, H.M., Hayward, C.J., Crosbie, P., Watts, M. and Nowak, B.F. (2008) Serological evidence of an antibody response in farmed southern bluefin tuna naturally infected with the blood fluke *Cardicola forsteri*. *Fish & Shellfish Immunology*, **25**, 66–75.

AKVA Group (2015) Net cleaning systems. Available at: www.akvagroup.com/products/cage-farming-aquaculture/net-cleaning-systems (accessed 30 November 2016).

Ali, H., Rico, A., Murshed-e-Jahan, K. and Belton, B. (2016) An assessment of chemical and biological product use in aquaculture in Bangladesh. *Aquaculture*, **454**, 199–209.

Ali, M.A. (2009) Light and scanning electron microscopy (SEM) of *Ortholinea africanus* Abdel-Ghaffar *et al.*, 2008 (Myxozoa: Myxosporea) infecting tilapia fish *Oreochromis niloticus* (Osteichthyes: Cichlidae) with description of preparation of coelozoic Myxosporea for SEM. *Acta Protozoologica*, **48**, 185–190.

Alvarez-Pellitero, P. (2008) Fish immunity and parasite infections: from innate immunity to immunoprophylactic prospects. *Veterinary Immunology and Immunopathology*, **126**, 171–198.

Amin, O.M. (1985) Classification, in *Biology of the Acanthocephala* (eds D.W.T. Crompton and B.B. Nickol), Cambridge University Press, London, pp. 27–72.

Amin, O.M. (1987) Key to the families and subfamilies of Acanthocephala, with the erection of a new class (Polyacanthocephala) and a new order (Polyacanthorhynchida). *Journal of Parasitology*, **73**, 1216–1219.

Amin, O.M. (2000) Acanthocephala in the Neotropical region, in *Metazoan Parasites in the Neotropics: A Systematic and Ecological Approach* (eds G. Salgado-Maldonado, A.N. García Aldrete and V.M. Vidal Martínez), Instituto de Biología, Universidad Nacional Autonóma de México, Mexico, pp. 167–174.

Amin, O.M. (2013) Classification of the Acanthocephala. *Folia Parasitologica*, **60**, 273–305.

Anderson, R.C. (2000) *Nematode Parasites of Vertebrates: Their Development and Transmission*, 2nd edn, CABI International, Wallingford.

Anderson, R.C., Chabaud, A.G. and Willmott, S. (2009) *Keys to the Nematode Parasites of Vertebrates, archival volume*, CABI International, Wallingford.

Anonymous (1996) Pumping with SILKSTREAM removes lice. *Fish Farming International*, **23**(9), 21.

Anonymous (2014) Chilean Firm wins Global Aquaculture Innovation and Leadership Award. Available at: http://gaalliance.org/news-events/newsroom/chilean-firm-wins-global-aquaculture-innovation-leadership-award/ (accessed 30 November 2016).

Aohagl, Y., Shibahara, T., Machlda, N., Vamaga, V. and Kagota, K. (1992) *Clinostomum complanatum* (Trematoda: Clinostomatidae) in five new fish hosts in Japan. *Journal of Wildlife Diseases*, **28**, 467–469.

Arai, H.P. (1989) Acanthocephala, in *Guide to the Parasites of Fishes of Canada. Part III* (eds L. Margolis and Z. Kabata), Canadian Special Publication of Fisheries and Aquatic Sciences.

Arkush, K.D., Mendoza, L., Adkison, M.A. and Hedrick, R.P. (2003) Observations on the life stages of *Sphaerothecum destruens* n. g., n. sp., a mesomycetozoean fish pathogen formally referred to as the rosette agent. *Journal of Eukaryotic Microbiology*, **50**, 430–438.

Arzul, I. and Carnegie, R.B. (2015) New perspective on the haplosporidian parasites of molluscs. *Journal of Invertebrate Pathology*, **131**, 32–42.

Athanassopoulou, F., Ragias, V., Tavla, J., Christofilogiannis, P. and Liberis, N. (2001) Preliminary trials on the efficacy and toxicity of ivermectin against *Lernanthropus kroyeri* van Beneden, 1851 in cultured sea bass *Dicentrarchus labrax* L. *Aquaculture Research*, **32**, 77–79.

Athanassopoulou, F., Pappas, I.S. and Bitchava, K. (2009) An overview of the treatments for parasitic disease in Mediterranean aquaculture, in *The Use of Veterinary Drugs and Vaccines in Mediterranean Aquaculture. Options Méditerranéennes : Série A* (eds C. Rogers and B. Basurco), Séminaires Méditerranéens, Zaragoza, Spain, pp. 65–83.

Atkinson, S.D., Foott, J.S. and Bartholomew, J.L. (2014) Erection of *Ceratonova* n. gen. (Myxosporea: Ceratomyxidae) to encompass freshwater species *C. gasterostea* n. sp. from threespine stickleback (*Gasterosteus aculeatus*) and *C. shasta* n. comb. from salmonid fishes. *Journal of Parasitology*, **100**, 640–645.

Atkinson, S.D., Bartošová-Sojková, P., Whipps, C.M. and Bartholomew, J.L. (2015) Approaches for characterising myxozoan species, in *Myxozoan Evolution, Ecology and Development* 02 (eds B. Okamura, A. Gruhl and J.L. Bartholomew), Springer International Publishing, Cham, Switzerland, pp. 111–123.

Bandyopadhyay, A.K. and Nandy, A. (1986) A preliminary observation on the prevalence of echinostomes in a tribal community near Calcutta. *Annals of Tropical Medicine and Parasitology*, **80**, 373–375.

Baohua, W. and Suo, L. (2000) *Fauna Sinica Platyhelminthes Monogenea*, Science Press, Beijing, pp. 1–756.

Barber, I. and Huntingford, F.A. (1995) The effect of *Schistocephalus solidus* (Cestoda: Pseudophyllidea) on the foraging and shoaling behaviour of three-spined sticklebacks, *Gasterosteus aculeatus*. *Behaviour*, **132**, 1223–1240.

Barber, I., Huntingford, F.A. and Crompton, D.W.T. (1995) The effect of hunger and cestode parasitism on the shoaling decisions of small freshwater fish. *Journal of Fish Biology*, **47**, 524–536.

Barber, I., Wright, H.A., Arnott, S.A. and Wootton, R.J. (2008) Growth and energetics in the stickleback–*Schistocephalus* host–parasite system: a review of experimental infection studies. *Behaviour*, **145**, 647–668.

Barnard, K.H. (1955) South African parasitic Copepoda. *Annals of the South African Museum*, **41**, 223–312.

Bartošová, P., Fiala, I. and Hypsa, V. (2009) Concatenated SSU and LSU rDNA data confirm the main evolutionary trends within myxosporeans (Myxozoa: Myxosporea) and provide an effective tool for their molecular phylogenetics. *Molecular Phylogenetics and Evolution*, **53**, 81–93.

Bartošová-Sojková, P., Kodádková, A., Pecková, H., Kuchta, R. and Reed, C.C. (2015) Morphology and phylogeny of two new species of *Sphaeromyxa* Thélohan, 1892 (Cnidaria: Myxozoa) from marine fish (Clinidae and Trachichthyidae). *Parasitology*, **142**, 660–674.

Basch, P.F. (1991) *Schistosomes: Development, Reproduction and Host Relations*, Oxford University Press, New York.

Bass, D., Stentiford, G.D., Littlewood, D.T.J. and Hartikainen, H. (2015) Diverse applications of environmental DNA methods in parasitology. *Trends in Parasitology*, **31**, 499–513.

Bass, H.S. and LeFlore, W.B. (1984) *In vitro* excystment of the metacercaria of *Acanthoparyphium spinulosum* (Trematoda: Echinostomatidae). *Proceedings of the Helminthological Society of Washington*, **51**, 149–153.

Baticados, M.C.L. and Paclibare, J.O. (1992) The use of chemotherapeutic agents in aquaculture in the Philippines, in *Diseases in Asian Aquaculture I* (eds M. Shariff, R.P. Subasinghe and J.R. Arthur), Asian Fisheries Society, Fish Health Section, Bali, Indonesia, pp. 531–546.

Bauer, O.N. (1970) *The Ecology of Parasites of Freshwater Fish. Parasites of Freshwater Fish and the Biological Basis of their Control, vol.* **XLIX**. Bulletin of the State Scientific Research Institute of Lake and Fisheries, Nauka, Leningrad.

Bauer, O.N. (1984) *Key to Parasites of Freshwater Fishes of USSR*, Nauka, Leningrad.

Baxa, D.V., El-Matbouli, M., Andree, K.B., *et al.* (2002) *In situ* hybridization: a detection tool for fish pathogens and its application on recent advances on whirling disease research, in *Diseases in Asian Aquaculture IV* (eds C.R. Lavilla-Pitogo and E.R. Cruz-Lacierda), Fish Health Section, Asian Fisheries Society, Manila, Philippines, pp. 293–300.

Berthe, F.C.J., Le Roux, F., Adlard, R.D. and Figueras, A. (2004) Marteiliosis in molluscs: a review. *Aquatic Living Resources*, **17**, 433–448.

Beverley-Burton, M. (1984) Monogenea and Turbellaria, in *Guide to the Parasites of Fishes of Canada. Part III* (eds L. Margolis and Z. Kabata), Canadian Special Publication of Fisheries and Aquatic Sciences.

Biswas, G. and Sakai, M. (2014) Loop-mediated isothermal amplification (LAMP) assays for detection and identification of aquaculture pathogens: current state and perspectives. *Applied Microbiology and Biotechnology*, **98**, 2881–2895.

Blanco-Bercial, L., Cornils, A., Copley, N. and Bucklin, A. (2014) DNA barcoding of marine copepods: assessment of analytical approaches to species identification. *PLoS Currents*, **6**, ecurrents.tol.cdf8b74881f87e3b01d56b43791626d2.

Blank, C. (2015) Salmon Farm to be Built on World's Largest Ship. Available at: www.seafoodsource.com/news/aquaculture/salmon-farm-to-be-built-on-world-s-largest-ship (accessed 30 November 2016).

Boeger, W.A. and Kritsky, D.C. (1993) Phylogeny and a revised classification of the Monogenoidea Bychowsky, 1937 (Platyhelminthes). *Systematic Parasitology*, **26**, 1–32.

Boeger, W.A. and Kritsky, D.C. (1997) Coevolution of the Monogenoidea (Platyhelminthes) based on a revised hypothesis of parasite phylogeny. *International Journal of Parasitology*, **27**, 1495–1511.

Boeger, W.A. and Kritsky, D.C. (2001) Phylogenetic relationships of the Monogenoidea, in *Interrelationships of the Platyhelminthes* (eds D.T.J. Littlewood and R.A Bray), Taylor and Francis Group, London, pp. 92–102.

Boreham, R.E., Hendrick, S., O'Donoghue, P.J. and Stenzel, D.J. (1998) Incidental finding of *Myxobolus* spores (Protozoa: Myxozoa) in stool samples from patients with gastrointestinal symptoms. *Journal of Clinical Microbiology*, **36**, 3728–3730.

Born-Torrijos, A., Kostadinova, A., Raga, J.A. and Holzer, A.S. (2012) Molecular and morphological identification of larval opecoelids (Digenea: Opecoelidae) parasitising prosobranch snails in a Western Mediterranean lagoon. *Parasitology International*, **61**, 450–460.

Bousfield, E.L. and Kabata, Z. (1988) Amphipoda, Crustacea in *Guide to the Parasites of Fishes of Canada. Part III* (eds L. Margolis and Z. Kabata), Canadian Special Publication of Fisheries and Aquatic Sciences, pp. 149–163.

Bower, S.M., McGladdery, S.E. and Price, I.M. (1994) Synopsis of infectious diseases and parasites of commercially exploited shellfish. *Annual Review of Fish Diseases*, **4**, 1–199.

Boxshall, G.A. (1974) Infections with parasitic copepods in North Sea marine fishes. *Journal of the Marine Biological Association of the United Kingdom*, **54**, 355–372.

Boxshall, G.A. (2005a) Branchiura (fish lice), in *Marine Parasitology* (ed. K. Rohde), CABI Publishing, Wallingford, pp. 145–147.

Boxshall, G.A. (2005b) Copepoda (copepods), in *Marine Parasitology* (ed. K. Rohde), CABI Publishing, Wallingford, pp. 123–138.

Boxshall, G.A. (2005c) Tantulocarida (tantulocarids), in *Marine Parasitology* (ed. K. Rohde), CABI Publishing, Wallingford, pp. 147–149.

Boxshall, G.A. and Defaye, D. (1993) *Pathogens of Wild and Farmed Fish: Sea Lice*, Ellis Horwood, Chichester.

Boxshall, G.A. and Halsey, S.H. (2004) *An Introduction to Copepod Diversity*, Ray Society, London.

Boxshall, G.A. and Montú, M.A. (1997) *Copepods Parasitic on Brazilian Coastal Fishes: A Handbook*, Nauplius, pp. 1–225.

Boxshall, G.A., Kihara, T.C. and Huys, R. (2016) Collecting and processing non-planktonic copepods. *Journal of Crustacean Biology*, **36**, 576–583.

Bragoni, G., Romestand, B. and Trilles, J.-P. (1984) Parasitoses a cymothoadien chez le loup, *Dicentrarchus labrax* (Linnaeus, 1758) en élevage. I. Écologie parasitaire dans le cas de l'étang de Diana (Haute-Corse) (Isopoda, Cymothoidae). *Crustaceana*, **47**, 44–51.

Brandt, A. (1990) *Antarctic Valviferans (Crustacea, Isopoda, Valvifera): New Genera, New Species, and Redescriptions*, E.J. Brill, Leiden.

Brannelly, L.A., McMahon, T.A., Hinton, M., Lenger, D. and Richards-Zawacki, C.L. (2015) *Batrachochytrium dendrobatidis* in natural and farmed Louisiana crayfish populations: prevalence and implications. *Disease of Aquatic Organisms*, **112**, 229–235.

Bray, R.A. and Cribb, T.H. (1998) Lepocreadiidae (Digenea) of Australian coastal fishes: new species of *Opechona* Looss, 1907, *Lepotrema* Ozaki, 1932 and *Bianium* Stunkard, 1930 and comments on other species reported for the first time or poorly known in Australian waters. *Systematic Parasitology*, **41**, 123–148.

Bray, R.A. and Justine, J.-L. (2014) A review of the Zoogonidae (Digenea: Microphalloidea) from fishes of the waters around New Caledonia, with the description of *Overstreetia cribbi* n. sp. *PeerJ*, **2**, e292.

Bray, R.A., Gibson, D.I. and Jones, A. (2008) *Keys to the Trematoda*, vol. **3**, CABI Publishing, London.

Bron, J.E., Sommerville, C., Wootten, R. and Rae, G.H. (1993) Fallowing of marine Atlantic salmon, *Salmo salar* L., farms as a method for the control of sea lice, *Lepeophtheirus salmonis* (Kroyer, 1837). *Journal of Fish Diseases*, **16**, 487–493.

Bron, J.E., Frisch, D., Goetze, E., Johnson, S.C., Lee, C.E. and Wyngaard, G.A. (2011) Observing copepods through a genomic lens. *Frontiers in Zoology*, **8**, 22.

Brooker, A.J., Shinn, A.P. and Bron, J.E. (2007) A review of the biology of the parasitic copepod *Lernaeocera branchialis* (L., 1767) (Copepoda: Pennellidae). *Advances in Parasitology*, **65**, 297–341.

Brooker, A.J., Grano Maldonado, M.I., Irving, S., Bron, J.E., Longshaw, M. and Shinn, A.P. (2011) The effect of octopaminergic compounds on the behaviour and transmission of *Gyrodactylus*. *Parasites and Vectors*, **4**, 207.

Brooker, A.J., Shinn, A.P. and Bron, J.E. (2012) Use of laser scanning confocal microscopy for morphological taxonomy and the potential for digital type specimens (e-types). *Aquatic Biology*, **14**, 165–173.

Brown, A.F., Chubb, J.C. and Veltkamp, C.J. (1986) A key to the species of Acanthocephala parasitic in British freshwater fishes. *Journal of Fish Biology*, **28**, 327–334.

Brown, L. (1993) *Aquaculture for Veterinarians: Fish Husbandry and Medicine*, Pergamon Press, Oxford.

Bruce, N.L. (1987) Australian species of *Nerocila* Leach, 1818, and *Creniola* n. gen. (Isopoda: Cymothoidae), crustacean parasites of marine fishes. *Records of the Australian Museum*, **39**, 355–412.

Bucci, C., Gallotta, S., Morra, I., Fortunato, A., Ciacci, C. and Iovino, P. (2013) *Anisakis*, just think about it in an emergency. *International Journal of Infectious Diseases*, **17**, e1071–e1072.

Buchmann, K. and Nielsen, M.E. (1999) Chemoattraction of *Ichthyophthirius multifiliis* (Ciliophora) theronts to host molecules. *International Journal of Parasitology*, **29**, 1415–1423.

Bucklin, A., Steinke, D. and Blanco-Bercial, L. (2011) DNA barcoding of marine Metazoa. *Annual Review of Marine Science*, **3**, 471–508.

Bunkley-Williams, L. and Williams, E.H.J. (1998) Isopods associated with fishes: a synopsis and corrections. *Journal of Parasitology*, **84**, 893–896.

Burreson, E.M. and Ford, S.E. (2004) A review of recent information on the Haplosporidia, with special reference to *Haplosporidium nelsoni* (MSX disease). *Aquatic Living Resources*, **17**, 499–517.

Bychowsky, B.E. (1957) *Monogenetic Trematodes, their Classification and Phylogeny*, Academy of Sciences, Moscow.

Caffara, M., Locke, S.A., Gustinelli, A., Marcogliese, D.J. and Fioravanti, M.L. (2011) Morphological and molecular differentiation of *Clinostomum complanatum* and *Clinostomum marginatum* (Digenea: Clinostomidae) metacercariae and adults. *Journal of Parasitology*, **97**, 884–891.

Callaway, R., Shinn, A.P., Grenfell, S.E., *et al.* (2012) Review of climate change impacts on marine aquaculture in the UK and Ireland. *Aquatic Conservation: Marine and Freshwater Ecosystems*, **22**, 389–421.

Canning, E.U. and Okamura, B. (2003) Biodiversity and evolution of the Myxozoa. *Advances in Parasitology*, **56**, 43–131.

Carnegie, R.B., Hill, K.M., Stokes, N.A. and Burreson, E.M. (2014) The haplosporidian *Bonamia exitiosa* is present in Australia, but the identity of the parasite described as *Bonamia* (formerly *Mikrocytos*) *roughleyi* is uncertain. *Journal of Invertebrate Pathology*, **115**, 33–40.

Castellanos-Martínez, S., Pérez-Losada, M. and Gestal, C. (2013) Molecular phylogenetic analysis of the coccidian cephalopod parasites *Aggregata octopiana* and *Aggregata eberthi* (Apicomplexa: Aggregatidae) from the NE Atlantic coast using 18S rRNA sequences. *European Journal of Protistology*, **49**, 373–380.

Cavaleiro, F.I., Pina, S., Russell-Pinto, F., *et al.* (2012) Morphology, ultrastructure, genetics, and morphometrics of *Diplostomum* sp. (Digenea: Diplostomidae) metacercariae infecting the European flounder, *Platichthys flesus* (L.) (Teleostei: Pleuronectidae), off the northwest coast of Portugal. *Parasitology Research*, **110**, 81–93.

Chai, J.-Y. (2007) Intestinal flukes, in *Food-Borne Parasitic Zoonoses: Fish and Plant-Borne Parasites* (eds K.D. Murrell and B. Fried), Springer Science, New York, pp. 53–116.

Chai, J.-Y., Shin, E.-H., Lee, S.-H. and Rim, H.-J. (2009) Foodborne intestinal flukes in Southeast Asia. *Korean Journal of Parasitology*, **47**, 69–102.

Choudhury, A. and Nelson, P.A. (2000) Redescription of *Crepidostomum opeongoensis* Caira, 1985 (Trematoda: Allocreadiidae) from fish hosts *Hiodon alosoides* and *Hiodon tergisus* (Osteichthyes: Hiodontidae). *Journal of Parasitology*, **86**, 1305–1312.

Cole, R.A. (1999) Eustrongylidosis, in *Field Manual of Wildlife Diseases: General Field Procedures and Diseases of Birds* (eds M. Friend and J.C. Franson), Washington, DC, pp. 223–228.

Colorni, A. (1985) Aspects of the biology of *Cryptocaryon irritans*, and hyposalinity as a control measure in cultured gilt-head sea bream *Sparus aurata*. *Disease of Aquatic Organisms*, **1**, 19–22.

Colorni, A. and Burgess, P. (1997) *Cryptocaryon irritans* Brown 1951, the cause of 'white spot disease' in marine fish: an update. *Aquarium Sciences and Conservation*, **1**, 217–238.

Cone, D.K. and Wiles, M. (1984) *Ichthyobodo necator* (Henneguy, 1883) from winter flounder, *Pseudopleuronectes americanus* (Walbaum), in the north-west Atlantic Ocean. *Journal of Fish Diseases*, **7**, 87–89.

Cone, D.K., Horner, R.W. and Hoffman, G.L. (1990) Description of *Myxobolus corneus* (Myxosporea): a new species from the eyes of bluegills from Illinois. *Journal of Aquatic Animal Health*, **2**, 132–134.

Corradi, N. and Slamovits, C.H. (2011) The intriguing nature of microsporidian genomes. *Briefings in Functional Genomics*, **10**, 115–124.

Crespo, S., Grau, A. and Padros, F. (1992) Sanguinicoliasis in the cultured amberjack *Seriola dumerili* Risso, from the Spanish Mediterranean area. *Bulletin of the European Association of Fish Pathologists*, **12**, 157–159.

Cressey, R.F. (1978) Marine Flora and Fauna of the Northeastern United States. Crustacea: Branchiura. *NOAA Technical Report NMFS Circular* **413**, pp. 1–10.

Cribb, T.H. and Bray, R.A. (2010) Gut wash, body soak, blender and heat-fixation: approaches to the effective collection, fixation and preservation of trematodes of fishes. *Systematic Parasitology*, **76**, 1–7.

Cribb, T.H., Daintith, M. and Munday, B. (2000) A new blood-fluke, *Cardicola forsteri* (Digenea: Sanguinicolidae) of southern bluefin tuna (*Thunnus maccoyii*) in aquaculture. *Transactions of the Royal Society of South Australia*, **124**, 117–120.

Cribb, T.H., Bray, R.A., Olson, P.D. and Littlewood, D.T.J. (2003) Life cycle evolution in the Digenea: a new perspective from phylogeny. *Advances in Parasitology*, **54**, 197–254.

Cribb, T.H., Adlard, R.D., Hayward, C.J., *et al.* (2011) The life cycle of *Cardicola forsteri* (Trematoda: Aporocotylidae), a pathogen of ranched southern bluefin tuna, *Thunnus maccoyii*. *International Journal of Parasitology*, **41**, 861–870.

Crosbie, P.B.B., Bridle, A.R., Cadoret, K. and Nowak, B.F. (2012) *In vitro* cultured *Neoparamoeba perurans* causes amoebic gill disease in Atlantic salmon and fulfils Koch's postulates. *International Journal of Parasitology*, **42**, 511–515.

Davies, A. and Johnston, M.R. (2000) The biology of some intraerythrocytic parasites of fishes, amphibia and reptiles. *Advances in Parasitology*, **45**, 1–107.

Dawes, B. (1968) *The Trematoda*, Cambridge University Press, London.

De Iuliis, G. and Pulerá, D. (2011) *The Dissection of Vertebrates*, 2nd edn, Academic Press, London.

Dempster, T., Korsøen, Ø., Folkedal, O., Juell, J.-E. and Oppedal, F. (2009) Submergence of Atlantic salmon (*Salmo salar* L.) in commercial scale sea-cages: a potential short-term solution to poor surface conditions. *Aquaculture*, **288**, 254–263.

Desser, S.S. and Bower, S.M. (1997) *Margolisiella kabatai* gen. *et* sp. n. (Apicomplexa: Eimeriidae), a parasite of native littleneck clams, *Protothaca staminea*, from British Columbia, Canada, with a taxonomic revision of the coccidian parasites of bivalves (Mollusca: Bivalvia). *Folia Parasitologica*, **44**, 241–247.

Dezfuli, B.S., Giari, L., Simoni, E., Bosi, G. and Manera, M. (2002) Histopathology, immunohistochemistry and ultrastructure of the intestine of *Leuciscus cephalus* (L.) naturally infected with *Pomphorhynchus laevis* (Acanthocephala). *Journal of Fish Diseases*, **25**, 7–14.

Dezfuli, B.S., Giari, L., Konecny, R., Jaeger, P. and Manera, M. (2003) Immunohistochemistry, ultrastructure and pathology of gills of *Abramis brama* from Lake Mondsee, Austria, infected with *Ergasilus sieboldi* (Copepoda). *Disease of Aquatic Organisms*, **53**, 257–262.

Dezfuli, B.S., Giari, L. and Shinn, A.P. (2007) The role of rodlet cells in the inflammatory response in *Diplostomum* infected *Phoxinus phoxinus* brains. *Fish & Shellfish Immunology*, **23**, 300–304.

Dezfuli, B.S., Giari, L., Squerzanti, S., *et al.* (2011) Histological damage and inflammatory response elicited by *Monobothrium wageneri* (Cestoda) in the intestine of *Tinca tinca* (Cyprinidae). *Parasites and Vectors*, **4**, 225.

Dezfuli, B.S., Lui, A., Pironi, F., Manera, M., Shinn, A.P. and Lorenzoni, M. (2013) Cell types and structures involved in tench, *Tinca tinca* (L.), defence mechanisms against a systemic digenean infection. *Journal of Fish Diseases*, **36**, 577–585.

Diaz, J.H. (2015) Gnathostomiasis: an emerging infection of raw fish consumers in *Gnathostoma* nematode-endemic and nonendemic countries. *Journal of Travel Medicine*, **22**, 318–324.

Diéguez-Uribeondo, J., García, M.A., Cerenius, L., *et al.* (2009) Phylogenetic relationships among plant and animal parasites, and saprotrophs in *Aphanomyces* (Oomycetes). *Fungal Genetics and Biology*, **46**, 365–376.

Direkbusarakom, S. (2004) Application of medicinal herbs to aquaculture in Asia. *Walailak Journal of Science and Technology*, **1**, 7–14.

Dojiri, M. and Ho, J.S. (2013) *Systematics of the Caligidae, Copepods Parasitic on Marine Fishes. Crustaceana Monographs, 18*. Brill, Boston.

Duszynski, D.W., Bolek, M.G. and Upton, S.J. (2007) Coccidia (Apicomplexa: Eimeriidae) of amphibians of the world. *Zootaxa*, **1667**, 1–77.

Dwyer, W.P. and Smith, C.E. (1989) Metacercariae of *Diplostomum spathaceum* in the eyes of fishes from Yellowstone lake, Wyoming. *Journal of Wildlife Diseases*, **25**, 126–129.

Dyková, I. and Lom, J. (1988) Review of pathogenic myxosporeans in intensive culture of carp (*Cyprinus carpio*) in Europe. *Folia Parasitologica*, **35**, 289–307.

Dyková, I. and Lom, J. (2004) Advances in the knowledge of amphizoic amoebae infecting fish. *Folia Parasitologica*, **51**, 81–97.

Dyková, I. and Lom, J. (2007) *Histopathology of Protistan and Myxozoan Infections in Fishes. An Atlas*, Academia, Prague.

Dyková, I. and Tyml, T. (2016) Testate amoeba *Rhogostoma minus* Belar, 1921, associated with nodular gill disease of rainbow trout, *Oncorhynchus mykiss* (Walbaum). *Journal of Fish Diseases*, **39**, 539–546.

Dyková, I., Kostka, M., Wortberg, F., Nardy, E. and Pecková, H. (2010) New data on aetiology of nodular gill disease in rainbow trout, *Oncorhynchus mykiss*. *Folia Parasitologica*, **57**, 157–163.

Dzikowski, R., Levy, M.G., Poore, M.F., Flowers, J.R. and Paperna, I. (2004) Use of rDNA polymorphism for identification of Heterophyidae infecting freshwater fishes. *Diseases of Aquatic Organisms*, **59**, 35–41.

Eiras, J.C. and Adriano, E.A. (2012) A checklist of new species of *Henneguya* Thélohan, 1892 (Myxozoa: Myxosporea, Myxobolidae) described between 2002 and 2012. *Systematic Parasitology*, **83**, 95–104.

Eiras, J.C., Takemoto, R.M., Pavanelli, G.C. and Luque, J.L. (2012a) Checklist of protozoan parasites of fishes from Brazil. *Zootaxa*, **3221**, 1–25.

Eiras, J.C., Lu, Y.S., Gibson, D.I., *et al.* (2012b) Synopsis of the species of *Chloromyxum* Mingazinni, 1890 (Myxozoa: Myxosporea: Chloromyxidae). *Systematic Parasitology*, **83**, 203–225.

Eiras, J.C., Zhang, J. and Molnár, K. (2014) Synopsis of the species of *Myxobolus* Bütschli, 1882 (Myxozoa: Myxosporea, Myxobolidae) described between 2005 and 2013. *Systematic Parasitology*, **88**, 11–36.

El-Matbouli, M. and Soliman, H. (2005) Rapid diagnosis of *Tetracapsuloides bryosalmonae*, the causative agent of proliferative kidney disease (PKD) in salmonid fish by a novel DNA amplification method, loop-mediated isothermal amplification (LAMP). *Parasitology Research*, **96**, 277–284.

Elston, R.A. (1993) Infectious diseases of the Pacific oyster, *Crassostrea gigas*. *Annual Review of Fish Diseases*, **3**, 259–276.

Engelsma, M.Y., Culloty, S.C., Lynch, S.A., Arzul, I. and Carnegie, R.B. (2014) *Bonamia* parasites: a rapidly changing perspective on a genus of important mollusc pathogens. *Diseases of Aquatic Organisms*, **110**, 5–23.

Er, A. and Kayiş, Ş. (2015) Intensity and prevalence of some crustacean fish parasites in Turkey and their molecular identification. *Turkish Journal of Zoology*, **39**, 1142–1150.

Estensoro, I., Redondo, M.J., Alvarez-Pellitero, P. and Sitjà-Bobadilla, A. (2010) Novel horizontal transmission route for *Enteromyxum leei* (Myxozoa) by anal intubation of gilthead sea bream *Sparus aurata*. *Diseases of Aquatic Organisms*, **92**, 51–58.

Eszterbauer, E. (2002) Molecular biology can differentiate morphologically indistinguishable myxosporean species: *Myxobolus elegans* and *M. hungaricus*. *Acta Veterinaria Hungarica*, **50**, 59–62.

Eszterbauer, E., Benko, M., Dán, A. and Molnár, K. (2001) Identification of fish-parasitic *Myxobolus* (Myxosporea) species using a combined PCR-RFLP method. *Diseases of Aquatic Organisms*, **44**, 35–39.

EWOS (2016) Functional Feeds: Tackling the Sea Lice Issue. Available at: www.ewos.com/wps/wcm/connect/ewos-content-innovation/ewos-innovation/research-areas/functional-feeds/ (accessed 30 November 2016).

Fannes, W., Vanhove, M.P.M., Huyse, T. and Paladini, G. (2015) A scanning electron microscope technique for studying the sclerites of *Cichlidogyrus*. *Parasitology Research*, **114**, 2031–2034.

Feehan, C.J., Johnson-Mackinnon, J., Scheibling, R.E., Lauzon-Guay, J.-S. and Simpson, A.G.B. (2013) Validating the identity of *Paramoeba invadens*, the causative agent of recurrent mass mortality of sea urchins in Nova Scotia, Canada. *Diseases of Aquatic Organisms*, **103**, 209–227.

Feist, S.W., Hine, P.M., Bateman, K.S., Stentiford, G.D. and Longshaw, M. (2009) *Paramarteilia canceri* sp. n. (Cercozoa) in the European edible crab (*Cancer pagurus*) with a proposal for the revision of the order Paramyxida Chatton, 1911. *Folia Parasitologica*, **56**, 73–85.

Ferguson, H.W. (2006) *Systemic Pathology of Fish. A Text and Atlas of Normal Tissues in Teleosts and their Responses in Disease*, Scotian Press, London.

Fiala, I. (2006) The phylogeny of Myxosporea (Myxozoa) based on small subunit ribosomal RNA gene analysis. *International Journal of Parasitology*, **36**, 1521–1534.

Fiala, I. and Bartosová, P. (2010) History of myxozoan character evolution on the basis of rDNA and EF-2 data. *BMC Evolutionary Biology*, **10**, 228.

Foissner, W. (2014) An update of 'basic light and scanning electron microscopic methods for taxonomic studies of ciliated Protozoa.' *International Journal of Systematic and Evolutionary Microbiology*, **64**, 271–292.

Fonseka, S., Lim, C.S.H., Bandara, U.N. and Dissanayake, M. (2011) New contrast stain for the rapid diagnosis of dermatophytosis and pityriasis versicolor. *Labmedicine*, **42**, 649–652.

Ford, S.E., Fugueras, A.J. and Haskin, H.H. (1990) Influence of selective breeding, geographic origin, and disease on gametogenesis and sex ratios of oysters, *Crassostrea virginica*, exposed to the parasite *Haplosporidium nelsoni* (MSX). *Aquaculture*, **88**(3-4), 285–301.

Freeman, M.A., Bell, A.S. and Sommerville, C. (2003) A hyperparasitic microsporidian infecting the salmon louse, *Lepeophtheirus salmonis*: an rDNA-based molecular phylogenetic study. *Journal of Fish Diseases*, **26**, 667–676.

Frenzl, B., Stien, L.H., Cockerill, D., *et al.* (2014a) Manipulation of farmed Atlantic salmon swimming behaviour through the adjustment of lighting and feeding regimes as a tool for salmon lice control. *Aquaculture*, **424**, 183–188.

Frenzl, B., Migaud, H., Fjelldal, P.G., *et al.* (2014b) Triploid and diploid Atlantic salmon show similar susceptibility to infection with salmon lice *Lepeophtheirus salmonis*. *Pest Management Science*, **70**(6), 982–988.

Fried, B., Graczyk, T.K. and Tamang, L. (2004) Food-borne intestinal trematodiases in humans. *Parasitology Research*, **93**, 159–170.

Fryer, G. (1968) The parasitic Crustacea of African freshwater fishes; their biology and distribution. *Journal of Zoology*, **156**, 45–95.

Fryer, G. (1982) *The Parasitic Copepoda and Branchiura of British Freshwater Fishes. A Handbook and Key*, Freshwater Biological Association Scientific Publication No. 46.

Gaevskaya, A.V. (2004) *Parasites and Diseases of Marine and Oceanic Fishes in Natural and Culture Conditions*, ÉKOSI-Gidrofizika, Sevastopol, Crimea.

Galaktionov, K.V. and Dobrovolskij, A.A. (2003) *The Biology and Evolution of Trematodes*. Springer-Science+Business Media, St Petersburg.

García-Vásquez, A., Shinn, A.P. and Bron, J.E. (2012) Development of a light microscopy stain for the sclerites of *Gyrodactylus* von Nordmann, 1832 (Monogenea) and related genera. *Parasitology Research*, **110**, 1639–1648.

Gaughan, D.J. (2002) Disease-translocation across geographic boundaries must be recognized as a risk even in the absence of disease identification: the case with Australian *Sardinops*. *Reviews in Fish Biology and Fisheries*, **11**, 113–123.

Gault, N.F.S., Kilpatrick, D.J. and Stewart, M.T. (2002) Biological control of the fish louse in a rainbow trout fishery. *Journal of Fish Biology*, **60**, 226–237.

Gaze, W.H. and Wootten, R. (1998) Ectoparasitic species of the genus *Trichodina* (Ciliophora: Peritrichida) parasitising British freshwater fish. *Folia Parasitologica*, **45**, 177–190.

Georgiev, B., Biserkov, V. and Genov, T. (1986) *In toto* staining method for cestodes with iron acetocarmine. *Helminthologia*, **23**, 279–281.

Gestal, C., Guerra, A., Pascual, S. and Azevedo, C. (2002) On the life cycle of *Aggregata eberthi* and observations on *Aggregata octopiana* (Apicomplexa, Aggregatidae) from Galicia (NE Atlantic). *European Journal of Protistology*, **37**, 427–435.

Gharbi, K., Matthews, L., Bron, J., Roberts, R., Tinch, A. and Stear, M. (2015) The control of sea lice in Atlantic salmon by selective breeding. *Journal of the Royal Socieity Interface* **12**, 21050574.

Ghimire, T.R. (2010) Redescription of genera of family Eimeriidae Minchin, 1903. *International Journal of Life Sciences*, **4**, 26–47.

Giangaspero, A., Papini, R., Marangi, M., Koehler, A. V. and Gasser, R.B. (2014) *Cryptosporidium parvum* genotype IIa and *Giardia duodenalis* assemblage A in *Mytilus galloprovincialis* on sale at local food markets. *International Journal of Food Microbiology*, **171**, 62–67.

Gibbons, L.M. (2010) *Keys to the Nematode Parasites of Vertebrates, supplementary volume*, CABI, Wallingford.

Gibson, D.I. (1996) Trematoda, in *Guide to the Parasites of Fishes of Canada. Part IV* (eds L. Margolis and Z. Kabata), Canadian Special Publication of Fisheries and Aquatic Sciences.

Gibson, D.I., Jones, A. and Bray, R.A. (2002) *Keys to the Trematoda*, vol. **1**, CABI Publishing, London.

Gill, E.E. and Fast, N.M. (2006) Assessing the Microsporidia-fungi relationship: combined phylogenetic analysis of eight genes. *Gene*, **375**, 103–109.

Gioia, I. and Silva Cordeiro, N. (1996) Brazilian myxosporidians' check-list (Myxozoa). *Acta Protozoologica*, **35**, 137–149.

Glockling, S.L., Marshall, W.L. and Gleason, F.H. (2013) Phylogenetic interpretations and ecological potentials of the Mesomycetozoea (Ichthyosporea). *Fungal Ecology*, **6**, 237–247.

Goggin, C.L. and Lester, R.J.G. (1995) *Perkinsus*, a protistan parasite of abalone in Australia: a review. *Marine and Freshwater Research*, **46**, 639–646.

Golvan, Y.J. (1969) Systematique des acanthocephales (Acanthocephala Rudolphi, 1801). Part I. L'ordes des Palaeacanthocephala Meyer, 1931. Volume 1. La super-famillille des

Echinorhynchoidea (Cobbold, 1876) Golvan *et* Houin, 1963. *Mémoires du Muséum National d'Histoire Naturelle*, **57**, 1–373.

Gopko, M., Mikheev, V.N. and Taskinen, J. (2015) Changes in host behaviour caused by immature larvae of the eye fluke: evidence supporting the predation suppression hypothesis. *Behavioral Ecology and Sociobiology*, **69**, 1723–1730.

Gozlan, R.E., Marshall, W.L., Liljc, O., Jessop, C.N., Gleason, F.H. and Andreou, D. (2014) Current ecological understanding of fungal-like pathogens of fish: what lies beneath? *Frontiers in Microbiology*, **5**, 62.

Grabda, J. (1991) *Phylum Arthropoda, in Marine Fish Parasitology: An Outline*, PWN-Polish Scientific Publishers, Warszawa, pp. 179–227.

Gratzek, J.B., Gilbert, J.P., Lohr, A.L., Shotts, E.B. and Brown, J. (1983) Ultraviolet light control of *Ichthyophthirius multifiliis* Fouquet in a closed fish culture recirculation system. *Journal of Fish Diseases*, **6**, 145–153.

Grutter, A.S. (1995) Comparison of methods for sampling ectoparasites from coral reef fishes. *Marine and Freshwater Research*, **46**, 897–903.

Grygier, M.J. and Høeg, J.T. (2005) Asothoracida (ascothoracids), in *Marine Parasitology* (ed. K. Rohde), CABI Publishing, Wallingford, pp. 149–154.

Gupta, T. and Mullins, M.C. (2010) Dissection of organs from the adult zebrafish. *Journal of Visualized Experiments*, **37**, 1717.

Gurney, R. (1934) The development of certain parasitic Copepoda of the families Caligidae and Clavellidae. *Proceedings of the Zoological Society of London*, 177–217.

Gusev, A.V. (1985) *Key to the Parasites of the Freshwater Fish Fauna of the USSR II. Parasitic Monogeneans,* Izdat Nauka, Leningrad.

Hansell, E., Braschi, S., Medzihradszky, K.F., *et al.* (2008) Proteomic analysis of skin invasion by blood fluke larvae. *PLoS Neglected Tropical Diseases*, **2**, e262.

Hardy-Smith, P., Ellis, D., Humphrey, J., *et al.* (2012) *In vitro* and *in vivo* efficacy of anthelmintic compounds against blood fluke (*Cardicola forsteri*). *Aquaculture*, **334-337**, 39–44.

Harikrishnan, R., Kim, J.-S., Kim, M.-C., Balasundaram, C. and Heo, M.-S. (2011) *Prunella vulgaris* enhances the non-specific immune response and disease resistance of *Paralichthys olivaceus* against *Uronema marinum*. *Aquaculture*, **318**, 61–66.

Hauge Aqua (2016) Addressing Key Challenges Through New Innovative Technology. Available at: www.haugeaqua.com/Technology/ (accessed 30 November 2016).

Hayward, C.J., Aiken, H.M. and Nowak, B.F. (2008) An epizootic of *Caligus chiastos* on farmed southern bluefin tuna *Thunnus maccoyii* off South Australia. *Diseases of Aquatic Organisms*, **79**, 57–63.

Heasman, M.P., O'Connor, W.A. and Frazer, A.W.J. (1996) Digenean (Bucephalidae) infections in commercial scallops, *Pecten fumatus* Reeve, and doughboy scallops, *Chlamys* (*Mimachlamys*) *asperrima* (Lamarck), in Jervis Bay, New South Wales. *Journal of Fish Diseases*, **19**, 333–339.

Hedrick, R.P., Baxa, D. V., de Kinkelin, P. and Okamura, B. (2004) Malacosporean-like spores in urine of rainbow trout react with antibody and DNA probes to *Tetracapsuloides bryosalmonae*. *Parasitology Research*, **92**, 81–88.

Heegaard, P. (1962) Parasitic Copepoda from Australian waters. *Records of the Australian Museum*, **25**, 149–233.

Heinecke, R.D. and Buchmann, K. (2009) Control of *Ichthyophthirius multifiliis* using a combination of water filtration and sodium percarbonate: dose-response studies. *Aquaculture*, **288**, 32–35.

Herman, R.L. (1970) Chemotherapy of fish diseases: a review. *Journal of Wildlife Diseases*, **6**, 31–34.

Herwig, N. (1979) *Handbook of Drugs and Chemicals Used in the Treatment of Fish Diseases: A Manual of Fish Pharmacology and Materia Medica*, Charles C. Thomas, London.

Hewitt, G.C. (1963) Some New Zealand parasitic Copepoda of the family Caligidae. *Transactions of the Royal Society of New Zealand*, **4**, 61–115.

Hine, P.M., Carnegie, R.B., Burreson, E.M. and Engelsma, M.Y. (2009) Inter-relationships of haplosporidians deduced from ultrastructural studies. *Diseases of Aquatic Organisms*, **83**, 247–256.

Hirt, R.P., Logsdon, J.M., Healy, B., Dorey, M.W., Doolittle, W.F. and Embley, T.M. (1999) Microsporidia are related to Fungi: evidence from the largest subunit of RNA polymerase II and other proteins. *Proceedings of the National Academy of Sciences USA*, **96**, 580–585.

Ho, J.S. (1990) Phylogenetic analysis of copepod orders. *Journal of Crustacean Biology*, **10**, 528–536.

Ho, J.S. and Kim, I.H. (1991) Copepod parasites of commercial bivalves in Korea. *II. Copepods from cultured bivalves. Bulletin of the Korean Fisheries Society*, **24**, 369–396.

Ho, J.S. and Lin, C.L. (2004) *Sea Lice of Taiwan (Copepoda: Siphonostomatoida: Caligidae)*, Sueichan Press, Taiwan.

Ho, J.S. and Zheng, G.X. (1994) *Ostrincola koe* (Copepoda, Myicolidae) and mass mortality of cultured hard clam (*Meretrix meretrix*) in China. *Hydrobiologia*, **284**, 169–173.

Hochberg, F.G. (1990) Diseases of Mollusca: Cephalopoda, in *Diseases of Marine Animals, vol. III. Cephalopoda to Urochordata* (ed. O. Kinne), Biologische Anstalt Helgoland, Hamburg, pp. 47–227.

Høeg, J.T., Glenner, H. and Shields, J.D. (2005) Cirripedia Thoracica and Rhizocephala (barnacles), in *Marine Parasitology* (ed. K. Rohde), CABI Publishing, Wallingford, pp. 154–165.

Hoffman, G.L. (1977) *Argulus*, a branchiuran parasite of freshwater fishes. *US Fish and Wildlife Publication No.* **49**, pp. 1–9.

Hoffman, G.L. (1999) *Parasites of North American Freshwater Fishes*, Cornell University Press, London.

Höglund, J. and Thuvander, A. (1990) Indications of non-specific protective mechanisms in rainbow trout *Oncorhynchus mykiss* with diplostomosis. *Diseases of Aquatic Organisms*, **8**, 91–97.

Holzer, A.S., Montero, F.E., Repullés, A., *et al.* (2008) *Cardicola aurata* sp. n. (Digenea: Sanguinicolidae) from Mediterranean *Sparus aurata* L. (Teleostei: Sparidae) and its unexpected phylogenetic relationship with *Paradeontacylix* McIntosh, 1934. *Parasitology International*, **57**, 472–482.

Horton, T. (2000) *Ceratothoa steindachneri* (Isopoda: Cymothoidae) new to British waters with a key to north-east Atlantic and Mediterranean *Ceratothoa*. *Journal of the Marine Biological Association of the United Kingdom*, **80**, 1041–1052.

Horton, T. and Okamura, B. (2003) Post-haemorrhagic anaemia in sea bass, *Dicentrarchus labrax* (L.), caused by blood feeding of *Ceratothoa oestroides* (Isopoda: Cymothoidae). *Journal of Fish Diseases*, **26**, 401–406.

Humason, G.L. (1979) *Animal Tissue Techniques*, 4th edn, W.H. Freeman, San Francisco.

Humes, A.G. and Gooding, R.U. (1964) A method for studying the external anatomy of copepods. *Crustaceana*, **6**, 238–240.

Igboeli, O.O., Burka, J.F. and Fast, M.D. (2013) *Lepeophtheirus salmonis*: a persisting challenge for salmon aquaculture. *Animal Frontiers*, **4**, 22–32.

Iglesias, R., Paramá, A., Alvarez, M.F., Leiro, J. and Sanmartín, M.L. (2002) Antiprotozoals effective *in vitro* against the scuticociliate fish pathogen *Philasterides dicentrarchi*. *Diseases of Aquatic Organisms*, **49**, 191–197.

Imsland, A.K., Reynolds, P., Eliassen, G., *et al.* (2014) The use of lumpfish (*Cyclopterus lumpus* L.) to control sea lice (*Lepeophtheirus salmonis* Krøyer) infestations in intensively farmed Atlantic salmon (*Salmo salar* L.). *Aquaculture*, **424-425**, 18–23.

Ingvarsdóttir, A., Birkett, M.A., Duce, I., *et al.* (2002) Role of semiochemicals in mate location by parasitic sea louse, *Lepeophtheirus salmonis*. *Journal of Chemical Ecology*, **28**, 2107–2117.

IRAC (2016) www.irac-online.org/modes-of-action/ (accessed 30 November 2016]).

Isaksen, T.E., Karlsbakk, E., Watanabe, K. and Nylund, A. (2011) *Ichthyobodo salmonis* sp. n. (Ichthyobodonidae, Kinetoplastida), an euryhaline ectoparasite infecting Atlantic salmon (*Salmo salar* L.). *Parasitology*, **138**, 1164–1175.

Isaksen, T.E., Karlsbakk, E., Repstad, O. and Nylund, A. (2012) Molecular tools for the detection and identification of *Ichthyobodo* spp. (Kinetoplastida), important fish parasites. *Parasitology International*, **61**, 675–683.

Iwashita, Y., Kamijo, Y., Nakahashi, S., *et al.* (2013) Food poisoning associated with *Kudoa septempunctata*. *Journal of Emergency Medicine*, **44**, 943–945.

Izawa, K. (1973) On the development of parasitic Copepoda I. *Sarcotaces pacificus* Komai (Cyclopoida: Philichthyidae). *Publications of the Seto Marine Biological Laboratory*, **21**, 77–86.

Jain, S. (2012) *Dermatology: Illustrated Study Guide and Comprehensive Board Review*, Springer, New York.

Jankovská, I., Miholová, D., Petrtýl, M., *et al.* (2011) Intestinal parasite *Acanthocephalus lucii* (Acanthocephala) from European perch (*Perca fluviatilis*) as a bioindicator for lead pollution in the stream 'Jevanský potok' near Prague, Czech Republic. *Bulletin of Environmental Contamination and Toxicology*, **86**, 342–346.

Jansen, P.A., Kristoffersen, A.B., Viljugrein, H., Jimenez, D., Aldrin, M. and Stien, A. (2012) Sea lice as a density-dependent constraint to salmonid farming. *Proceedings of the Royal Society B*, **279**, 2330–2338.

Jaysari, M. and Hoffman, G.L. (1982) Review of *Myxidium* (Protozoa: Myxozoa: Myxosporea). *Protozoology Abstracts*, **6**, 61–91.

Jiang, B., Li, Y.W., Abdullahi, A.Y., *et al.* (2016) Placemat and rotational culturing: a novel method to control *Cryptocaryon irritans* infection by removing tomonts. *Aquaculture*, **459**, 84–88.

Jirků, M., Bartošová, P., Kodádková, A. and Mutschmann, F. (2011) Another chloromyxid lineage: molecular phylogeny and redescription of *Chloromyxum careni* from the Asian horned frog *Megophrys nasuta*. *Journal of Eukaryotic Microbiology*, **58**, 50–59.

Johansen, P.-O. and Brattegard, T. (1998) Observations on behaviour and distribution of *Natatolana borealis* (Lilljeborg) (Crustacea, Isopoda). *Sarsia*, **83**, 347–360.

Johnson, P.T. (1977) Paramoebiasis in the blue crab, *Callinectes sapidus*. *Journal of Invertebrate Pathology*, **29**, 308–320.

Johnson, S.C., Treasurer, J.W., Bravo, S., Nagasawa, K. and Kabata, Z. (2004) A review of the impact of parasitic copepods on marine aquaculture. *Zoological Studies*, **43**, 229–243.

Jones, A., Bray, R.A. and Gibson, D.I. (2005) *Keys to the Trematoda*, vol. **2**, CABI Publishing, London.

Jones, J.B. (1988) New Zealand parasitic Copepoda; genus *Caligus* Müller, 1785 (Siphonostomatoida: Caligidae). *New Zealand Journal of Zoology*, **15**, 397–413.

Jones, M.W., Sommerville, C. and Bron, J.E. (1990) The histopathology associated with the juvenile stages of *Lepeophtheirus salmonis* on the Atlantic salmon, *Salmo salar* L. *Journal of Fish Diseases*, **13**, 303–310.

Jones, S.R.M. (2001) The occurrence and mechanisms of innate immunity against parasites in fish. *Developmental and Comparative Immunology*, **25**(8-9), 841-852.

Jørgensen, A. and Sterud, E. (2006) The marine pathogenic genotype of *Spironucleus barkhanus* from farmed salmonids redescribed as *Spironucleus salmonicida* n. sp. *Journal of Eukaryotic Microbiology*, **53**, 531–541.

Jørgensen, A. and Sterud, E. (2007) Phylogeny of *Spironucleus* (Eopharyngia: Diplomonadida: Hexamitinae). *Protist*, **158**, 247–254.

Jørgensen, T.R., Larsen, T.B. and Buchmann, K. (2009) Parasite infections in recirculated rainbow trout (*Oncorhynchus mykiss*) farms. *Aquaculture*, **289**, 91–94.

Justine, J.L. (2005) Species of *Pseudorhabdosynochus* Yamaguti, 1958 (Monogenea: Diplectanidae) from *Epinephelus fasciatus* and *E. merra* (Perciformes: Serranidae) off New Caledonia and other parts of the Indo-Pacific Ocean, with a comparison of measurements of specimens prepare. *Systematic Parasitology*, **62**, 1–37.

Kabata, Z. (1970) Crustacea as enemies of fishes, in *Diseases of Fishes* (eds S.F. Snieszko and R.R. Axelrod), T.F.R. Publications, Jersey City.

Kabata, Z. (1979) *Parasitic Copepoda of British Fishes*, Ray Society, London.

Kabata, Z. (1981) Copepoda (Crustacea) parasitic on fishes: problems and perspectives. *Advances in Parasitology*, **19**, 1–71.

Kabata, Z. (1984) Diseases caused by metazoans: crustaceans, in *Diseases of Marine Animals, vol. IV, Part 1. Introduction, Pisces* (ed. O. Kinne), Biologische Anstatt Helgoland, Hamburg, pp. 321–399.

Kabata, Z. (1988) Copepoda and Branchiura, in *Guide to the Parasites of Fishes of Canada. Part II. Crustacea* (eds L. Margolis and Z. Kabata), Canadian Special Publication of Fisheries and Aquatic Sciences, pp. 3–127.

Kabata, Z. (2003) *Copepods Parasitic on Fishes. Keys and Notes for the Identification of British Species. Synopses of the British Fauna (New Series), No. 47*, Linnean Society of London and the Estuarine and Coastal Sciences Association Field Studies Council, London.

Karlsson, J.D. (1991) Parasites of the bay scallop, *Argopecten irradians* (Lamarck, 1819), in *International Compendium of Scallop Biology and Culture* (eds S.E. Shumway and P.A. Sandifer), World Aquaculture Society, Baton Rouge, pp. 180–190.

Karvonen, A., Paukku, S., Valtonen, E.T. and Hudson, P.J. (2003) Transmission, infectivity and survival of *Diplostomum spathaceum* cercariae. *Parasitology*, **127**, 217–224.

Kazachenko, V.N. (2001) *Key to Families and Genera of Parasitic Copepods (Crustacea: Copepoda) of Fishes, Parts I and II*, Vladivostok.

Keable, S.J. (2006) Taxonomic revision of *Natatolana* (Crustacea: Isopoda: Cirolanidae). *Records of the Australian Museum*, **58**, 133–244.

Keable, S.J. and Bruce, N.L. (1997) Redescription of the North Atlantic and Mediterranean species of *Natatolana* (Crustacea: Isopoda: Cirolanidae). *Journal of the Marine Biological Association of the United Kingdom*, **77**, 655–705.

Kearn, G.C. (1986) The eggs of monogeneans. *Advances in Parasitology*, **25**, 175–273.

Kearn, G.C. (1998) *Parasitism and Platyhelminths*, Chapman and Hall, London.

Kearn, G.C. (2005) *Leeches, Lice and Lampreys. A Natural History of Skin and Gill Parasites of Fishes*, Springer, Dordrecht.

Keiser, J. and Utzinger, J. (2005) Emerging foodborne trematodiasis. *Emerging Infectious Diseases*,**11**, 1507–1514.

Kennedy, C.R. (1999) Post-cyclic transmission in *Pomphorhynchus laevis* (Acanthocephala). *Folia Parasitologica*, **46**, 111–116.

Kennedy, C.R. (2006) *Ecology of the Acanthocephala*, Cambridge University Press, Cambridge.

Kensley, B. and Grindley, J.R. (1973) South African parasitic Copepoda. *Annals of the South African Museum*, **62**, 69–130.

Kent, M.L., Andree, K.B., Bartholomew, J.L., *et al.* (2001) Recent advances in our knowledge of the Myxozoa. *Journal of Eukaryotic Microbiology*, **48**, 395–413.

Khalil, L.F., Jones, A. and Bray, R.A. (1994) *Keys to the Cestode Parasites of Vertebrates*, CABI International, Wallingford.

Khan, R.A., Lee, E.M. and Barker, D. (1990) *Lernaeocera branchialis*: a potential pathogen to cod ranching. *Journal of Parasitology*, **76**, 913–917.

Khatoon, N. and Bilqees, F.M. (2011) *Acanthocephala of Vertebrates. A World Record*, VDM Verlag, Saarbrücken.

Khotenovsky, I.A. (1985) *Suborder Octomacrinea Khotenovsky*, Nauka, Leningrad.

Kilburn, R., Bricknell, I.R., Cook, P., Pert, C.C., Dunn, J. and Matějusová, I. (2010) Design and application of a portable, automated plankton sampler for the capture of the parasitic copepods *Lepeophtheirus salmonis* (Krøyer 1837) and *Caligus elongatus* (Von Nordmann 1832). *Journal of Plankton Research*, **32**, 967–970.

Kimura, M. and Endo, M. (1979) Whirling Disease caused by metacercaria of a fluke. *Fish Pathology*, **13**, 211–213.

King, C.H. (2011) Schistosomiasis: challenges and opportunities, in *The Causes and Impacts of Neglected Tropical and Zoonotic Diseases: Opportunities for Integrated Intervention Strategies*, National Academies Press, Washington, DC, pp. 323–341.

Kirchhoff, N.T., Rough, K.M. and Nowak, B.F. (2011) Moving cages further offshore: effects on Southern bluefin tuna, *T. maccoyii*, parasites, health and performance. *PLoS One*, **6**, e23705.

Klein, B.M. (1943) Das Silberlinien- oder neuroformative System der Ciliaten. *Eine zusammenfassende Darstellung unter Berücksichtigung eines homologen und eines analogen Zwischensystems bei den Metazoen. Annales des Naturhistorischen Museums Wien*, **53**, 156–336.

Knudsen, G.M., Medzihradszky, K.F., Lim, K.-C., Hansell, E. and McKerrow, J.H. (2005) Proteomic analysis of *Schistosoma mansoni* cercarial secretions. *Molecular and Cellular Proteomics*, **4**, 1862–1875.

Kohn, A. and Justo, M.C.N. (2008) *Didymocystis lamotheargumedoi* n. sp. (Digenea: Didymozoidae) a parasite of three species of scombrid fishes. *Revista Mexicana de Biodiversidad*, **79**, 9S-14S.

Koinari, M., Karl, S., Ng-Hublin, J., Lymbery, A.J. and Ryan, U.M. (2013) Identification of novel and zoonotic *Cryptosporidium* species in fish from Papua New Guinea. *Veterinary Parasitology*, **198**, 1–9.

Kolstad, K., Heuch, P.A., Gjerde, B., Gjedrem, T. and Salte, R. (2005) Genetic variation in resistance of Atlantic salmon (*Salmo salar*) to the salmon louse *Lepeophtheirus salmonis. Aquaculture*, **247**(1-4), 145–151.

Kostadinova, A., Power, A.M., Fernández, M., Balbuena, J.A., Raga, J.A. and Gibson, D.I. (2003) Three species of *Magnibursatus* Naidenova, 1969 (Digenea: Derogenidae) from Atlantic and Black Sea marine teleosts. *Folia Parasitologica*, **50**, 202–210.

Kozubíková-Balcarová, E., Koukol, O., Martín, M.P., Svoboda, J., Petrusek, A. and Diéguez-Uribeondo, J. (2013) The diversity of oomycetes on crayfish: morphological vs. molecular identification of cultures obtained while isolating the crayfish plague pathogen. *Fungal Biology*, **117**, 682–691.

Kristoffersen, A.B., Rees, E.E., Stryhn, H., *et al.* (2013) Understanding sources of sea lice for salmon farms in Chile. *Preventive Veterinary Medicine*, **111**, 165–175.

Kristoffersen, R. (1992) Occurrence of the digenean *Cryptocotyle lingua* in farmed Arctic charr *Salvelinus alpinus* and periwinkles *Littorina littorea* sampled close to charr farms in northern Norway. *Diseases of Aquatic Organisms*, **12**, 59–65.

Kritsky, D.C., Leiby, P.D. and Kayton, R.J. (1978) A rapid stain technique for the haptoral bars of *Gyrodactylus* species (Monogenea). *Journal of Parasitology*, **64**, 172–174.

Kuchta, R., Scholz, T. and Bray, R.A. (2008) Revision of the order Bothriocephalidea Kuchta, Scholz, Brabec and Bray, 2008 (Eucestoda) with amended generic diagnoses and keys to families and genera. *Systematic Parasitology*, **71**, 81–136.

Kudryavtsev, A., Pawlowski, J. and Hausmann, K. (2011) Description of *Paramoeba atlantica* n. sp. (Amoebozoa, Dactylopodida) - a marine amoeba from the eastern Atlantic, with emendation of the dactylopodid. *Acta Protozoologica*, **50**, 239–253.

Lafferty, K.D., Harvell, C.D., Conrad, J.M., *et al.* (2015) Infectious diseases affect marine fisheries and aquaculture economics. *Annual Review of Marine Science*, **7**, 471–496.

Lane, R.L. and Morris, J.E. (2000) Biology, prevention, and effects of common grubs (digenetic trematodes) in freshwater fish. *Technical Bulletin Series*, **115**, 1–6.

Lankester, M.W. and Smith, J.D. (1980) Host specificity and distribution of the swim-bladder nematodes, *Cystidicola farionis* Fischer, 1798 and *C. cristivomeri* White, 1941 (Habronematoidea), in salmonid fishes of Ontario. *Canadian Journal of Zoology*, **58**, 1298–1305.

Larsen, A.H., Bresciani, J. and Buchmann, K. (2005) Pathogenicity of *Diplostomum* cercariae in rainbow trout, and alternative measures to prevent diplostomosis in fish farms. *Bulletin of the European Association of Fish Pathologists*, **25**, 20–27.

Lauckner, G. (1983) Diseases of Mollusca: Bivalvia, in *Diseases of Marine Animals*, vol. **II**, Biologische Anstalt Helgoland, Hamburg, pp. 805–817.

Lauridsen, J.H. and Buchmann, K. (2010) Effects of short- and long-term glucan feeding of rainbow trout (Salmonidae) on the susceptibility to *Ichthyophthirius multifiliis* infections. *Acta Ichthyologica et Piscatoria*, **40**, 61–66.

Lebedev, B.I. (1988) Monogenea in the light of new evidence and their position among platyhelminths. *Angewandte Parasitologie*, **29**, 149–167.

Leclercq, E., Davie, A. and Migaud, H. (2014) Delousing efficiency of farmed ballan wrasse (*Labrus bergylta*) against *Lepeophtheirus salmonis* infecting Atlantic salmon (*Salmo salar*) post-smolts. *Pest Management Science*,**70**, 1274–1282.

Lee, J.J., Leedale, G.F. and Bradbury, P. (2000) *An Illustrated Guide to the Protozoa*, 2nd edn, Allen Press, Kansas.

Lee, S.C., Corradi, N., Byrnes, E.J., *et al.* (2008) Microsporidia evolved from ancestral sexual Fungi. *Current Biology*, **18**, 1675–1679.

Lee, S.H., Chai, J.Y. and Hong, S.T. (1993) *Gymnophalloides seoi* n. sp. (Digenea: Gymnophallidae), the first report of human infection by a gymnophallid. *Journal of Parasitology*, **79**, 677–680.

Lefebvre, F., Wielgoss, S., Nagasawa, K. and Moravec, F. (2012) On the origin of *Anguillicoloides crassus*, the invasive nematode of anguillid eels. *Aquatic Invasions* **7**, 443–453.

Leiro, J., Paniagua, E., Ortega, M., Paramá, A., Fernández, J. and Sanmartín, M.L. (1998) An amoeba associated with gill disease in turbot, *Scophthalmus maximus* (L.). *Journal of Fish Diseases*, **21**, 281–288.

Lester, R.J.G. (2005) Isopoda (isopods), in *Marine Parasitology* (ed. K. Rohde), CABI Publishing, Wallingford, pp. 138–144.

Lester, R.J.G. and Hayward, C.J. (2006) Phylum Arthropoda, in *Fish Diseases and Disorders. Volume 1: Protozoan and Metazoan Infections*, 2nd edn (ed. P.T.K. Woo), CABI Publishing, Wallingford, pp. 466–565.

Levine, N.D. (1985) Phylum II. Apicomplexa Levine, 1970, in *An Illustrated Guide to the Protozoa* (eds J.J. Lee, S.H. Hutner and E.C. Bovee), Society of Protozoologists, Lawrence, pp. 302–374.

Levri, E.P. and Lively, C.M. (1996) The effects of size, reproductive condition, and parasitism on foraging behaviour in a freshwater snail, *Potamopyrgus antipodarum*. *Animal Behavior*, **51**, 891–901.

Levy, M.G., Flowers, J.R., Poore, M.F., *et al.* (2006) Morphologic, pathologic, and genetic investigations of *Bolbophorus* species affecting cultured channel catfish in the Mississippi delta. *Journal of Aquatic Animal Health*, **18**, 235–246.

Lewbart, G.A. (2011) *Invertebrate Medicine*, 2nd edn, Wiley-Blackwell, London.

Li, Y.-C., Sato, H., Tanaka, S., Ohnishi, T., Kamata, Y. and Sugita-Konishi, Y. (2013) Characterization of the ribosomal RNA gene of *Kudoa neothunni* (Myxosporea: Multivalvulida) in tunas (*Thunnus* spp.) and *Kudoa scomberi* n. sp. in a chub mackerel (*Scomber japonicus*). *Parasitology Research*, **112**, 1991–2003.

Li, Y.-C., Zhang, Y., Siriguleng and Sato, H. (2015) *Henneguya doneci* (Myxosporea: Bivalvulida) in the gill filaments of Prussian carp *Carassius gibelio* (Bloch) from the upper Yellow River running through Inner Mongolia, China. *Journal of Veterinary Medical Science*, **77**, 1001–1005.

Lima dos Santos, C.A.M. and Howgate, P. (2011) Fishborne zoonotic parasites and aquaculture: a review. *Aquaculture*, **318**, 253–261.

Lin, C.L. (1989) A new species of *Caligus* (Copepoda, Caligidae) parasitic on milk fish *Chanos chanos*. *Crustaceana*, **57**, 225–246.

Lin, C.-L. and Ho, J.-S. (1998) Two new species of ergasilid copepods parasitic on fishes cultured in brackish water in Taiwan. *Proceedings of the Biological Society of Washington*, **111**, 15–27.

Lin, C.-L., Ho, J.-S. and Chen, S.-N. (1994) Two species of *Caligus* (Copepoda: Caligidae) parasitic on black seabream (*Acanthopagrus schlegeli*) cultured in Taiwan. *Fish Pathology*, **29**, 253–264.

Linton, E. (1915) Note on trematode sporocysts and cercariae in marine mollusks of the Woods Hole region. *Biological Bulletin*, **28**, 198–209.

Littlewood, D.T.J. and Bray, R.A. (2001) *Interrelationships of the Platyhelminthes*, Taylor and Francis, London.

Liu, Q., Wei, F., Liu, W., Yang, S. and Zhang, X. (2008) Paragonimiasis: an important food-borne zoonosis in China. *Trends in Parasitology*, **24**, 318–323.

Lom, J. and Arthur, J.R. (1989) A guideline for the preparation of species descriptions in Myxosporea. *Journal of Fish Diseases*, **12**, 151–156.

Lom, J. and Dyková, I. (1992) *Protozoan Parasites of Fishes. Developments in Aquaculture and Fisheries, 26*, Elsevier, Amsterdam.

Lom, J. and Dyková, I. (1993) Scanning electron microscopic revision of common species of the genus *Chloromyxum* (Myxozoa: Myxosporea) infecting European freshwater fishes. *Folia Parasitologica*, **40**, 161–174.

Lom, J. and Dyková, I. (2006) Myxozoan genera: definition and notes on taxonomy, life-cycle terminology and pathogenic species. *Folia Parasitologica*, **53**, 1–36.

Lom, J. and Nilsen, F. (2003) Fish Microsporidia: fine structural diversity and phylogeny. *International Journal of Parasitology*, **33**, 107–127.

Lom, J., Dyková, I. and Pavlaskova, M. (1983) 'Unidentified' mobile protozoans from the blood of carp and some unsolved problems of myxosporean life cycles. *Journal of Protozoology*, **30**, 497–508.

Lom, J., McGeorge, J., Feist, S.W., Morris, D. and Adams, A. (1997) Guidelines for the uniform characterisation of the actinosporean stages of parasites of the phylum Myxozoa. *Diseases of Aquatic Organisms*, **30**, 1–9.

Longshaw, M., Frear, P. and Feist, S.W. (2003) *Myxobolus buckei* sp. n. (Myxozoa), a new pathogenic parasite from the spinal column of three cyprinid fishes from the United Kingdom. *Folia Parasitologica*, **50**, 251–262.

Longshaw, M., Frear, P.A. and Feist, S.W. (2005) Descriptions, development and pathogenicity of myxozoan (Myxozoa: Myxosporea) parasites of juvenile cyprinids (Pisces: Cyprinidae). *Journal of Fish Diseases*, **28**, 489–508.

Longshaw, M., Stone, D.M., Wood, G., Green, M.J. and White, P. (2013) Detection of *Bonamia exitiosa* (Haplosporidia) in European flat oysters *Ostrea edulis* cultivated in mainland Britain. *Diseases of Aquatic Organisms*, **106**, 173–179.

Lützen, J. (2005) Amphipoda (amphipods), in *Marine Parasitology* (ed. K. Rohde), CABI Publishing, Wallingford, pp. 165–169.

Lynn, D.H. (2011) *The Ciliated Protozoa: Characterization, Classification, and Guide to the Literature*, 3rd edn, Springer, London.

Mackiewicz, J.S. (1972) Caryophyllidea (Cestoidea): a review. *Experimental Parasitology*, **31**, 417–512.

Malmberg, G. (1957) On the occurrence of *Gyrodactylus* on Swedish fishes. *Skrifter Utgivna av Södra Sveriges Fiskeriförening Årsskrift*, 19–76.

Malmberg, G. (1970) The excretory systems and the marginal hooks as a basis for the systematics of *Gyrodactylus* (Trematoda, Monogenea). *Arkiv för Zoologi*, **23**, 1–235.

Manera, M. and Dezfuli, B.S. (2003) *Lernanthropus kroyeri* infections in farmed sea bass *Dicentrarchus labrax*: pathological features. *Diseases of Aquatic Organisms*, **57**, 177–180.

Marin de Mateo, M., Adams, A., Richards, R.H., Castagnaro, M. and Hedrick, R.P. (1993) Monoclonal antibody and lectin probes recognize developmental and sporogonic stages of PKX, the causative agent of proliferative kidney disease in European and North American salmonid fish. *Diseases of Aquatic Organisms*, **15**, 23–29.

Marino, F., Giannetto, S., Cavallaro, M., Paradiso, M.L., Bottari, T. and de Vico, G. (2003) *Unitubulotestis sardae* (Trematoda: Didymozoidae) infection in Atlantic bonito *Sarda sarda* (Perciformes: Scomberomoridae) in the Ionian and Tyrrhenian Seas: histopathological and SEM investigations. *Journal of Submicroscopic Cytology and Pathology*, **35**, 215–220.

Martin, J.W. and Davis, G.E. (2001) *An Updated Classification of the Recent Crustacea. No. 30 Science Series*, Natural History Museum of Los Angeles County.

Martin, M.F. (1932) 37. On the morphology and classification of *Argulus* (Crustacea). *Proceedings of the Zoological Society of London*, **102**, 771–806.

Martínez de Velasco, G., Rodero, M., Cuéllar, C., Chivato, T., Mateos, J.M. and Laguna, R. (2008) Skin prick test of *Kudoa* sp. antigens in patients with gastrointestinal and/or allergic symptoms related to fish ingestion. *Parasitology Research*, **103**, 713–715.

Mathis, A., Weber, R. and Deplazes, P. (2005) Zoonotic potential of the Microsporidia. *Clinical Microbiology Review*, **18**, 423–445.

Matthews, R.A. (2005) *Ichthyophthirius multifiliis* Fouquet and ichthyophthiriosis in freshwater teleosts. *Advances in Parasitology*, **59**, 159–241.

Mattiucci, S. and Nascetti, G. (2008) Advances and trends in the molecular systematics of anisakid nematodes, with implications for their evolutionary ecology and host-parasite co-evolutionary processes. *Advances in Parasitology*, **66**, 47–148.

Mazzoni, R. (2003) Emerging pathogen of wild amphibians in frogs (*Rana catesbeiana*) farmed for international trade. *Emerging Infectious Diseases*, **9**, 995–998.

McClelland, R.S., Murphy, D.M. and Cone, D.K. (1997) Report of spores of *Henneguya salminicola* (Myxozoa) in human stool specimens: possible source of confusion with human spermatozoa. *Journal of Clinical Microbiology*, **35**, 2815–2818.

McClymont, H.E., Dunn, A.M., Terry, R.S., Rollinson, D., Littlewood, D.T.J. and Smith, J.E. (2005) Molecular data suggest that microsporidian parasites in freshwater snails are diverse. *International Journal of Parasitology*, **35**, 1071–1078.

McGladdery, S.E., Murphy, L., Hicks, B.D. and Wagner, S.K. (1990) The effect of *Stephanostomum tenue* (Digenea: Acanthocolpidae) on marine aquaculture of the rainbow trout, *Salmo gairdneri*, in *Pathology in Marine Science* (eds T.C. Chen and F.O. Perkins), Academic Press, London, pp. 305–315.

McKerrow, J. and Salter, J. (2002) Invasion of skin by *Schistosoma* cercariae. *Trends in Parasitology*, **18**, 193–195.

McLaughlin, D. and Spatafora, J. (2014) *The Mycota VII. Systematics and Evolution Part A*, 2nd edn, Springer-Verlag, Berlin.

McRobbie, A.S. and Shinn, A.P. (2011) A modular, mechanical rotary device for the cleaning of commercial-scale, circular tanks used in aquaculture. *Aquaculture*, **317**, 16–19.

Meehan, O.L. (1940) A review of the parasitic Crustacea of the genus *Argulus* in the collections of the United States National Museum. *Proceedings of the United States National Museum*, **88**, 459–522.

Mehlhorn, H., Schmahl, G. and Haberkorn, A. (1988) Toltrazuril effective against a broad spectrum of protozoan parasites. *Parasitology Research*, **75**, 64–66.

Mendoza, L., Taylor, J.W. and Ajello, L. (2002) The class Mesomycetozoea: a heterogeneous group of microorganisms at the animal-fungal boundary. *Annual Review of Microbiology*, **56**, 315–344.

Mendoza-Palmero, C., Blasco-Costa, I. and Scholz, T. (2015) Molecular phylogeny of Neotropical monogeneans (Platyhelminthes: Monogenea) from catfishes (Siluriformes). *Parasites and Vectors*, **8**, 164.

Messu Mandeng, F.D., Bilong Bilong, C.F., Pariselle, A., Vanhove, M.P.M., Bitja Nyom A.R. and Agnèse, J.F. 2015. A phylogeny of *Cichlidogyrus* spp. (Monogenea, Dactylogyridea) clarifies a host-switch between fish families and reveals an adaptive component to attachment organ morphology of this parasite genus. *Parasites and Vectors*, **8**, 582.

Mikheev, V.N., Pasternak, A.F., Taskinen, J. and Valtonen, E.T. (2010) Parasite-induced aggression and impaired contest ability in a fish host. *Parasites and Vectors*, **3**, 17.

Milne, S.J. and Avenant-Oldewage, A. (2006) The fluorescent detection of *Paradiplozoon* sp. (Monogenea: Diplozoidae) attachment clamps' sclerites and integumental proteins. *Onderstepoort Journal of Veterinary Research*, **73**, 149–152.

Minchew, C.D. and Sleight, B.H. (1977) *Henneguya episclera* sp. n. (Protozoa: Myxosporida), a new myxosporidan from the eye of the pumpkinseed sunfish. *Journal of Parasitology*, **63**, 667–668.

Mitchell, A.J., Overstreet, R.M., Goodwin, A.E. and Brandt, T.M. (2005) Spread of an exotic fish-gill trematode: a far-reaching and complex problem. *Fisheries*, **30**, 11–16.

Mitchell, S.O. and Rodger, H.D. (2011) A review of infectious gill disease in marine salmonid fish. *Journal of Fish Diseases*, **34**, 411–432.

Mladineo, I. (2003) Life cycle of *Ceratothoa oestroides*, a cymothoid isopod parasite from sea bass *Dicentrarchus labrax* and sea bream *Sparus aurata*. *Diseases of Aquatic Organisms*, **57**, 97–101.

Mladineo, I. (2006) Histopathology of five species of *Didymocystis* spp. (Digenea: Didymozoidae) in cage-reared Atlantic bluefin tuna (*Thunnus thynnus thynnus*). *Veterinary Research Communications*, **30**, 475–484.

Mladineo, I. and Block, B.A. (2010) Expression of cytokines IL-1β and TNF-α in tissues and cysts surrounding *Didymocystis wedli* (Digenea, Didymozoidae) in the Pacific bluefin tuna (*Thunnus orientalis*). *Fish and Shellfish Immunology*, **29**, 487–493.

Mladineo, I. and Jozić, M. (2005) *Aggregata* infection in the common octopus, *Octopus vulgaris* (Linnaeus, 1758), Cephalopoda: Octopodidae, reared in a flow-through system. *Acta Adriatica*, **46**, 193–199.

Mladineo, I. and Tudor, M. (2004) Digenea of Adriatic cage-reared northern bluefin tuna (*Thunnus thynnus thynnus*). *Bulletin of the European Association of Fish Pathologists*, **24**, 144–153.

Moestrup, Ø., Hansen, G., Daugbjerg, N., *et al.* (2014) The dinoflagellates *Pfiesteria shumwayae* and *Luciella masanensis* cause fish kills in recirculation fish farms in Denmark. *Harmful Algae*, **32**, 33–39.

Möller, H. and Anders, K. (1986) *Diseases and Parasites of Marine Fishes*, Möller, Kiel.

Molnár, K. (2002a) Site preference of myxosporean spp. on the fins of some Hungarian fish species. *Diseases of Aquatic Organisms*, **52**, 123–128.

Molnár, K. (2002b) Site preference of fish myxosporeans in the gill. *Diseases of Aquatic Organisms*, **48**, 197–207.

Molnár, K. (2007) Site preference of myxozoans in the kidneys of Hungarian fishes. *Diseases of Aquatic Organisms*, **78**, 45–53.

Molnár, K. and Székely, C. (2014) Tissue preference of some myxobolids (Myxozoa: Myxosporea) from the musculature of European freshwater fishes. *Diseases of Aquatic Organisms*, **107**, 191–198.

Molnár, K., Székely, C. and Baska, F. (1991) Mass mortality of eel in Lake Balaton due to *Anguillicola crassus* infection. *Bulletin of the European Association of Fish Pathologists*, **11**, 211–212.

Morado, J.F. and Small, E.B. (1995) Ciliate parasites and related diseases of Crustacea: a review. *Reviews in Fisheries Science*, **3**, 275–354.

Moran, J.D.W., Whitaker, D.J. and Kent, M.L. (1999) A review of the myxosporean genus *Kudoa* Meglitsch, 1947, and its impact on the international aquaculture industry and commercial fisheries. *Aquaculture*, **172**, 163–196.

Morant, M.P., Prpich, G., Peeler, E., Thrush, M., Rocks, S.A. and Pollard, S.J.T. (2013) Assessment of consequences of notifiable fish disease incursions in England and Wales. *Human and Ecological Risk Assessment*, **19**, 278–290.

Moravec, F. (1994) *Parasitic Nematodes of Freshwater Fishes of Europe*, Kluwer Academic Publishers, London.

Moravec, F. (1998) *Nematodes of Freshwater Fishes of the Neotropical Region*, Academia, Prague.

Moravec, F. (2001) *Trichinelloid Nematodes Parasitic in Cold-blooded Vertebrates*, Academia, Prague.

Moravec, F. (2002) *Dracunculoid and Anguillicoloid Nematodes Parasitic in Vertebrates*, Academia, Prague.

Moravec, F. (2004) Some aspects of the taxonomy and biology of dracunculoid nematodes parasitic in fishes: a review. *Folia Parasitologica*, **51**, 1–13.

Moravec, F. and van As, L.L. (2015) Studies on ascarid, oxyurid and enoplid nematodes (Nematoda) from fishes of the Okavango River, Botswana. *Folia Parasitologica*, **62**, 039.

Moravec, F., Chaabane, A., Justine, J.-L. and Neifar, L. (2016) Two gonad-infecting species of *Philometra* (Nematoda: Philometridae) from groupers (Serranidae) off Tunisia, with a key to *Philometra* species infecting serranid gonads. *Parasite*, **23**, 8.

Morris, D.J. (2012) Towards an *in vitro* culture method for the rainbow trout pathogen *Tetracapsuloides bryosalmonae*. *Journal of Fish Diseases*, **35**, 941–944.

Morris, D.J, Adams, A. and Richards, R.H. (1997) Studies of the PKX parasite in rainbow trout *via* immunohistochemistry and immunogold electron microscopy. *Journal of Aquatic Animal Health*, **9**, 265–272.

Muñoz, P., Palenzuela, O., Alvarez-Pellitero, P. and Sitjà-Bobadilla, A. (1999) Comparative studies on carbohydrates of several myxosporean parasites of fish using lectin histochemical methods. *Folia Parasitologica*, **46**, 241–247.

Murray, A.G., Marcos-Lopez, M., Collet, B. and Munro, L.A. (2012) A review of the risk posed to Scottish mollusc aquaculture from *Bonamia*, *Marteilia* and oyster herpesvirus. *Aquaculture*, **370**, 7–13.

Nachev, M. and Sures, B. (2016) Seasonal profile of metal accumulation in the acanthocephalan *Pomphorhynchus laevis*: a valuable tool to study infection dynamics and implications for metal monitoring. *Parasites and Vectors*, **9**, 300.

Nachev, M., Schertzinger, G. and Sures, B. (2013) Comparison of the metal accumulation capacity between the acanthocephalan *Pomphorhynchus laevis* and larval nematodes of the genus *Eustrongylides* sp. infecting barbel (*Barbus barbus*). *Parasites and Vectors*, **6**, 21.

Nagasawa, K. (2015) Parasitic copepods of marine fish cultured in Japan: a review. *Journal of Natural History*, **49**, 2891–2903.

Nagasawa, K. and Nagata, M. (1992) Effects of *Pectenophilus ornatus* (Copepoda) on the biomass of cultured Japanese scallop *Patinopecten yessoensis*. *Journal of Parasitology*, **78**, 552–554.

Nascimento Justo, M.C., Kohn, A., de Souza Pereira, C. and Flores-Lopes, F. (2013) Histopathology and autoecology of *Didymocylindrus simplex* (Digenea: Didymozoidae), parasite of *Katsuwonus pelamis* (Scombridae) in the southwestern Atlantic Ocean, off South America. *Zoologia*, **30**, 312–316.

Nell, J.A. and Perkins, B. (2006) Evaluation of the progeny of third-generation Sydney rock oyster *Saccostrea glomerata* (Gould, 1850) breeding lines for resistance to QX disease *Marteilia sydneyi* and winter mortality *Bonamia roughleyi*. *Aquaculture Research*, **37**(7), 693–700.

Niewiadomska, K. (1986) Verification of the life-cycles of *Diplostomum spathaceum* (Rudolphi, 1819) and *D. pseudospathaceum* Niewiadomska, 1984 (Trematoda, Diplostomidae). *Systematic Parasitology*, **8**, 23–31.

Noble, A.C. (1996) Major diseases encountered in rainbow trout reared in recirculating systems, in *Successes and Failures in Commercial Recirculating Aquaculture*, Virginia Polytechnic Institute and State University, Roanoke, pp. 17–27.

Noble, A.C., Herman, R.L., Noga, E.J. and Bullock, G.L. (1997) Recurrent amoebic gill infestation in rainbow trout cultured in a semiclosed water recirculation system. *Journal of Aquatic Animal Health*, **9**, 64–69.

Noga, E.J. (2010) *Fish Disease: Diagnosis and Treatment*, 2nd edn, Wiley-Blackwell, Ames.

Ogawa, K. (2015) Diseases of cultured marine fishes caused by Platyhelminthes (Monogenea, Digenea, Cestoda). *Parasitology*, **142**, 178–195.

Ogawa, K. and Fukudome, M. (1994) Mass mortality caused by blood fluke (*Paradeontacylix*) among amberjack (*Seriola dumerili*) imported to Japan. *Fish Pathology*, **29**, 265–269.

Ogawa, K., Hattori, K., Hatai, K. and Kubota, S.S. (1989) Histopathology of cultured marine fish, *Seriola purpurascens* (Carangidae) infected with *Paradeontacylix* spp. (Trematoda: Sanguinicolidae) in its vascular system. *Fish Pathology*, **24**, 75–81.

Ogawa, K., Andoh, H. and Yamaguchi, M. (1993) Some biological aspects of *Paradeontacylix* (Trematoda: Sanguinicolidae) infection in cultured marine fish *Seriola dumerili*. *Gyobyo Kenkyu*, **28**, 177–180.

Ogawa, K., Bondad-Reantaso, M. and Wakabayashi, H. (1995) Redescription of *Benedenia epinepheli* (Yamaguti, 1937) Meserve, 1938 (Monogenea: Capsalidae) from cultured and aquarium marine fishes of Japan. *Canadian Journal of Fisheries and Aquatic Sciences*, **52**(Suppl. 1), 62–70.

Ogedengbe, J.D., Hanner, R.H. and Barta, J.R. (2011) DNA barcoding identifies *Eimeria* species and contributes to the phylogenetics of coccidian parasites (Eimeriorina, Apicomplexa, Alveolata). *International Journal of Parasitology*, **41**, 843–850.

Olsen, O.W. (1974) *Animal Parasites: Their Life Cycles and Ecology*, 3rd edn, Dover, New York.

Olson, P.D. and Littlewood, D.T.J. (2002) Phylogenetics of the Monogenea – evidence from a medley of molecules. *International Journal of Parasitology*, **32**, 233–244.

Olson, P.D., Cribb, T.H., Tkach, V. V, Bray, R.A. and Littlewood, D.T.J. (2003) Phylogeny and classification of the Digenea (Platyhelminthes: Trematoda). *International Journal of Parasitology*, **33**, 733–755.

Ondracková, M., Simková, A., Gelnar, M. and Jurajda, P. (2004) *Posthodiplostomum cuticola* (Digenea: Diplostomatidae) in intermediate fish hosts: factors contributing to the parasite infection and prey selection by the definitive bird host. *Parasitology*, **129**, 761–770.

Overstreet, R.M. (1976) A redescription of *Crassicutis archosargi*, a digenean exhibiting an unusual tegumental attachment. *Journal of Parasitology*, **62**, 702–708.

Overstreet, R.M., Dyková, I. and Hawkins, W.E. (1992a) Branchiura, in *Microscopic Anatomy of the Invertebrates, vol. 9: Crustacea* (eds F.W. Harrison and A.G. Humes), Wiley-Liss, New York, pp. 385–413.

Overstreet, R.M., Heard, R.W. and Lotz, J.M. (1992b) *Microphallus fonti* sp. n. (Digenea: Microphallidae) from the Red Swamp Crawfish in Southern United States. *Memorias do Instituto Oswaldo Cruz*, **87**, 175–178.

Overstreet, R.M., Curran, S.S., Pote, L.M., King, D.T., Blend, C.K. and Grater, W.D. (2002) *Bolbophorus damnificus* n. sp. (Digenea: Bolbophoridae) from the channel catfish *Ictalurus punctatus* and American white pelican *Pelecanus erythrorhynchos* in the USA based on life-cycle and molecular data. *Systematic Parasitology*, **52**, 81–96.

Page, F.C. (1970) Two new species of *Paramoeba* from Maine. *Journal of Protozoology*, **17**, 421–427.

Page, R. (1983) Description of a new species of *Pinnotheres*, and redescription of *P. novaezelandiae* (Brachyura: Pinnotheridae). *New Zealand Journal of Zoology*, **10**, 151–162.

Paladini, G., Cable, J., Fioravanti, M.L., Faria, P.J., di Cave, D. and Shinn, A.P. (2009a) *Gyrodactylus orecchiae* sp. n. (Monogenea: Gyrodactylidae) from farmed populations of gilthead seabream (*Sparus aurata*) in the Adriatic Sea. *Folia Parasitologica*, **56**, 21–28.

Paladini, G., Gustinelli, A., Fioravanti, M.L., Hansen, H. and Shinn, A.P. (2009b) The first report of *Gyrodactylus salaris* Malmberg, 1957 (Platyhelminthes, Monogenea) on Italian cultured stocks of rainbow trout (*Oncorhynchus mykiss* Walbaum). *Veterinary Parasitology*, **165**, 290–297.

Paladini, G., Huyse, T. and Shinn, A.P. (2011) *Gyrodactylus salinae* n. sp. (Platyhelminthes: Monogenea) infecting the south European toothcarp *Aphanius fasciatus* (Valenciennes) (Teleostei, Cyprinodontidae) from a hypersaline environment in Italy. *Parasites and Vectors*, **4**, 100.

Palenzuela, O., Redondo, M. and Alvarez-Pellitero, P. (2002) Description of *Enteromyxum scophthalmi* gen. nov., sp. nov. (Myxozoa), an intestinal parasite of turbot (*Scophthalmus maximus* L.) using morphological and ribosomal RNA sequence data. *Parasitology*, **124**, 369–379.

Palm, H.W. (2004) *The Trypanorhyncha Diesing, 1863*, PKSPL-IPB Press, Bogor, Indonesia.

Pandey, K.C. and Agrawal, N. (2008) *An Encyclopaedia of Indian Monogenoidea*, Vitasta, New Delhi.

Papapanagiotou, E.P. and Trilles, J.P. (2001) Cymothoid parasite *Ceratothoa parallela* inflicts great losses on cultured gilthead sea bream *Sparus aurata* in Greece. *Diseases of Aquatic Organisms*, **45**, 237–239.

Papapanagiotou, E.P., Trilles, J.P. and Photis, G. (1999) First record of *Emetha audouini*, a cymothoid isopod parasite, from cultured sea bass *Dicentrarchus labrax* in Greece. *Diseases of Aquatic Organisms*, **38**, 235–237.

Paperna, I. (1975) Parasites and diseases of the grey mullet (Mugilidae) with special reference to the seas of the Near East. *Aquaculture*, **5**, 65–80.

Paperna, I. (1991) Diseases caused by parasites in the aquaculture of warm water fish. *Annual Review of Fish Diseases*, **1**, 155–194.

Paperna, I. and Lahav, M. (1974) Mortality among grey mullets in a seawater pond due to caligid parasitic copepod epizootic. *Bamidgeh*, **26**, 12–15.

Park, C.-W., Kim, J.-S., Joo, H.-S. and Kim, J. (2009) A human case of *Clinostomum complanatum* infection in Korea. *Korean Journal of Parasitology*, **47**, 401–404.

Parker, J.D. and Warner, M.C. (1970) Effects of fixation, dehydration and staining on dimensions of myxosporidan and microsporidan spores. *Journal of Wildlife Diseases*, **6**, 448–456.

Pérez-Urbiola, J.C. and Martínez-Diaz, S.F. (2001) *Stephanostomum* sp. (Trematoda: Acanthocolpidae), the cause of 'pimientilla' disease in Catarina scallop *Argopecten ventricosus* (circularis) (Sowerby II, 1842) in Baja California Sur, México. *Journal of Shellfish Research*, **20**, 107–109.

Peterson, T.S., Spitsbergen, J.M., Feist, S.W. and Kent, M.L. (2011) Luna stain, an improved selective stain for detection of microsporidian spores in histologic sections. *Diseases of Aquatic Organisms*, **95**, 175–180.

Piasecki, W., Goodwin, A.E., Eiras, J.C. and Nowak, B.F. (2004) Importance of Copepoda in freshwater aquaculture. *Zoological Studies*, **43**, 193–205.

Picón-Camacho, S.M., Leclercq, E., Bron, J.E. and Shinn, A.P. (2012a) The potential utility of the leopard pleco (*Glyptoperichthys gibbiceps*) as a biological control of the ciliate protozoan *Ichthyophthirius multifiliis*. *Pest Management Science*, **68**, 557–563.

Picón-Camacho, S.M., Marcos-Lopez, M., Beljean, A., Debeaume, S. and Shinn, A.P. (2012b) *In vitro* assessment of the chemotherapeutic action of a specific hydrogen peroxide, peracetic,

acetic, and peroctanoic acid-based formulation against the free-living stages of *Ichthyophthirius multifiliis* (Ciliophora). *Parasitology Research*, **110**, 1029–1032.

Pike, A.W. and Wadsworth, S.L. (1999) Sealice on salmonids: their biology and control. *Advances in Parasitology*, **44**, 233–337.

Pina, S., Russell-Pinto, F. and Rodrigues, P. (2011) Morphological and molecular study of *Microphallus primas* (Digenea: Microphallidae) metacercaria, infecting the shore crab *Carcinus maenas* from northern Portugal. *Folia Parasitologica*, **58**, 48–54.

Pinto, H.A. and Melo, A.L. (2012) Metacercariae of *Centrocestus formosanus* (Trematoda: Heterophyidae) in *Australoheros facetus* (Pisces: Cichlidae) in Brazil. *Revista Brasiliera Parasitologia Veterinária*, **21**, 334–337.

Pinto, H.A., Mati, V.L.T. and Melo, A.L. (2014) Metacercarial infection of wild Nile tilapia (*Oreochromis niloticus*) from Brazil. *Scientific World Journal*, 1–7.

Pogoda, B., Jungblut, S., Buck, B.H. and Hagen, W. (2012) Infestation of oysters and mussels by mytilicolid copepods: differences between natural coastal habitats and two offshore cultivation sites in the German Bight. *Journal of Applied Ichthyology*, **28**, 756–765.

Poléo, A.B.S., Schjolden, J., Hansen, H., *et al.* (2004) The effect of various metals on *Gyrodactylus salaris* (Platyhelminthes, Monogenea) infections in Atlantic salmon (*Salmo salar*). *Parasitology*, **128**, 169–177.

Poulin, R. (2010) Parasite manipulation of host behavior: an update and frequently asked questions. *Advances in the Study of Behavior*, **41**, 151–186.

Pouyaud, L., Desmarais, E., Deveney, M. and Pariselle, A. (2006) Phylogenetic relationships among monogenean gill parasites (Dactylogyridea, Ancyrocephalidae) infesting tilapiine hosts (Cichlidae): Systematic and evolutionary implications. *Molecular Phylogenetics and Evolution*, **38**, 241–249.

Poynton, S.L., Fard, M.R.S., Jenkins, J. and Ferguson, H.W. (2004) Ultrastructure of *Spironucleus salmonis* n. comb. (formerly *Octomitus salmonis sensu* Moore 1922, Davis 1926, and *Hexamita salmonis sensu* Ferguson 1979), with a guide to *Spironucleus* species. *Diseases of Aquatic Organisms*, **60**, 49–64.

Printrakoon, C. and Purivirojkul, W. (2012) Infection of speckled shrimp *Metapenaeus monoceros* (Decapoda: Penaeidae) by the branchial parasite *Orbione bonnieri* (Epicardidea: Bopyridae). *Vie Milieu*, **62**, 17–22.

Pugachev, O.N., Gerasev, P.I., Gussev, A. V, Ergens, R. and Khotenowsky, I. (2009) *Guide to the Monogenoidea of Freshwater Fish of Palaeartic and Amur Regions*, Ledizioni, Milan.

Quaglio, F., Perolo, A., Bronzatti, P., *et al.* (2016) Nodular gill disease in farmed rainbow trout (*Oncorhynchus mykiss*) in Italy. *Journal of Fish Diseases*, **39**(9), 1139–1142.

Quignard, J.P. (1968) Rapport entre la présence d'une 'gibbosité frontale' chez les Labridae (Poissons, Téléostéens) et le parasite *Leposphilus labrei* Hesse, 1866 (Copépode Philichthyidae). *Annales Parasitologie Humaine et Comparee*, **43**, 51–57.

Rae, G.H. (2002) Sea louse control in Scotland, past and present. *Pest Management Science*, **58**, 515–520.

Rafi, F. (1988) Isopoda, in *Guide to the Parasites of Fishes of Canada. Part II. Crustacea* (eds L. Margolis and Z. Kabata), Canadian Special Publication of Fisheries and Aquatic Sciences, pp. 129–148.

Ragan, M.A., Goggin, C.L., Cawthorn, R.J., *et al.* (1996) A novel clade of protistan parasites near the animal-fungal divergence. *Proceedings of the National Academy of Sciences USA*, **93**, 11907–11912.

Redondo, M.J., Palenzuela, O. and Alvarez-Pellitero, P. (2003) *In vitro* studies on viability and proliferation of *Enteromyxum scophthalmi* (Myxozoa), an enteric parasite of cultured turbot *Scophthalmus maximus*. *Diseases of Aquatic Organisms*, **55**, 133–144.

Reed, C.C., Basson, L. and van As, L.L. (2002) *Myxobolus* species (Myxozoa), parasites of fishes in the Okavango River and Delta, Botswana, including descriptions of two new species. *Folia Parasitologica*, **49**, 81–88.

Regidor, S.E. and Arthur, J.R. (1986) Parasites of juvenile milkfish, *Chanos chanos*, in *The First Asian Fisheries Forum*, vol. **1**, Asian Fisheries Society, Manila, pp. 261–264.

Reid, A., Lymbery, A., Ng, J., Tweedle, S. and Ryan, U. (2010) Identification of novel and zoonotic *Cryptosporidium* species in marine fish. *Veterinary Parasitology*, **168**, 190–195.

Reimschuessel, R., Gieseker, C. and Poynton, S. (2011) *In vitro* effect of seven antiparasitics on *Acolpenteron ureteroecetes* (Dactylogyridae) from largemouth bass *Micropterus salmoides* (Centrarchidae). *Diseases of Aquatic Organisms*, **94**, 59–72.

Repullés-Albelda, A., Montero, F.E., Holzer, A.S., Ogawa, K., Hutson, K.S. and Raga, J.A. (2008) Speciation of the *Paradeontacylix* spp. (Sanguinicolidae) of *Seriola dumerili*. Two new species of the genus *Paradeontacylix* from the Mediterranean. *Parasitology International*, **57**, 405–414.

Reverter, M., Bontemps, N., Lecchini, D., Banaigs, B. and Sasal, P. (2014) Use of plant extracts in fish aquaculture as an alternative to chemotherapy: current status and future perspectives. *Aquaculture*, **433**, 50–61.

Rigby, M.C., Font, W.F. and Deardorf, T.L. (1997) Redescription of *Camallanus cotti* Fujita, 1927 (Nematoda: Camallanidae) from Hawai'i. *Journal of Parasitology*, **83**, 1161–1164.

Roberts, L.S. and Janovy Jr, J. (2009) *Gerald D. Schmidt and Larry S. Roberts' Foundations of Parasitology*, 8th edn, McGraw Hill Higher Education, New York.

Robledo, J.A.F., Santarém, M.M. and Figueras, A. (1994) Parasite loads of rafted blue mussels (*Mytilus galloprovincialis*) in Spain with special reference to the copepod, *Mytilicola intestinalis*. *Aquaculture*, **127**, 287–302.

Rodger, H.D., Henry, L. and Mitchell, S.O. (2011) Non-infectious gill disorders of marine salmonid fish. *Reviews in Fish Biology and Fisheries*, **21**, 423–440.

Rohde, K. (2005) *Marine Parasitology*, CABI Publishing, London.

Rosser, T.G., Griffin, M.J., Quiniou, S.M.A., *et al.* (2015) Small subunit ribosomal RNA sequence links the myxospore stage of *Henneguya mississippiensis* n. sp. from channel catfish *Ictalurus punctatus* to an actinospore released by the benthic oligochaete *Dero digitata*. *Parasitology Research*, **114**, 1595–1602.

Roth, M. (2000) The availability and use of chemotherapeutic sea lice control products. *Contributions to Zoology*, **69**, 109–118.

Roubal, F.R. (1989) Comparative pathology of some monogenean and copepod ectoparasites on the gills of *Acanthopagrus australis* (Family Sparidae). *Journal of Fish Biology*, **34**, 503–514.

Rowley, J.J.L., Gleason, F.H., Andreou, D., Marshall, W.L., Lilje, O. and Gozlan, R. (2013) Impacts of mesomycetozoean parasites on amphibian and freshwater fish populations. *Fungal Biology Review*, **27**, 100–111.

Salim, K.Y. and Desser, S.S. (2000) Descriptions and phylogenetic systematics of *Myxobolus* spp. from cyprinids in Algonquin Park, Ontario. *Journal of Eukaryotic Microbiology*, **47**, 309–318.

Sanders, M.J. and Lester, R.J.G. (1981) Further observations on a bucephalid trematode infection in scallops (*Pecten alba*) in Port Phillip Bay, Victoria. *Australian Journal of Marine and Freshwater Research*, **32**, 475–478.

Sanil, N.K., Vikas, P.A., Ratheesh, T.B., George, K.C. and Vijayan, K.K. (2009) Mortalities caused by the crustacean isopod, *Cirolana fluviatilis*, in tropical, cage-cultured Asian seabass, *Lates calcarifer*: a case study from the southwest coast of India. *Aquaculture Research*, **40**, 1626–1633.

Santos, M.J., Cavaleiro, F., Campos, P., Sousa, A., Teixeira, F. and Martins, M. (2010) Impact of amoeba and scuticociliatidia infections on the aquaculture European sea bass (*Dicentrarchus labrax* L.) in Portugal. *Veterinary Parasitology*, **171**, 15–21.

Sarker, S., Kallert, D.M., Hedrick, R.P. and El-Matbouli, M. (2015) Whirling disease revisited: pathogenesis, parasite biology and disease intervention. *Diseases of Aquatic Organisms*, **114**, 155–175.

Šarušic, G. (1999) Preliminary report of infestation by isopod *Ceratothoa oestroides* (Risso, 1826), in marine cultured fish. *Bulletin of the European Association of Fish Pathologists*, **19**, 110–112.

Sayer, M.D.J., Treasurer, J.W. and Costello, M.J. (1996) *Wrasse: Biology and Use in Aquaculture*, Fishing News Books, Oxford.

Schafer da Silva, A., Gonzalez Monteiro, S., Laureano Doyle, R., de Araújo Pedron, F., da Silva Filipetto, J.E. and Radünz Neto, J. (2008) Ocorrência de *Clinostomum complanatum* em diferentes espécies de peixes de uma piscicultura do município de Santa Maria. *Veterinária e Zootecnia*, **15**, 27–32.

Schäperclaus, W. (1992) *Fish Diseases*, vols 1 and 2, A.A. Balkema, Rotterdam.

Schelkle, B., Shinn, A.P., Peeler, E. and Cable, J. (2009) Treatment of gyrodactylid infections in fish. *Diseases of Aquatic Organisms*, **86**, 65–75.

Schelkle, B., Doetjes, R. and Cable, J. (2011) The salt myth revealed: Treatment of gyrodactylid infections on ornamental guppies, *Poecilia reticulata*. *Aquaculture*, **311**, 74–79.

Schell, S.C. (1985) *Handbook of the Trematodes of North America North of Mexico*, University Press of Idaho, Moscow, Idaho.

Schmahl, G. (1991) The chemotherapy of monogeneans which parasitize fish: a review. *Folia Parasitologica*, **38**, 97–106.

Schmahl, G. (1993) Treatment of fish parasites. 10. Effects of a new triazine derivative, HOE 092 V, on Monogenea: a light and transmission electron microscopy study. *Parasitology Research*, **79**, 559–566.

Schmahl, G. and Taraschewski, H. (1987) Treatment of fish parasites. 2. Effects of praziquantel, niclosamide, levamisole-HCl, and metrifonate on monogenea (*Gyrodactylus aculeati*, *Diplozoon paradoxum*). *Parasitology Research*, **73**, 341–351.

Schmidt, G.D. (1971) Acanthocephalan infections of man, with two new records. *Journal of Parasitology*, **57**, 582–584.

Schmidt, G.D. (1986) *CRC Handbook of Tapeworm Identification*, CABI International, Wallingford.

Schmidt, G.D. and Nickol, B.B. (1985) Development and life cycles, in *Biology of the Acanthocephala* (eds D.W.T. Crompton and B.B. Nickol), Cambridge University Press, Cambridge, pp. 273–305.

Scholz, T. (1999a) Parasites in cultured and feral fish. *Veterinary Parasitology*, **84**, 317–335.

Scholz, T. (1999b) Life cycles of species of *Proteocephalus*, parasites of fishes in the Palearctic region: a review. *Journal of Helminthology*, **73**, 1–19.

Scholz, T. and Hanzelová, V. (1999) Species of *Proteocephalus* Weinland, 1858 (Cestoda: Proteocephalidae) from cyprinid fishes in North America. *Journal of Parasitology*, **85**, 150–154.

Scholz, T., Garcia, H.H., Kuchta, R. and Wicht, B. (2009) Update on the human broad tapeworm (genus *Diphyllobothrium*), including clinical relevance. *Clinical Microbiology Review*, **22**, 146–160.

Scholz, T., Brabec, J., Král'ová-Hromadová, I., *et al.* (2011) Revision of *Khawia* spp. (Cestoda: Caryophyllidea), parasites of cyprinid fish, including a key to their identification and molecular phylogeny. *Folia Parasitologica*, **58**, 197–223.

Scott, T. and Scott, A. (1913) *The British Parasitic Copepoda*, vols 1 and 2,. Ray Society, London.

Seppälä, O., Karvonen, A. and Tellervo Valtonen, E. (2012) Behavioural mechanisms underlying 'specific' host manipulation by a trophically transmitted parasite. *Evolutionary Ecology Research*, **14**, 73–81.

Shariff, M. and Roberts, R.J. (1989) The experimental histopathology of *Lernaea polymorpha* Yu, 1938 infection in naive *Aristichthys nobilis* (Richardson) and a comparison with the lesion in naturally infected clinically resistant fish. *Journal of Fish Diseases*, **12**, 405–414.

Shiino, S.M. (1932) *Ichthyotaces pteroisicola* n. g. *et* n. sp. a copepod on the fish *Pterois lunulata* Temm *et* Schl. *Annotationes Zoologicae Japonenses*, **13**, 417–433.

Shimazu, T. (2013) Digeneans parasitic in freshwater fishes (Osteichthyes) of Japan. I. Aporocotylidae, Bivesiculidae and Haploporidae. *Bulletin of the National Museum of Natural Science Series A*, **39**, 167–184.

Shinn, A.P. and Bron, J.E. (2012) Considerations for the use of anti-parasitic drugs in aquaculture, in *Infectious Disease in Aquaculture, Prevention and Control* (ed. B. Austin), Woodhead Publishing, Cambridge, pp. 190–217.

Shinn, A.P., Gibson, D.I. and Sommerville, C. (1993) An SEM study of the haptoral sclerites of the genus *Gyrodactylus* Nordmann, 1832 (Monogenea) following extraction by digestion and sonication techniques. *Systematic Parasitology*, **25**, 135–144.

Shinn, A.P., Wootten, R., Côté, I. and Sommerville, C. (2003) Efficacy of selected oral chemotherapeutants against *Ichthyophthirius multifiliis* (Ciliophora: Ophyroglenidae) infecting rainbow trout *Oncorhynchus mykiss*. *Diseases of Aquatic Organisms*, **55**, 17–22.

Shinn, A.P., Picon-Camacho, S.M., Bawden, R. and Taylor, N.G.H. (2009) Mechanical control of *Ichthyophthirius multifiliis* Fouquet, 1876 (Ciliophora) in a rainbow trout hatchery. *Aquacultural Engineering*, **41**, 152–157.

Shinn, A.P., Pratoomyot, J., Bron, J.E., Paladini, G., Brooker, E.E. and Brooker, A.J. (2015a) Economic costs of protistan and metazoan parasites to global mariculture. *Parasitology*, **142**, 196–270.

Shinn, A.P., Pratoomyot, J., Bron, J.E., Paladini, G., Brooker, E.E. and Brooker, A.J. (2015b) Economic impacts of aquatic parasites on global finfish production. *Global Aquaculture Advocate*, Sept/Oct, 82–84.

Shirakashi, S., Andrews, M., Kishimoto, Y., *et al.* (2012a) Oral treatment of praziquantel as an effective control measure against blood fluke infection in Pacific bluefin tuna (*Thunnus orientalis*). *Aquaculture*, **326-329**, 15–19.

Shirakashi, S., Kishimoto, Y., Kinami, R., *et al.* (2012b) Morphology and distribution of blood fluke eggs and associated pathology in the gills of cultured Pacific bluefin tuna, *Thunnus orientalis*. *Parasitology International*, **61**, 242–249.

Sievers, G., Lobos, C., Inostroza, R. and Ernst, S. (1996) The effect of the isopod parasite *Ceratothoa gaudichaudii* on the body weight of farmed *Salmo salar* in southern Chile. *Aquaculture*, **143**, 1–6.

Smith, J.L., Wootten, R. and Sommerville, C. (2007) The pathology of the early stages of the crustacean parasite, *Lernaeocera branchialis* (L.), on Atlantic cod, *Gadus morhua* L. *Journal of Fish Diseases*, **30**, 1–11.

Smyth, J.D. (1994) *Introduction to Animal Parasitology*, 3rd edn, Cambridge University Press, London.

Sommerville, C. (2012) Advances in non-chemical methods for parasite prevention and control in fish, in *Infectious Disease in Aquaculture* (ed. B. Austin), Woodhead Publishing, Cambridge, pp. 480–512.

Špakulová, M., Perrot-Minnot, M. and Neuhaus, B. (2011) Resurrection of *Pomphorhynchus tereticollis* (Rudolphi, 1809) (Acanthocephala: Pomphorhynchidae) based on new morphological and molecular data. *Helminthologia*, **48**, 268–277.

Stebbing, P., Longshaw, M. and Scott, A. (2014) Review of methods for the management of non-indigenous crayfish, with particular reference to Great Britain. *Ethology, Ecology and Evolution*, **26**, 204–231.

Stentiford, G.D. (2008) Diseases of the European edible crab (*Cancer pagurus*): a review. *ICES Journal of Marine Science*, **65**, 1578–1592.

Stien, L.H., Nilsson, J., Hevrøy, E.M., *et al.* (2012) Skirt around a salmon sea cage to reduce infestation of salmon lice resulted in low oxygen levels. *Aquaculture Engineering*, **51**, 21–25.

Stien, L.H., Dempster, T., Bui, S., *et al.* (2016) 'Snorkel' sea lice barrier technology reduces sea lice loads on harvest-sized Atlantic salmon with minimal welfare impacts. *Aquaculture*, **458**, 29–37.

Stingray Marine Solutions AS (2016) Available at: http://en.stingray.no/ (accessed 30 November 2016).

Stoskopf, M.K. (1993) *Fish Medicine*, W.B. Saunders, London.

Stunkard, H.W. (1938) The morphology and life cycle of the trematode *Himasthla quissetensis* (Miller and Northup, 1926). *Biological Bulletin of the Marine Biological Laboratory*, **75**, 145–164.

Sturrock, R.F. (2001) Schistosomiasis epidemiology and control: how did we get here and where should we go? *Memorias do Instituto Oswaldo Cruz*, **96**, 17–27.

Sugihara, Y., Yamada, T., Tamaki, A., Yamanishi, R. and Kanai, K. (2014) Larval stages of the bluefin tuna blood fluke *Cardicola opisthorchis* (Trematoda: Aporocotylidae) found from *Terebella* sp. (Polychaeta: Terebellidae). *Parasitology International*, **63**, 295–299.

Summerfelt, S.T. (2003) Ozonation and UV irradiation – an introduction and examples of current applications. *Aquaculture Engineering*, **28**, 21–36.

Sures, B. (2001) The use of fish parasites as bioindicators of heavy metals in aquatic ecosystems: a review. *Aquatic Ecology*, **35**, 245–255.

Tada, I., Otsuji, Y., Kamiya, H., Mimori, T., Sakaguchi, Y. and Makizumi, S. (1983) The first case of a human infected with an acanthocephalan parasite, *Bolbosoma* sp. *Journal of Parasitology*, **69**, 205–208.

Tang, D., Andrews, M. and Cobcroft, J.M. (2007) The first chondracanthid (Copepoda: Cyclopoida) reported from cultured finfish, with a revised key to the species of *Chondracanthus*. *Journal of Parasitology*, **93**, 788–795.

Taraschewski, H. (2000) Host-parasite interactions in Acanthocephala: a morphological approach. *Advances in Parasitology*, **46**, 1–179.

Tenter, A.M., Barta, J.R., Beveridge, I., *et al.* (2002) The conceptual basis for a new classification of the coccidia. *International Journal of Parasitology*, **32**, 595–616.

Thatcher, V.E. (1987) Hope for HYP. *Monoculus Copepod Newsletter*, **15**, 20–23.

Thomas, P.A., Kaliamurthy, J., Jesudasan, C.A.N. and Geraldine, P. (2008) Use of chlorazol black E mounts of corneal scrapes for diagnosis of filamentous fungal keratitis. *American Journal of Ophthalmology*, **145**, 971–976.

Thoney, D.A. and Hargis, W.J. (1991) Monogenea (Platyhelminthes) as hazards for fish in confinement. *Annual Review of Fish Diseases*, **1**, 133–153.

Todal, J.A., Karlsbakk, E., Isaksen, T.E., *et al.* (2004) *Ichthyobodo necator* (Kinetoplastida) - a complex of sibling species. *Diseases of Aquatic Organisms*, **58**, 9–16.

Toledo, R., Esteban, J.-G. and Fried, B. (2006) Immunology and pathology of intestinal trematodes in their definitive hosts. *Advances in Parasitology*, **63**, 285–365.

Tossavi, N.D., Gbankoto, A., Yessoufou, A., *et al.* (2015) Histopathological and ultrastructural studies of a *Henneguya* species (Myxozoa: Myxosporea) infesting the intestine of *Clarias gariepinus* from Benin (West Africa). *Parasitology Research*, **114**, 861–872.

Tran, T.K.C., Murrell, K.D., Madsen, H., Nguyen, V.K. and Dalsgaard, A. (2009) Fishborne zoonotic trematodes in raw fish dishes served in restaurants in Nam Dinh Province and Hanoi, Vietnam. *Journal of Food Protection*, **72**, 2394–2399.

Treves-Brown, K.M. (2000) *Applied Fish Pharmacology*, Springer, London.

Trottier, O., Walker, D. and Jeffs, A.G. (2012) Impact of the parasitic pea crab *Pinnotheres novaezelandiae* on aquacultured New Zealand green-lipped mussels, *Perna canaliculus*. *Aquaculture*, **344**, 23–29.

Urawa, S. and Kato, T. (1991) Heavy infections of *Caligus orientalis* (Copepoda: Caligidae) on caged rainbow trout *Oncorhynchus mykiss* in brackish water. *Fish Pathology*, **26**, 161–162.

Urawa, S., Ueki, N. and Karlsbakk, E. (1998) A review of *Ichthyobodo* infection in marine fishes. *Fish Pathology*, **33**, 311–320.

Urawa, S., Lida, Y., Freeman, M.A., Yanagida, T., Karlsbakk, E. and Yokoyama, H. (2009) Morphological and molecular comparisons of *Myxobolus* spp. in the nerve tissues of salmonid fishes with the description of *Myxobolus murakamii* n. sp., the causative agent of myxosporean sleeping disease. *Fish Pathology*, **44**, 72–80.

Urawa, S., Freeman, M.A., Johnson, S.C., Jones, S.R.M. and Yokoyama, H. (2011) Geographical variation in spore morphology, gene sequences, and host specificity of *Myxobolus arcticus* (Myxozoa) infecting salmonid nerve tissues. *Diseases of Aquatic Organisms*, **96**, 229–237.

Urquhart, K., Pert, C.C., Fryer, R.J., *et al.* (2010) A survey of pathogens and metazoan parasites on wild sea trout (*Salmo trutta*) in Scottish waters. *ICES Journal of Marine Science*, **67**, 444–453.

Vagianou, S., Athanassopoulou, F., Ragias, V., di Cave, D., Leontides, L. and Golomazou, E. (2006) Prevalence and pathology of ectoparasites of Mediterranean sea bream and sea bass reared under different environmental and aquaculture conditions. *Bamidgeh*, **58**, 78–88.

Valencia, V. and George-Nascimento, M. (2013) Farming systems as an ecological refuge against the parasitism by *Edotia doellojurdoi* (Isopoda: Idoteidae) on *Mytilus edulis* (Mollusca: Mytilidae) in Aysén, Chile. *Revista Chilena de Historia Natural*, **86**, 153–159.

Van As, J.G. and Basson, L. (1989) A further contribution to the taxonomy of the Trichodinidae (Ciliophora: Peritrichia) and a review of the taxonomic status of some fish ectoparasitic trichodinids. *Systematic Parasitology*, **14**, 157–179.

Villalba, A., Mourelle, S.G., Carballal, M.J. and Lopez, C. (1997) Symbionts and diseases of farmed mussels *Mytilus galloprovincialis* throughout the culture process in the Rías of Galicia (NW Spain). *Diseases of Aquatic Organisms*, **31**, 127–139.

Villalba, A., Reece, K.S., Camino Ordás, M., Casas, S.M. and Figueras, A. (2004) Perkinsosis in molluscs: a review. *Aquatic Living Resources*, **17**, 411–432.

Vo, D.T., Murrell, D., Dalsgaard, A., *et al.* (2008) Prevalence of zoonotic metacercariae in two species of grouper, *Epinephelus coioides* and *Epinephelus bleekeri*, and flathead mullet, *Mugil cephalus*, in Vietnam. *Korean Journal of Parasitology*, **46**, 77–82.

Vo, D.T., Bristow, G.A., Vo, D.T., *et al.* (2011) Digenean trematodes of cultured grouper (*Epinephelus coioides* and *E. bleekeri*) in Khanh Hoa Province, Vietnam, in *Diseases in Asian*

Aquaculture VII (eds M.G. Bondad-Reantaso, J.B. Jones, F. Corsin and T. Aoki), Fish Health Section, Asian Fisheries Society, Selangor, pp. 39–52.

Vrålstad, T., Strand, D.A., Grandjean, F., *et al.* (2014) Molecular detection and genotyping of *Aphanomyces astaci* directly from preserved crayfish samples uncovers the Norwegian crayfish plague disease history. *Veterinary Microbiology*, **173**, 66–75.

Wanstall, S.T., Robotham, P.W. and Thomas, J.S. (1982) Changes in the energy reserves of two species of freshwater fish during infection by *Pomphorhynchus laevis*. *Proceedings of the British Society for Parasitology*, **85**, 27.

Wanstall, S.T., Robotham, P.W. and Thomas, J.S. (1986. Pathological changes induced by *Pomphorhynchus laevis* Muller (Acanthocephala) in the gut of rainbow trout, *Salmo gairdneri* Richardson. *Zeitschrift für Parasitenkunde*, **72**, 105–114.

Whittington, I.D., Chisholm, L.A. and Rohde, K. (2000) The larvae of Monogenea (Platyhelminthes). *Advances in Parasitology*, **44**, 139–232.

Whyte, S.K., Allan, J.C., Secombes, C.J. and Chappell, L.H. (1987) Cercariae and diplostomules of *Diplostomum spathaceum* (Digenea) elicit an immune response in rainbow trout, *Salmo gairdneri* Richardson. *Journal of Fish Biology*, **31**, 185–190.

Whyte, S.K., Secombes, C.J. and Chappell, L.H. (1991) Studies on the infectivity of *Diplostomum spathaceum* in rainbow trout (*Oncorhynchus mykiss*). *Journal of Helminthology*, **65**, 169–78.

Willemse, J.J. (1979) Guide to the internal morphology of the European eel, *Anguilla anguilla* (L.) (Pisces, Teleostei). *Aquaculture*, **17**, 91–103.

Willis, J.E., McClure, J.T., Davidson, J., McClure, C. and Greenwood, S.J. (2013) Global occurrence of *Cryptosporidium* and *Giardia* in shellfish: Should Canada take a closer look? *Food Research International*, **52**, 119–135.

Wilson, C.B. (1905) North American parasitic copepods belonging to the family Caligidae. Part 1. The Caliginae. *Proceedings of the United States National Museum*, **28**, 479–672.

Wilson, C.B. (1915) North American parasitic copepods belonging to the Lernaeopodidae, with a revision of the entire family. *Proceedings of the United States National Museum*, **47**, 565–729.

Wilson, C.B. (1917) North American parasitic copepods belonging to the Lernaeidae, with a revision of the entire family. *Proceedings of the United States National Museum*, **53**, 1–150.

Winters, A.D., Langohr, I.M., Souza, M.D.E.A., Colodel, E.M., Soares, M.P. and Faisal, M. (2016) Ultrastructure and molecular phylogeny of *Pleistophora hyphessobryconis* (Microsporidia) infecting hybrid jundiara (*Leiarius marmoratus* × *Pseudoplatystoma reticulatum*) in a Brazilian aquaculture facility. *Parasitology*, **143**, 41–49.

Wolf, K. and Markiw, M.E. (1976) *Myxosoma cerebralis*: in vitro sporulation of the myxosporidan of salmonid whirling disease. *Journal of Protozoology*, **23**, 425–427.

Woo, P.T.K. (2006) *Fish Diseases and Disorders*, 2nd edn, CABI International, Wallingford.

World Organisation for Animal Health (OIE) (2016) OIE-Listed diseases, infections and infestations in force in 2016. Available at: www.oie.int/animal-health-in-the-world/oie-listed-diseases-2016/ (accessed 30 November 2016).

Yamaguti, S. (1958) *Systema Helminthum. Vol. I. The Digenetic Trematodes of Vertebrates.* Interscience Wiley, New York.

Yamaguti, S. (1959) *Systema Helminthum. Vol. II. The Cestodes of Vertebrates*, Interscience Wiley, New York.

Yamaguti, S. (1962) *Systema Helminthum. Vol. III. The Nematodes of Vertebrates*, Interscience Wiley, New York.

Yamaguti, S. (1963a) *Systema Helminthum. Vol. IV. Monogenea and Aspidocotylea*, Interscience Wiley, New York.

Yamaguti, S. (1963b) *Systema Helminthum. Vol. V. Acanthocephala*, Interscience Wiley, New York.

Yamaguti, S. (1963c) *Parasitic Copepoda and Branchiura of Fishes*, Interscience Wiley, New York.

Yanmar (2016) Net cleaning robot. Available at: www.yanmarmarine.eu/Products/Net-Cleaning-Robot/ (accessed 30 November 2016).

Yasunaga, N., Ogawa, S., Hirakawa, E., Hatai, K., Yasumoto, S. and Yamamoto, H. (1981) On the marine-fish disease caused by *Galactosomum* sp. with special reference to its species and life cycle. *Bulletin of the Nagazaki Prefecture Institute of Fisheries*, 7, 65–76.

Yin, W.Y. (1962) Parasitic Copepoda and Branchiura of freshwater fishes from northeast China and Inner Mongolia. *Acta Hydrobiologica Sinica*, **1**, 31–46.

Yokoyama, H., Liyanage, Y.S., Sugai, A. and Wakabayashi, H. (1998) Hemorrhagic thelohanellosis of color carp caused by *Thelohanellus hovorkai* (Myxozoa: Myxosporea). *Fish Pathology*, **33**, 85–89.

Yokoyama, H., Shigehiko, U., Grabner, D. and Shirakashi, S. (2012) *Henneguya cartilaginis* n. sp. (Myxozoa: Myxosporea) in the head cartilage of masu salmon *Oncorhynchus masou masou*. *Parasitology International*, **61**, 594–598.

Yoshinaga, T., Tsutsumi, N., Hall, K.A. and Ogawa, K. (2009) Origin of the diclidophorid monogenean *Neoheterobothrium hirame* Ogawa, 1999, the causative agent of anemia in olive flounder *Paralichthys olivaceus*. *Fisheries Science*, **75**, 1167–1176.

Yost, M., Dorr, B.S. and Pote, L.M. (2005) Confirmation of *Bolbophorus damnificus* life cycle and characterization of all life stages. *Southeastern Biology*, **52**, 163.

Young, N.D., Crosbie, P.B.B., Adams, M.B., Nowak, B.F. and Morrison, R.N. (2007) *Neoparamoeba perurans* n. sp., an agent of amoebic gill disease of Atlantic salmon (*Salmo salar*). *International Journal of Parasitology*, **37**, 1469–1481.

Young, P.S. (1998) *Catalogue of Crustacea of Brazil, Série Livros* 6, Museo Nacional, Rio de Janeiro.

Yu, S.-H. and Mott, K.E. (1994) Epidemiology and morbidity of food-borne intestinal trematode infections. *Tropical Diseases Bulletin*, **91**, 125–152.

5

Modern Methods of Diagnosis

Ahran Kim, Thanh Luan Nguyen* and Do-Hyung Kim*

Department of Aquatic Life Medicine, Pukyong National University, Busan, Republic of Korea

Introduction

Fish and shellfish are susceptible to diverse pathogenic micro-organisms, including bacteria, viruses, parasites and fungi, some of which pose a major threat to the aquaculture industry. Unlike terrestrial animals, aquatic animals live in complex and dynamic environments and they are not readily visible. This makes control of fish and shellfish disease problematic so monitoring of the health status of aquatic animals is vital. Rapid and accurate diagnostic methods are useful, as early detection and diagnosis are critical for the management and control of infectious disease, especially in aquatic animals. Many diagnostic techniques have been developed, some of which are widely used for detection of pathogens. The diagnostic approaches used in aquaculture comprise conventional microbiological, immunoserological and molecular methods. Here we describe methods in each category and give some examples of applications of techniques with advantages and disadvantages.

The first section briefly describes conventional diagnostic methods (some of which have already been superseded by modern techniques), including traditional microbiology and histopathology for parasites, bacteria and viruses that affect aquaculture. In the subsequent section, immunoserological diagnostic tools based on highly specific and sensitive binding reaction between antigens and antibodies are described. Development of immunodiagnostic methods has revolutionized aquaculture diagnostics as they are more sensitive and specific than traditional approaches, and can be used at the farm level without the aid of instruments. Also, these methods can detect non-culturable micro-organisms. However, antibody selection is critical for acceptable results. Many monoclonal or polyclonal antibodies against fish pathogens are now available commercially, which are different in sensitivity and specificity. However, insufficient availability of antibodies against fish and shellfish pathogens still hampers fish immunodiagnostics. Western blotting and immunoblotting techniques are not used routinely as diagnostic methods, but can be useful for confirmation of certain pathogens, such as viral pathogens (e.g. white spot syndrome virus and yellow head virus in shrimp), that cannot be cultured in cell lines. Thus, we introduce commonly used immunological methods, such as ELISA and lateral flow immunoassays, which are important for detection of aquatic pathogens.

* Joint first authors

Diagnosis and Control of Diseases of Fish and Shellfish, First Edition. Edited by Brian Austin and Aweeda Newaj-Fyzul.

The limitations of conventional methods in terms of sensitivity and specificity led to the development and use of molecular techniques. Diverse molecular assays for the detection and identification of aquatic pathogens have been developed which significantly reduce the time to and improve the accuracy of the diagnosis. The majority of nucleic acid-based techniques in use are discussed in detail. These techniques can be used to identify and characterize the genotypes of the micro-organisms after isolation, and to exclude particular pathogens or detect pathogens in specimens without deteriorating the antigens and simultaneously reducing the risk of contamination with other microbes. Molecular techniques in this chapter are categorized into those based on hybridization, nucleic acid amplification and molecular typing. We briefly describe state-of-the-art clinical diagnostic approaches that may in future be routinely used in clinical laboratories. These include a technique based on nanoparticles, matrix-assisted laser desorption ionization time-of-flight (MALDI-TOF) mass spectrometry and next-generation sequencing technologies, which enables even more sensitive and rapid identification, detection and genetic characterization of micro-organisms.

Diagnostic Methods for Aquatic Diseases

Conventional Methods

Histopathology

Histopathology is assessment of tissue structure and function using a microscope, and has evolved together with the development of microscopy. Disease leads to histological changes in host tissues so histopathology has been utilized as a diagnostic tool for detection of pathogens in tissue sections. This facilitates assessment of the correlations and interactions between host tissue and pathogens. Observation of histopathological changes can support the results of other diagnostic methods, leading to confirmatory diagnosis. Indeed, several studies have used this technique as the primary method of detecting pathogens, especially parasites, or toxicopathic changes as a target endpoint in fish (Feist and Longshaw, 2008; Longshaw *et al.*, 2010; Rodnick *et al.*, 2008; Saksida *et al.*, 2012; Stentiford *et al.*, 2003). Moreover, histopathology facilitates detection of emerging pathogens for which diagnostic methods are not yet available. In general, however, histological techniques are less sensitive and specific than other methods, including culture-based and molecular techniques. Moreover, sensitivity in subclinical fish and shellfish is lower than that in a moribund subject showing clear signs of disease. In addition, histopathology requires complex sample preparation procedures, which are important for subsequent data analysis, and is time-consuming and costly. Nevertheless, collaboration between pathologists and microbiologists is of importance to provide precise diagnosis and determine optimal control measures. Various newly developed staining techniques will increase the importance of histopathology in the diagnosis of diseases of fish and shellfish.

Parasitology

A presumptive diagnosis of parasite infestation in fish is usually made on the basis of abnormal behaviour, such as lethargy, anaemia, whirling, scraping on wall and clinical signs (e.g. skin ulcers caused by *Miamiensis avidus*, and white cysts in muscle caused by *Myxobolus cerebralis*) on external or internal tissues, seen by the naked eye or by microscopy. For many years, microscopy has been the only tool available for detection of parasites in tissue specimens, including gills, skin, fins and internal organs, and blood smears. However, diagnosis by direct observation is greatly dependent on the presence of qualified clinicians. Freshly killed fish are of greater utility than subclinical fish and fixed or frozen tissues in terms of detection and identification of parasites. With the exception of helminths and parasitic crustaceans, the presence of parasites should be confirmed by microscopy in conjunction with other methods, including immunological and molecular techniques.

Bacteriology

Bacterial diseases can be identified using various diagnostic methods, including traditional microbiological, immunoserological and molecular techniques; these are discussed in the following section. Here, we briefly introduce conventional methods in common use, including Gram staining, biochemical, physiological and metabolic tests.

Samples are taken from freshly killed or moribund aquatic animals aseptically, and bacteria are grown on/in various non-selective media. If a target is a fastidious bacterium, it would require specific or complex nutrients and specific incubation conditions. Causal agents of disease can be recovered from lesions, blood and various tissues of diseased fish. Following growth of bacteria, various microbiological diagnostic methods can be applied. Phenotypic characterization of pure cultured bacteria is based on their biochemical, physiological and metabolic properties. Tests for biochemical characteristics are based on the different biochemical reactions that bacteria exhibit. A single-enzyme test determines the presence of a specific enzyme, such as oxidase, catalase and indole. Oxidation-fermentation, amino acid degradation and single substrate utilization tests are used to determine the metabolic pathways used and the products thereof. These tests require media containing specific substrates and indicators to detect changes in endproducts. Indeed, commercial kits are commonly used for bacterial identification in fish and shellfish diagnostic laboratories, as they are usually simple to use, time- and cost-effective and semi-automated. API kits (bioMérieux) for several bacterial species (e.g. for streptococci and vibrios) are widely used for identification of bacteria derived from aquatic animals. After incubation of target bacteria in a kit for 24–48 hours, results can be determined based on colour changes interpreted according to the manufacturer's reading table.

However, these methods have several drawbacks in terms of identification of aquatic pathogens:

- the presence of plasmids is not considered
- databases contain sparse information on fish and shellfish pathogens
- they have limited accuracy because they cannot distinguish subtypes or closely related bacterial species (e.g. the genera *Aeromonas* and *Vibrio*)
- there is the possibility of erroneous and ambiguous results (Austin, 2011; Topić Popović *et al*., 2007).

Although these phenotyping methods remain widely used for diagnosis of bacterial diseases, they are time-consuming and labour intensive and, more importantly, do not enable discrimination of several bacterial species important in aquaculture.

Virology

Diagnosis of viral infection has been based mainly on serological tests, the sensitivity and specificity of which vary depending on the antigens and techniques used. In recent years, molecular techniques in conjunction with histopathological examination are increasingly used for more sensitive and specific diagnosis. The diagnostic methods used for the major viral pathogens of aquatic animals are described in the *Manual of Diagnostic Tests for Aquatic Animals* (OIE, 2015). In this subsection, several conventional methods are introduced; immunological methods will be discussed in a subsequent section.

Virus can be detected directly through microscopic examination. Light microscopy can identify histological changes, such as inclusion bodies in the nucleus or cytoplasm or multinucleated giant cells, in a sample. Electron microscopy facilitates direct visualization of viral morphology, which represents its greatest advantage. However, this method is much less sensitive because a virus with a titre of $\geq 10^5$–10^6 plaque-forming units (PFU)/mL must be present. Detection of virus using light or electron microscopy is less sensitive compared to modern techniques, and electron microscopy requires expensive, specialized equipment and skilled technicians.

Cell culture is essential for virus isolation and identification because viruses are obligate intracellular parasites. In general, cell lines that can multiply continuously are used for cell culture. Virus-containing sample is inoculated into a cultured cell, and the resulting cytopathic effects (CPE) monitored. Cell culture facilitates virus isolation and detection but such techniques have limitations, particularly for fish and shellfish diagnostics.

- Virus may not grow in cell culture.
- CPE may not be specific.
- Culture of cells can take a long time, and some viruses (e.g. infectious salmon anaemia virus) grow slowly.
- Maintaining cell culture without contamination by bacteria or other agents can be problematic.
- Cultures can be susceptible to additives, including fetal calf serum (FCS) or toxicants.
- Sensitivity can be relatively low.
- Cell lines are not available for many viruses (e.g. for those pathogenic to shrimp and abalone).

Therefore, the presence of virus must be confirmed using additional diagnostic techniques, including serological methods. Agglutination tests are based on generation of precipitate visible to the naked eye or under a microscope due to formation of large antigen–antibody complexes (Figure 5.1a,b). Immunodiffusion tests are based on diffusion of proteins (e.g. antigen and antibody) through a solid phase (e.g. agar, agarose gel or acetate), and subsequent production of immunocomplexes (Figure 5.1c). Complement fixation tests detect the presence of a specific antigen or antibody in serum of infected fish, based on whether complement fixation occurs (Figure 5.1d). Neutralization tests detect and quantify neutralizing antibodies in serum after virus infection or vaccination. These are some examples of traditional specific tests for antibodies or antigens, and have now been superseded by newer techniques, including other immunological methods.

Immunoserological Methods

Monoclonal and Polyclonal Antibodies

The antibody used is critical for immunoserological diagnosis, and several monoclonal and polyclonal antibodies against fish pathogens are now available commercially. Monoclonal antibodies (mAbs) detect only one epitope on a single target antigen, and comprise a homogenous cloned immunoglobulin with high specificity. These antibodies are generated from hybridoma of antibody-producing cells and an immortalized cell line. Production

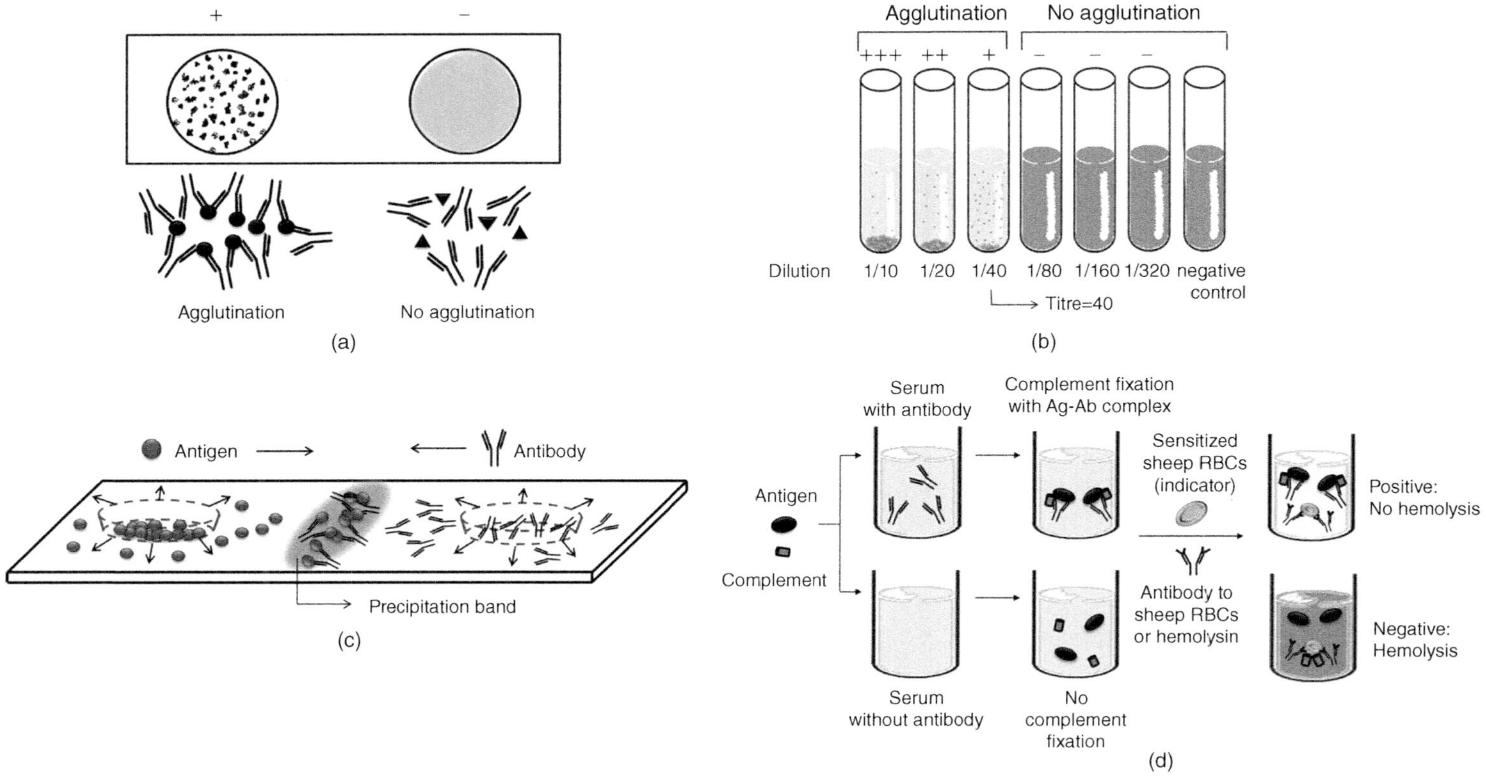

Figure 5.1 Conventional serological methods. Agglutination test uses the principles of precipitation occurring by formation of large antigen–antibody clumps visible with the naked eye or under microscope; (a) slide agglutination test; (b) tube agglutination test. The immunodiffusion test is based on characteristics of proteins (e.g. antigen or antibody) that can diffuse on solid phase (e.g. agar, agarose gel or acetate). This is to measure a precipitate band formed following reaction between antigen and antibody (c). Complement fixation test utilizes the properties of complement, a group of serum proteins that facilitates formation of antigen–antibody complexes to eliminate a pathogen (d).

of monoclonal antibodies requires a high level of technology and skilled staff. Although generation of a hybridoma is time-consuming and costly, mAbs can be produced continuously thereafter. mAbs are often used as primary antibodies due to their specificity. Use of a combination of two or more mAbs against a target pathogen would increase detection sensitivity. Polyclonal antibodies contain heterogeneous mixed immunoglobulin molecules that can recognize multiple epitopes on a single antigen. Therefore, polyclonal antibodies are superior for detection of pathogens due to their recognition of several epitopes of a target agent. Also, polyclonal antibodies are used for haemagglutination as binding of antibodies to multiple epitopes facilitates precipitation. In addition, when the exact nature of the antigen is unknown, polyclonal antibodies yield greater sensitivity. Polyclonal antibodies are generally used as secondary antibodies in indirect ELISAs and Western blots. Production of polyclonal antibodies is inexpensive, requires a shorter time and is less complicated than production of mAbs.

Enzyme-linked Immunosorbent Assay

Enzyme-linked immunosorbent assay (ELISA) involves detection of an antigen–antibody reaction by a change in colour or fluorescence due to byproduct of an enzymatic reaction. For ELISA, an antigen or antibody immobilized on a solid surface (usually microtitre plate), target substances (e.g. peptides, proteins or antibodies) and enzyme-conjugated detection antibody are required, and a visible signal is produced by enzymatic breakdown of an appropriate substrate. Horseradish peroxidase (HRP) and alkaline phosphatase (AP) are widely used for ELISA. There are four typical ELISA formats, depending on the sensitivity required and nature of the target (i.e. antigen/analyte or antibody): direct, indirect, sandwich and competitive ELISA. These are described briefly in Table 5.1 and Figure 5.2.

ELISA is a diagnostic technique widely used for aquatic animal diseases caused by viruses, including viral haemorrhagic septicaemia virus (VHSV) (Olesen and Jørgensen, 1991), infectious haematopoietic necrosis virus (IHNV) (Dixon and Hill, 1984), and epizootic haematopoietic necrosis virus (EHNV) (Whittington and Steiner, 1993). Antigen-capture ELISA based on the sandwich ELISA format is used to detect these pathogens, and either biotinylated polyclonal antibody or monoclonal antibody to target virus is used as the primary antibody. ELISA results are available in a short time (usually within three hours) and can quantify proteins of interest – including cytokines, growth factors, antibodies and antigens – with high sensitivity and specificity. Detection and identification of aquatic animal pathogens using ELISA are described in the *Manual of Diagnostic Tests for Aquatic Animals* (OIE, 2015). Commercial ELISA kits for detection of aquatic animal pathogens, such as the VHSV-IHNV diagnostic kit (Bio-X Diagnostics), are available.

ELISA techniques are advantageous in that they are specific, allow detection of toxins produced by pathogens, and can be automated to increase their time- and cost-effectiveness, although they are less sensitive than polymerase chain reaction (PCR)-based methods, can yield false-negative results and may exhibit cross-reactivity with closely related antigens (Law *et al.*, 2015). In addition, immunoserological tests do not distinguish between infected and vaccinated fish, and cannot be used in shellfish, as they do not produce antibodies.

Immunofluorescence Test

Immunofluorescence is a powerful technique that uses antibodies labelled with fluorophores such as fluorescein isothiocyanate (FITC) to detect specific antigens in clinical samples, cultured cells and formalin-fixed and paraffin-embedded (FFPE) tissue sections. Fluorescence

Table 5.1 ELISAs according to detection method.

Detection methods	Direct	Indirect	Sandwich	Competitive
Detection (in a given sample)	Ag level	Ab level	Ag level	Ag, Ab, small molecules (e.g. haptens)
Sensitivity/specificity	Low/low	High	High/high	High but less than that of sandwich ELISA
Advantages	· Simple and rapid · Suitable for specific antibody–antigen reactions · No cross-reactivity by secondary antibody	· Detection of very low concentrations of antibodies · Flexibility (various labelled secondary antibodies) · High immunoreactivity because primary antibody is not influenced by labelling · Signal amplification	· Possible to detect at very low concentration of antigens · High specificity and no purification using a purified specific antibody on antigens · Flexibility	· Detection in complex samples · Large-scale screening · Flexibility · No requirement for species-specific enzyme-labelled conjugates
Disadvantages	· Low immunoreactivity, time-consuming, expensive and inflexible due to direct labelling of primary antibody	· Cross-reactivity by secondary antibody · The method of antigen immobilization is not specific		

is generated when a fluorescently labelled antibody binds to its target antigen. Although this technique is sensitive and rapid, it generally requires skilled operators and specialized equipment (fluorescence microscope, confocal microscope or flow cytometer) to perform and interpret results. Fluorescence signals can be affected by the antibody quality and concentration and sample preparation method used (e.g. tissue sections) (Odell and Cook, 2013).

Direct Immunofluorescence (IF) Direct IF involves direct binding of fluorescently labelled antibodies to the target antigen. For pathogen detection, a fluorescently tagged primary antibody is used to detect the target pathogen (Figure 5.3). Direct IF is a rapid and specific technique, although less sensitive than other diagnostic methods; moreover, the lack of availability of antibodies is problematic (Odell and Cook, 2013).

Indirect Immunofluorescence Indirect IF is a two-step procedure. First, the primary unlabelled antibody binds to a specific antigen in the sample. After incubation, a secondary fluorescently labelled antibody is used to detect the primary antibody (see Figure 5.3). Indirect IF is more sensitive due to use of more than one secondary antibody for each primary antibody, which

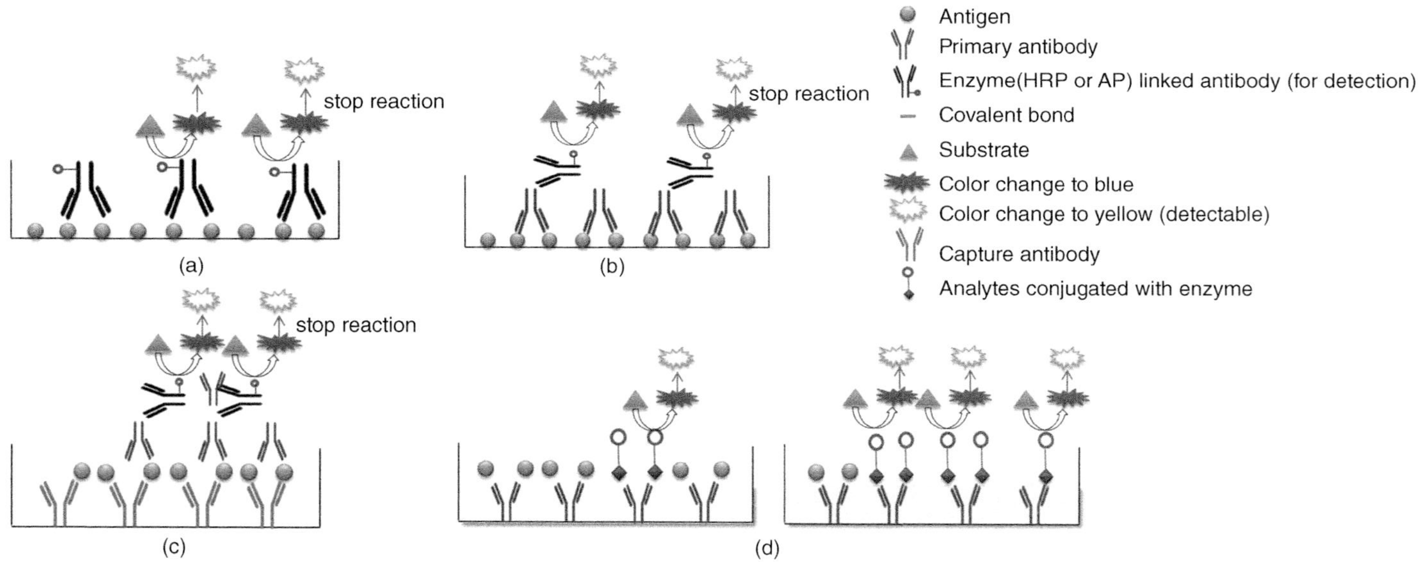

Figure 5.2 ELISAs according to detection method. (a) Direct ELISA; (b) indirect ELISA; (c) sandwich ELISA; (d) competitive ELISA. (*See plate section for the color representation of this figure.*)

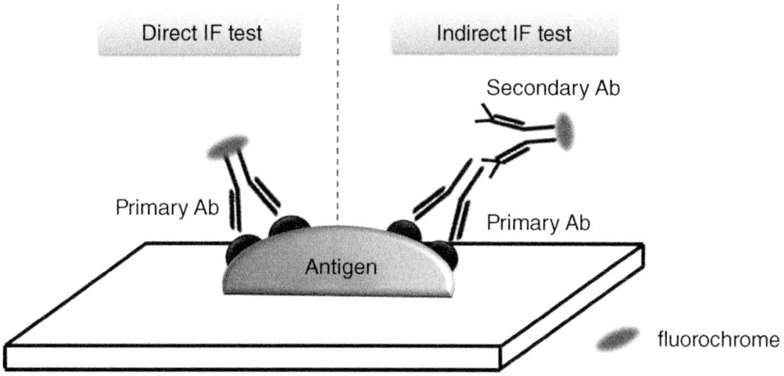

Figure 5.3 Direct and indirect immunofluorescent (IF) assay.

amplifies the fluorescent signal; however, it is complicated and time-consuming (Odell and Cook, 2013).

Immunohistochemistry (IHC)

Immunohistochemistry (IHC) is a powerful diagnostic technique based on antigen–antibody interactions that can be used to detect and localize specific antigens ranging from amino acids and proteins to infectious agents and specific cellular populations within cells or tissue sections from FFPE tissues with high sensitivity and specificity. This technique can confirm the results of other diagnostic methods by visualizing the presence of antigens. Use of an enzymatic label overcomes the limitations of immunofluorescence, for which specialized equipment is necessary. IHC can be used for semi-quantitative analysis in diagnostic and surgical pathology, and prognostic and predictive determinations.

A tissue section is first prepared from fixed organs as histological preparation. This requires elaborate techniques because false-negative results may result from improper tissue fixation, processing and pretreatment, leading to erroneous diagnosis. Furthermore, some tertiary and quaternary structures of antigenic epitopes can be denatured during fixation with formalin. This can be overcome by proteolytic digestion with trypsin or protease, and microwaving or heating of tissue sections to facilitate antigen retrieval (Schacht and Kern, 2015).

Second, antibody–antigen interactions can be divided into direct and indirect detection of antigen. In direct methods, an enzyme-labelled primary antibody binds directly to the antigen in FFPE tissues. Although this technique has advantages in terms of rapidity and ease of performance, a higher concentration of primary antibody is required and has lower sensitivity than other IHC methods. Indirect IHC methods utilize an enzyme-labelled secondary antibody to detect the primary antibody complex. Use of a secondary antibody that recognizes a wide range of unlabelled primary antibodies with high secificity and affinity increases the versatility of this method (Schacht and Kern, 2015). By interacting with the enzyme-conjugated reactant, the chromogen is oxidized and colour develops.

Avidin–biotin Complex Method The avidin–biotin complex (ABC) method utilizes the high-affinity binding between biotin and avidin or streptavidin, which is almost irreversible. A detection enzyme (e.g. HRP or AP) labelled with biotin is complexed with avidin in solution and ABC is then introduced to the biotinylated primary or secondary (that binds to

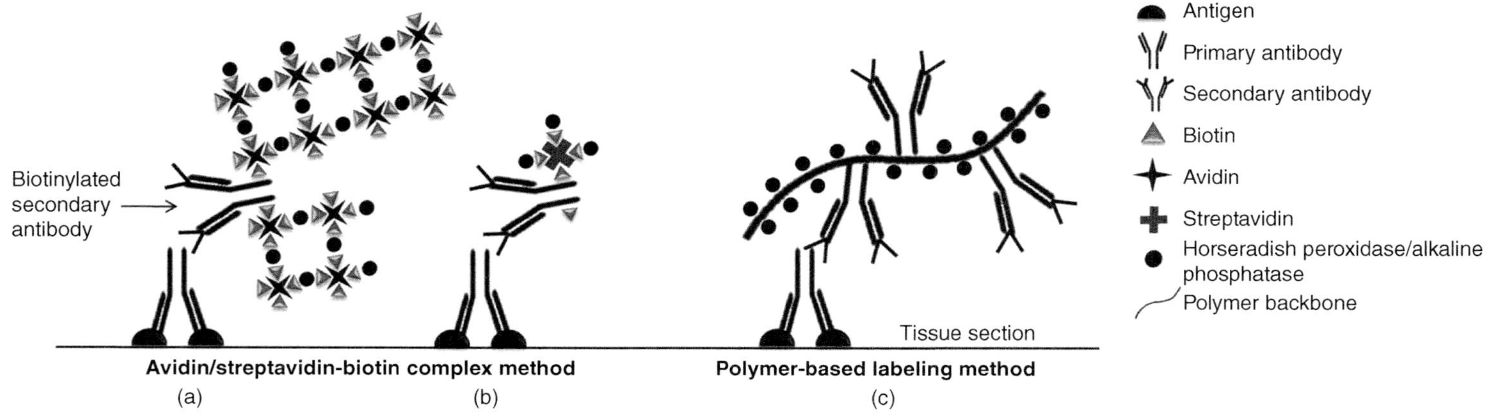

Figure 5.4 Indirect immunohistochemistry. (a) Avidin-biotin complex method; (b) streptavidin-biotin method; (c) polymer-based labelling method.

primary antibody-antigen sites) biotinylated antibody by a direct or indirect method, respectively. In this process, binding between enzyme-labelled avidin molecules and biotinylated antibodies enhances signal intensity, resulting in greater resolution (Figure 5.4a). However, avidin, a glycoprotein, has an isoelectric point (PI) of 10; therefore, it can non-specifically bind to lectin-like or negatively charged substances in tissues. To overcome this, the streptavidin-biotin method was developed based on the almost neutral isoelectric point of streptavidin, which, unlike avidin, does not contain carbohydrate (Figure 5.4b). The presence of endogenous biotin in normal tissues is problematic as it can lead to false positives by conjugating with avidin- or streptavidin-enzyme complex. This issue is worsened by the use of frozen tissue sections (Dabbs, 2013).

Polymer-based Labelling Method The limitations associated with the avidin-biotin system mentioned in the previous section led to the development of polymer-based labelling methods, which do not require a biotinylated antibody for signal amplification. The polymer chain comprises multiple antibodies and many enzyme molecules that are conjugated to a single polymer backbone (e.g. dextran, polypeptides, dendrimers and DNA branches) (Figure 5.4c) (Dabbs, 2013). The advantages of this method over ABC methods are simplicity compared with the multiple steps, equal or higher sensitivity due to the display of many ligands, and lack of background staining endogenous biotin or avidin (Ramos-Vara, 2005). Also, this technique enables detection of small amounts of antigen, and rapid assay of frozen sections with higher sensitivity and a higher working dilution of primary antibody. However, this technique is usually more expensive than ABC or labelled streptavidin-biotin methods.

Lateral Flow Immunoassay

Lateral flow immunoassays (LFIAs) enable rapid and convenient detection of target proteins – such as pathogens, antibodies or hormones – in small volumes of sample. LFIAs based on immunochromatographic strips have been developed for point-of-care testing. A LFIA strip comprises four components: the sample application pad, conjugate pad, nitrocellulose membrane and absorbent pad, which are arranged as shown in Figure 5.5. When the sample is loaded on the pad, the fluid migrates along the strip via capillary action. The sample interacts with the labelled (often colloidal gold or latex) analyte (i.e. antibody or antigen) (depending on the application) dried on a conjugate pad. The sample labelled with a particle passes the test line and control line upon which is immobilized antibody or antigen (Posthuma-Trumpie *et al.*, 2009). If the analyte is present in the sample, the antibody or antigen on the test line will bind to the antibody or antigen. A response at the control line confirms flow of the liquid across the strip.

The advantages of this technique are its rapidity (within minutes rather than hours or days), low cost and user-friendliness, as technicians or special equipment are not required (Adams and Thompson, 2008). However, it suffers from low reproducibility, low affinity of biomolecules for analytes, and a tendency to show cross-reactivity (Sajid *et al.*, 2014). Also, the analysis time depends on the nature of the sample (e.g. viscosity and surface tension). LFIAs comprise two basic formats: sandwich assay for analytes with several epitopes and competitive assay for analytes with a single epitope.

Pregnancy tests based on detection of HCG hormone in the urine of pregnant women are the best known diagnostic method based on lateral flow immunoassay. Antibody-coated GNPs immunoassay could detect specifically *Aeromonas salmonicida* in fish tissues down to 10^4 CFU/mL (with reddish purple agglutination) and results were obtained within 45 minutes

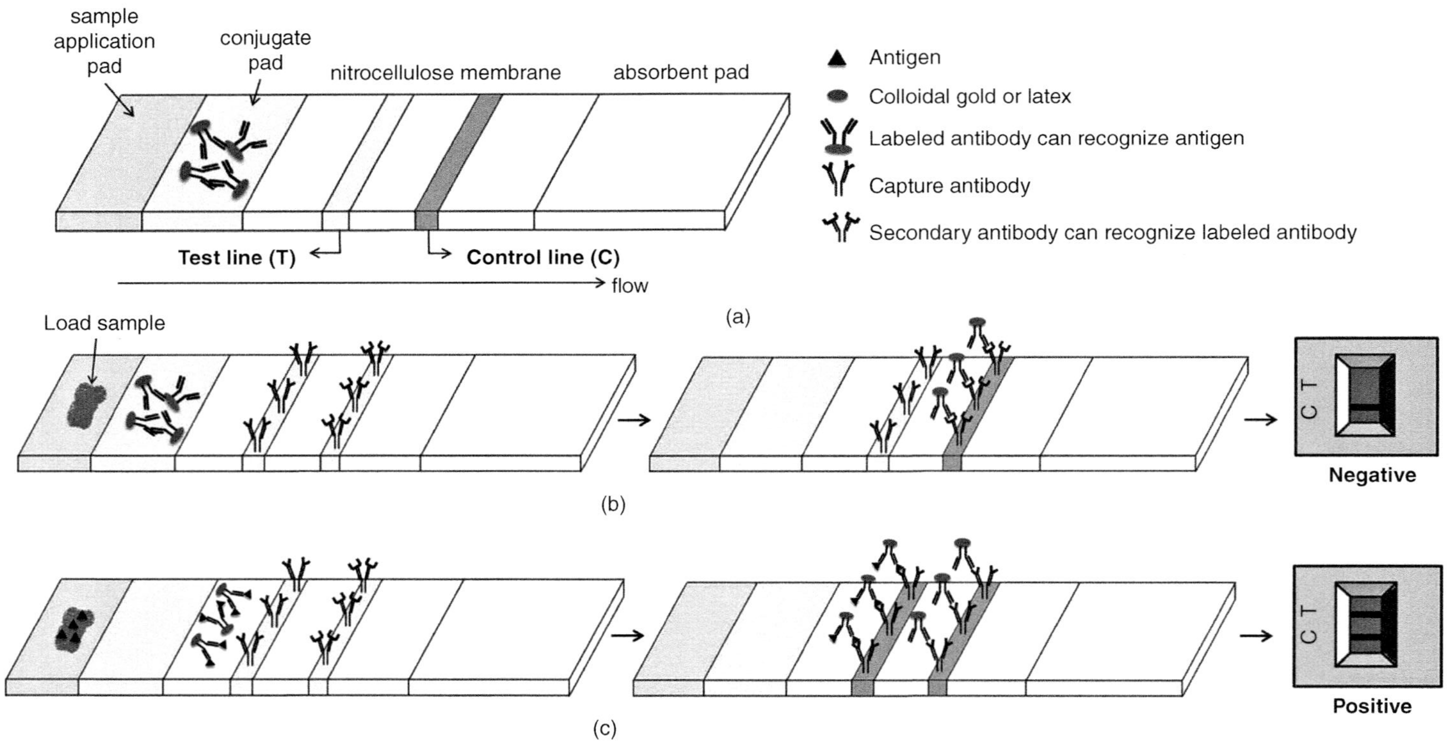

Figure 5.5 Lateral flow immunoassay (LFIA). (a) The LFIA strip comprises four components: sample application pad, conjugate pad, nitrocellulose membrane and absorbent pad; (b) negative reaction; (c) positive reaction.

(Saleh *et al.*, 2011). Also, examples of applications of LFIA include *Vibrio harveyi* (Sithigorngul *et al.*, 2007), *Vibrio anguillarum* (Zhao *et al.*, 2014) and *Edwardsiella tarda* (Liu *et al.*, 2015), YHV (Sithigorngul *et al.*, 2007), and ISAV (commercial kit is available; Aquatic Diagnostics Ltd).

Molecular Methods

Hybridization Methods

Fluorescence in situ Hybridization (FISH) *In situ* hybridization techniques involve detection of specific nucleic acid sequences in morphologically preserved chromosomes, tissues or cell preparations. When this technique was originally developed approximately 50 years ago, only radioisotopes labels for nucleic acids were available. Non-radioactive hybridization methods, either direct or indirect, are now commonplace. Indirect methods require the nucleic acid probe to contain a reporter molecule, such as digoxigenin (DIG) and biotin, which is detected using a specific antibody and streptavidin, respectively. Colorimetric *in situ* hybridization assays involve DIG-labelled probes, with detection by an anti-DIG antibody labelled with alkaline phosphatase, which reacts with 5-bromo-4-chloro-3-indolyl phosphate/nitroblue tetrazolium (BCIP/NBT) as a substrate. This method was developed to detect fish and shellfish pathogens, including PKX parasite, which causes proliferative kidney disease of salmonids (Morris *et al.*, 1999), infectious pancreatic necrosis virus (IPNV) (Biering and Bergh, 1996) and infectious salmon anaemia virus (Gregory, 2002).

In direct methods, a reporter molecule (e.g. fluorescein or other fluorochrome) is bound directly to the nucleic acid probe so that probe–target hybrids can be visualized by microscopy immediately following hybridization. Fluorescence *in situ* hybridization (FISH) relies on DNA or RNA probes labelled covalently at one end with a fluorescent dye designed to recognize a specific sequence of a particular organism. As mentioned above, FISH allows simultaneous direct visualization, identification and histological localization of micro-organisms in diverse samples. This technique also facilitates enumeration and/or quantification of micro-organisms by confocal microscopy, fluorescence microscopy or flow cytometry. In this way, FISH enhances understanding of correlations between the infection and any histopathological changes present.

While this straightforward technique has many advantages, it must be optimized for different samples and probes before use. For example, Gram-positive bacteria may require treatment with lysozyme or lysostaphin to remove peptidoglycan, which hampers probe penetration into bacterial cells (Cai *et al.*, 2014). In addition, a drawback of FISH in clinical diagnostics is the need for fluorescence microscopy, which is not present in most routine diagnostic laboratories. A FISH assay compatible with fluorescence IHC was developed for detection of IPNV in paraffin-embedded tissues of Atlantic salmon, *Salmo salar* (McCarthy *et al.*, 2008). Strepparava *et al.* (2012) developed a rapid and reliable qualitative FISH assay for *Flavobacterium psychrophilum* using species-specific, fluorescently labelled oligonucleotide probes. In addition, FISH has been used to detect pathogens in Caribbean spiny lobster (Li *et al.*, 2006) and freshwater crayfish (Ding *et al.*, 2015).

Tanner *et al.* (2000) first described the chromogenic *in situ* hybridization (CISH) method, which is an alternative to FISH for the detection of genetic alterations and microbes. In CISH, chromogenic visualization is mediated by detection of a DIG-labelled nucleic acid probe using enzyme-conjugated antibodies. Reaction of substrates with enzymes, such as horseradish peroxidase and/or alkaline phosphatase, leads to precipitation of the chromogen, which then can

Table 5.2 *In situ* hybridization-based methods.

Technique	Instrument/visualization method	Advantages
Chromogenic *in situ* hybridization (CISH)	Bright-field microscopy	Ability to visualize CISH signal and tissue morphology simultaneously More rapid than FISH Facilitates histopathological evaluation
Fluorescence *in situ* hybridization (FISH)	Fluorescence microscopy, flow cytometry	Visualization of multiple targets using multiple probes in the same sample Higher sensitivity than CISH
Peptide nucleic acid-fluorescence *in situ* hybridization (PNA-FISH)	Fluorescence microscopy, flow cytometry	No additional enzymatic permeabilization steps and required simpler fixation step Higher sensitivity and specificity than other ISH methods

be visualized by bright-field microscopy. CISH has several advantages over FISH in routine diagnostics (Tanner *et al.*, 2000). First, it is more rapid than FISH. Second, verification of histopathology can be performed simultaneously using CISH, while with FISH the cells for signal enumeration are selected based on nuclear DAPI staining, which is not sufficient for histopathological evaluation (Table 5.2).

Probe penetration of target cells can be enhanced by peptide–nucleic acid (PNA) probes, in which a neutral and achiral polyamide backbone comprising *N*-(2-aminoethyl) glycine units linked by peptide bonds replaces the charged deoxyribose-phosphate backbone of DNA. This is because PNA probes bind to DNA more strongly compared to natural oligonucleotides, particularly at low salt concentrations, and with a relative lack of electrostatic repulsion. However, the growing PNA oligomer can fold over itself during synthesis, PNA probes exhibit low solubility in organic solvents and purine-rich oligomers, and the probes are expensive.

DNA Microarrays DNA microarrays involve several thousand oligomeric DNA probes immobilized on planar surfaces, such as glass slides, and are used for the detection and identification of microbes in a single hybridization assay (Fukushima *et al.*, 2003). DNA microarray probe selection and design is important as it impacts the overall fidelity of the assay in terms of specificity and sensitivity (Loy and Bodrossy, 2006). This is because of the possibility of cross-hybridizations and orthogonal probe binding to target DNA, and achievement of uniformity of annealing temperatures for probes would be very difficult due to their different lengths and GC contents (Uttamchandani *et al.*, 2009). The occurrence of false positives and negatives is also problematic, although negative control probes with random sequences are included in some arrays to provide a threshold level for background noise correction. A microarray usually comprises 20–70-mer, single-stranded DNA oligonucleotide probes. This technique can be divided into two types, low- and high-density DNA microarrays, according to the number of probes used. In general, total DNA extracted from a pathogen of interest is labelled (chemically or by an enzymatic reaction) and then hybridized by base-pair matching to its cognate recognition probe on a DNA microarray. Non-specific target DNA is removed during washing steps of different stringency, and positive signals from successful hybridization are measured automatically by a scanner. Pathogen diversity is analysed using the included software.

DNA microarray coupled with broad-range PCR is commonly used to detect pathogens (Figure 5.6). Numerous targets amplified by universal primers that recognize conserved sequences flanking variable domains in housekeeping genes are discriminated after hybridization on the array. DNA microarrays have been used for the detection of bacterial and viral pathogens of fish and shellfish. González *et al.* (2004) first described use of a microarray for the detection of bacteria pathogenic for marine fish. The sensitivity and specificity of this method were suitable for preliminary diagnosis or confirmation of infection by five fish pathogens: *V. anguillarum*, *V. vulnificus*, *V. parahaemolyticus*, *Photobacterium damselae* subsp. *damselae* and *A. salmonicida*. Lua *et al.* (2005) developed a DNA microarray to monitor the transcription kinetics of red sea bream iridovirus during *in vitro* infection. A DNA array-based multiplex assay was developed to detect and identify cyprinid herpesviruses (CyHV-1, VyHV-2 and VyHV-3) and pathogenic *Flavobacterium* species including *F. branchiophilum*, *F. columnare* and *F. psychrophilum* (Lievens *et al.*, 2011). Chang *et al.* (2012) developed a microarray involving multiplex hybridization of 12 probes with DNA amplicons from mixtures of fish kidney and eight target pathogens. Targets annealed to the microarray probes react with streptavidin-conjugated alkaline phosphatase and NBT/BCIP, resulting in blue spots visible to the naked eye (Chang *et al.*, 2012). DNA microarrays are of great use for simultaneous pathogen detection, as fish and shellfish are often infected with several pathogens. This technique can also be very useful to monitor diverse pathogens in fish farm environments. However, DNA microarray technology is expensive and usually requires large amounts of nucleic acid. Data analysis must be completely automated, otherwise it is time-consuming and difficult to interpret. Furthermore, application of microarrays to microbial detection will require quality control procedures for manufacturing and processing, and data analysis and visualization methods that provide easily interpretable results.

Nucleic Acid Amplification Methods

Polymerase Chain Reaction Polymerase chain reaction (PCR) is the nucleic acid amplification technology used most frequently in microbiology laboratories. PCR-based techniques have revolutionized many areas of study based on amplification of specific sequences from either small quantities of genomic DNA or cDNA derived from RNA prepared from various samples. Therefore, PCR can detect infectious agents that are frequently impossible to isolate or culture under artificial conditions. Although PCR is a highly specific and sensitive method of detecting pathogens, given its complexity, an insufficient PCR product yield and occurrence of non-specific binding between primers and other DNAs in the mixture can hamper its utility. Several strategies can be used to overcome these problems. Hot-start PCR and touch-down PCR can be used to enhance amplification of desired target sequences and reduce non-specific binding and other PCR artefacts. In nested PCR, two different primer sets are used in two consecutive PCR reactions to increase the specificity and sensitivity of DNA amplification. The products generated in the first reaction are subjected to a second PCR reaction (the primer set of the second reaction amplifies a DNA sequence within the first reaction product). Nested PCR enabled detection of *Flavobacterium psychrophilum* at low densities in fish tissue and

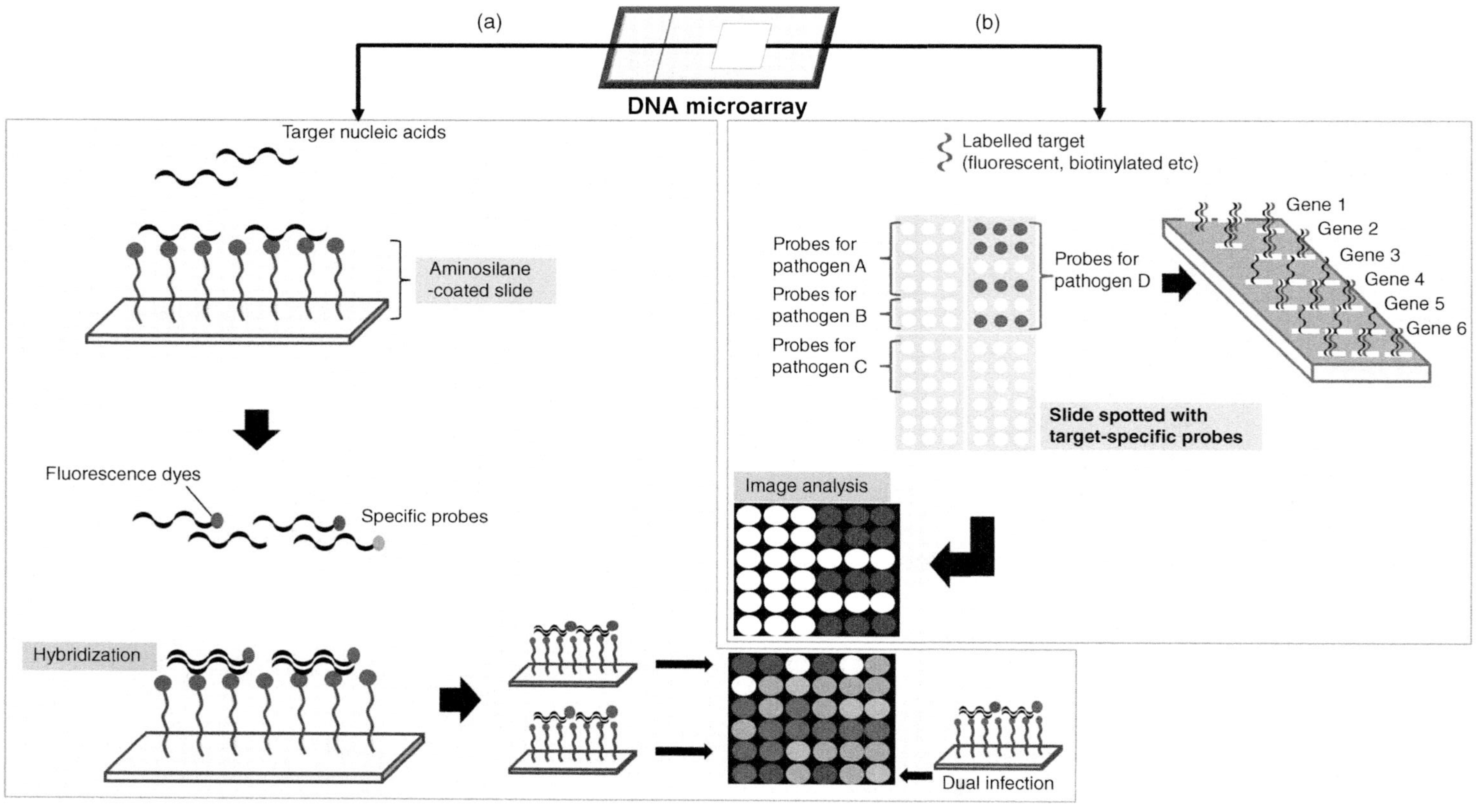

Figure 5.6 Schematic diagram of DNA microarray. (a) Nucleic acids (including cDNA through RT-PCR) extracted from the sample are printed on an aminosilane-coated slide. After UV cross-linking, specific fluorescent probes for targets are hybridized to the DNA microarray. (b) Labelled targets prepared by PCR amplification are hybridized to the microarray consisting of pathogen-specific probes (species or strain specific) immobilized onto a solid surface. This test can also detect the presence of specific virulence genes for a target (e.g. pathogen D). (*See plate section for the color representation of this figure.*)

water samples (Baliarda *et al.*, 2002; Crumlish *et al.*, 2007). A nested PCR following specific reverse transcriptase PCR was used to identify the spring viraemia of carp virus (SVCV) in carp (*Cyprinus carpio*) and zebrafish (*Danio rerio*) (Koutna *et al.*, 2003; Oreshkova *et al.*, 1999; Sanders *et al.*, 2003) tissue.

RNA targets such as RNA viruses can be detected using reverse transcriptase PCR (RT-PCR), which consists of an annealing step for a reverse primer or a mixture of random primers and an extension step during which the complementary DNA strand (cDNA) is synthesized, followed by a PCR assay. In the following subsections, other PCR-based techniques, such as multiplex PCR, real-time PCR, and loop mediated isothermal amplification (LAMP), as well as traditional molecular markers, including restriction fragment length polymorphism (RFLP), random amplified polymorphic DNA (RAPD) and amplified fragment length polymorphism (AFLP), will be discussed.

Multiplex PCR Using multiple primer pairs, multiplex PCR allows the amplification of more than one target of interest in a PCR, and yields specific amplicons of different sizes for the target organisms. This method has been used for diverse applications, for example for three bacterial fish pathogens (*F. columnare, Edwardsiella ictaluri* and *Aeromonas hydrophila*) by Panangala *et al.* (2007a) and for five pathogens (*A. hydrophila, A. salmonicida* subsp. *salmonicida, F. columnare, Renibacterium salmoninarum* and *Yersinia ruckeri*) (Altinok *et al.*, 2008), and did not generate non-specific amplification products when tested against 23 related species of bacteria. In addition, the fish pathogenic bacteria of the genera *Aeromonas, Vibrio, Edwardsiella* and *Streptococcus* can be diagnosed by means of a genus-specific multiplex PCR assay with detection limits of 50 colony-forming units (CFU) in pure culture and 100 CFU in fish tissue samples (Zhang *et al.*, 2014). Although a multiplex PCR approach can simultaneously identify several pathogens, incorporation of more than six target pathogens is problematic because of cross-reactions between probes and target DNA, and the challenges inherent in size discrimination among PCR products by conventional electrophoresis (Warsen *et al.*, 2004).

Real-time PCR Real-time PCR involves monitoring of PCR amplification by measuring fluorescence during the exponential phase of the reaction. Measuring the kinetics of the reaction in the early phases of PCR provides an advantage over traditional PCR assays, which are dependent on the results of agarose gel electrophoresis of endpoint reaction products. Non-specific DNA binding dyes, which emit fluorescence upon binding to double-stranded DNA, such as SYBR® Green and Eva Green®, enable determination of the presence or absence of an amplicon, without giving any information on the precise nature of the product.

Three types of labelled probe are used in real-time PCR: cleavage-based probes, molecular beacons and FRET (Förster resonance energy transfer) probes. Cleavage-based probes, also known as TaqMan® probes, are used most widely, and frequently incorporate a high-energy dye termed a reporter at the 5′ end, and a low-energy molecule termed a quencher (*e.g.* TAMRA) at the 3′ end. When the probe is cleaved by the 5′ to 3′ exonuclease activity of *Taq* DNA polymerase, the distance between the reporter and the quencher increases, causing the transfer of energy to stop. Thereby, the fluorescence of the reporter increases and that of the quencher decreases. Few FRET and molecular beacons have been applied to detection of fish and shellfish pathogens. Despite its high cost, the advantages of real-time PCR warrant its use for detection and quantification of aetiological agents in environmental samples or tissues. This technique enabled detection and quantification of various pathogens, such as *Aeromonas salmonicida* (Balcázar *et al.*, 2007), *Flavobacterium columnare* (Panangala *et al.*, 2007b), *Streptococcus parauberis* (Nguyen *et al.*, 2016), VHSV (Chico *et al.*, 2006), CyHV-2 (Goodwin *et al.*, 2006), alphavirus (Graham *et al.*, 2006), SPDV (Hodneland and Endresen, 2006), Pilchard herpesvirus (Crockford *et al.*, 2008) and SVCV (Yue *et al.*, 2008). Because real-time PCR can detect very low levels of nucleic acid in various types of specimen, including fish and shellfish tissue samples, it is a key diagnostic method in this field, and will probably remain so for the time being.

Loop-mediated Isothermal Amplification Loop-mediated isothermal amplification (LAMP) is a simple, rapid, specific and cost-effective nucleic acid amplification method. This technique employs a Bst DNA polymerase and a set of four primers (forward inner primer (FIP), forward outer primer (F3), backward inner primer (BIP), and backward outer primer (B3)) and two optional loop primers designed to recognize a total of six different sequences (F1, F2, F3; B1, B2 and B3) in the target gene. The inner primer (FIP or BIP) consists of a F2 (or B2) region at the 3′ end and a F1c (or B1c) region at the 5′ end. The F2 (or B2) region is complementary to the F2c (or B2c) region of the template sequence (Figure 5.7a). One of the most important components is the LAMP polymerase enzyme, which has 5′–3′ DNA polymerase and strand displacement activities, but lacks 5′–3′ exonuclease activity. Bst is the most frequently used LAMP polymerase (optimal activity at 66 °C), while Bsm is used less frequently (optimal activity at 63 °C); these are sourced from *Bacillus stearothermophilus* and *B. smithii*, respectively. The outer primers (F3 and B3) displace the FIP- and BIP-amplified strands, which then form a hairpin to create the starting loop for cyclic amplification. Amplification then proceeds in a cyclical manner, each previous strand being displaced during elongation, with the addition of extra loops during each round, resulting in generation of multiple products of predictable sizes. The amplified products are stem-loop DNA structures with several inverted repeats of the target and cauliflower-like structures with multiple loops, yielding >500 mg/mL of PCR products (Nagamine *et al.*, 2001).

LAMP has several advantages compared to conventional PCR-based methods because the reactions are performed under isothermal conditions (60–65 °C) using simple incubators (water bath or block heater) (Figure 5.7b); therefore, there is no time loss in thermal changes. This method is highly specific and enables highly efficient synthesis of amplified products, at least 50-fold greater than classic PCR reactions in identical volumes (Tomita *et al.*, 2008). In addition, high levels of insoluble salt of magnesium pyrophosphate accumulate in the reaction mixture, resulting in formation of a visible white precipitate. Thus, positive and negative reactions can be distinguished in real time by visualization using the naked eye (Mori *et al.*, 2001). Alternatively, DNA-intercalating dyes can be added to facilitate visualization of LAMP products, for example ethidium bromide, SYBR Green I, propidium iodide, Picogreen or metal-ion indicators such as hydroxynaphthol blue (HNB), $CuSO_4$ or calcein (Duan *et al.*, 2014). Therefore, no expensive instruments are required for the time-consuming postamplification detection step.

LAMP assays have been developed for rapid detection of *Edwardsiella tarda* (Savan *et al.*, 2004), *Vibrio anguillarum* (Kulkarni *et al.*, 2009), *Streptococcus iniae* (Han *et al.*, 2011), white spot syndrome virus (WSSV) (Caipang *et al.*, 2012; Kono *et al.*, 2004), infectious haematopoietic necrosis virus (IHNV) (Gunimaladevi *et al.*, 2005), *Macrobrachium rosenbergii* noda virus (Haridas *et al.*, 2010) and parasitic pathogens causing diseases in fish and shellfish such as *Clonorchis sinensis* and *Nucleospora salmonis* (Cai *et al.*, 2010; Sakai *et al.*, 2009). Triplex

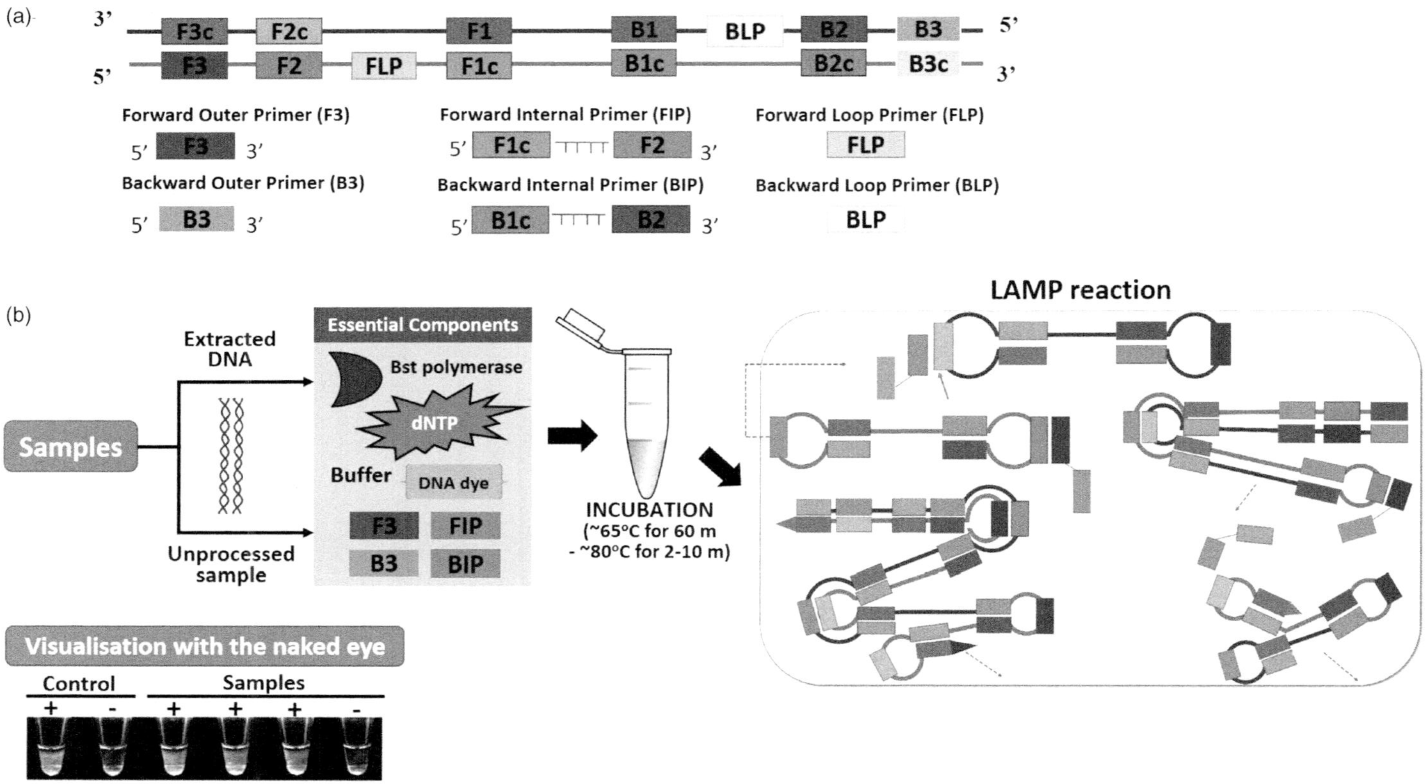

Figure 5.7 Schematic diagram of loop-mediated isothermal amplification (LAMP) diagnostics. (a) Primers used in the LAMP method, showing six primers (two optional: FLP and BLP) hybridizing to eight regions of a target gene. (b) LAMP assay protocol. (*See plate section for the color representation of this figure.*)

LAMP was developed to identify *V. harveyi*, *V. anguillarum* and *V. alginolyticus* using a combination of three sets of primers (four primers per set) in a single reaction by Yu *et al.* (2013). The sensitivity of the triplex LAMP assay was 10^2–10^3-fold higher than those of conventional PCR assays. Moreover, Soliman and El-Matbouli (2006) designed a one-step reverse transcription-LAMP targeting the G-protein sequence of VHSV using a set of six primers. A detection limit similar to that of a commonly used RT-PCR (VHSV RNA at a 10^{-6} dilution) suggested RT-LAMP to be suitable for use under field conditions for rapid diagnosis of VHS, which would facilitate implementation of expedited control and hygiene measures to prevent spread of infection. A commercial LAMP test kit is available for WSSV.

Various LAMP methods have been continuously adapted for diagnosis of various fish and shellfish pathogens; these include quantitative LAMP, LAMP-lateral flow dipstick, immunocapture/direct binding LAMP, fluorescence resonance energy transfer LAMP, LAMP-gold nanoparticles and reverse transcription-LAMP-nucleic acid lateral flow (Biswas and Sakai, 2014).

Although LAMP has many advantages, it is susceptible to false positives due to carry-over or cross-contamination. In addition, producing two long primers with HPLC-grade purity and designing primers (requirement for six primers) are problematic (Biswas and Sakai, 2014).

Molecular Typing Methods

Random Amplified Polymorphic DNA Random amplified polymorphic DNA (RAPD) typing is a reliable, reproducible, accurate and sensitive discriminatory method for epidemiological typing of various micro-organisms. RAPD involves use of arbitrary primers (typically 10-mers) to randomly amplify polymorphic segments of target DNA by PCR under low-stringency conditions (Wassenaar and Newell, 2000). RAPD does not require either prior information regarding the DNA sequence or DNA hybridization. This process generates a set of fingerprinting patterns, the sizes of which are species and strain specific. The amplified DNA fragments are separated by gel electrophoresis and the resulting banding pattern used for molecular profiling. Behura *et al.* (2015) showed that RAPD had sensitivity sufficient to reveal inter- and intraspecific genetic differences among *V. parahaemolyticus* and *V. anguillarum*, and was a rapid and convenient method of differentiating vibrios of the same and different serogroups. RAPD facilitated separation of *Tenacibaculum maritimum* strains into two major genetic groups, which were strongly correlated with the host species and O-antigen serotypes (Avendaño-Herrera *et al.*, 2004). Moreover, RAPD has been used to discriminate various fish and shellfish pathogens (e.g. Aznar *et al.*, 1993; Chakroun *et al.*, 1997; Magarinõs *et al.*, 2000; Romalde *et al.*, 1999). However, this method is labour intensive and time-consuming (typically requiring approximately three days).

Restriction Fragment Length Polymorphism Restriction fragment length polymorphism (RFLP) has been used to discriminate species and strains of pathogenic microbes. This technique is based on digestion of the genomic DNA of a target pathogen by specific restriction endonucleases into fragments that can be separated according to their size using gel electrophoresis. Depending on the frequency of restriction recognition sites in the genome, it is possible to compare digests of whole genomic DNAs among strains of the same species. In addition, mutations in the genome can lead to changes in the number of cleavage sites, and thus give rise to fragment-length polymorphisms. However, this method is not able to differentiate closely related species that have a similar or almost identical 16S rRNA gene sequence because all produce the same RFLP pattern (Beaz-Hidalgo *et al.*, 2010; Figueras *et al.*, 2011). Although this technique has been applied to genotyping of pathogens that affect aquaculture, such as *Flavobacterium columnare* (LaFrentz *et al.*, 2014) and *Aeromonas* strains (Beaz-Hidalgo *et al.*, 2010; Kozińska, 2007), use of RFLP-based typing has declined in the last decade as more effective assays have become available.

Amplified Fragment Length Polymorphism Amplified fragment length polymorphism (AFLP) technology employs PCR to selectively amplify restriction endonuclease-digested genomic DNA. In AFLP assay, the first step is restriction of genomic DNA and ligation of adaptors or linkers containing the restriction sites to both ends of the DNA fragments. Subsequent PCR involves two amplification steps using primers complementary to the adaptor sequences to amplify a selected subset of the restriction fragments. The number of amplicons generated in individual assays should be in a manageable range (e.g. 50–100 fragments of 50–500 bp). The primers used for amplification are labelled with radioactive or fluorescent markers and the patterns of polymorphisms can be visualised in acrylamide gels or by capillary electrophoresis. AFLP has been used for molecular typing of bacterial pathogens such as *Vibrio vulnificus* (Tao *et al.*, 2012) and *Photobacterium damselae* subsp. *damselae* (Botella *et al.*, 2002). However, this technique usually requires 3–4 days to complete and is expensive, although it has good reproducibility, discriminatory power and typing ability with no requirement for prior knowledge of genomic sequence information.

Multilocus Sequence Typing Multilocus sequence typing (MLST) makes use of the sequences of internal fragments of multiple, often seven, housekeeping genes and is considered the gold standard for bacterial typing and population analysis due to its discriminatory power. Approximately 450–500 bp internal fragments of each gene are used. The different sequences of each housekeeping gene within a bacterial species are assigned a random integer number, and a unique combination of alleles at each locus, an 'allelic profile', specifies the sequence type (ST). MLST allele sequence and ST profile databases are available at several curated host sites worldwide. The PubMLST site collects data from all databases and makes it easily accessible (http://pubmlst.org). This makes MLST typing data more suitable for global epidemiological studies (Adzitey *et al.*, 2013).

Nilsen *et al.* (2014) reported progress in mapping of the genetic diversity of *F. psychrophilum* globally and supported the existence of an epidemic population structure in which recombination is a significant driver of the evolution of *F. psychrophilum*. Likewise, MLST suggested the persistence of major *Y. ruckeri* (Calvez *et al.*, 2015) and *F. columnare* (Ashrafi *et al.*, 2015) sequence types and clonal complex(s) in diverse geographic regions, periods and aquatic hosts. Nevertheless, the MLST approach is not practical for use in a clinical laboratory, as it is time-consuming, labour intensive and costly. In addition, MLST lacks the ability to differentiate some bacterial strains, which can be overcome by using a multivirulence-locus sequence (Chen *et al.*, 2007).

Future Diagnostic Methods

Nanotechnology-based Strategies for Rapid Detection of Fish Pathogens

In recent years, the application of nanotechnology has expanded in diagnosis and therapeutics because of the unique properties of nanomaterials, such as high surface-to-volume ratios, translocation into cells and diverse binding abilities – nanoparticles can be designed to interact differently with targets of various sizes (e.g. peptides, nucleic acid, toxins, viruses and bacteria). Metal nanoparticles including gold, silver and iron nanoparticles have been applied in various fields.

Gold nanoparticles (GNPs) are frequently used in diagnosis, as they are inert and less cytotoxic. GNPs have a strong binding affinity to thiol groups; thus surface chemistries of GNPs can be modified by joining functionalized organic thiol molecules or thiol-containing polymers after stabilizing with ethylene glycol (Liao and Hafner, 2005) or polystyrene spheres (Huang *et al.*, 2007). In addition, thiolated functional molecules facilitate conjugation with various biomolecules. Therefore, GNPs can be used to detect various biomolecules after conjugating with antibodies, nucleic acids and similar molecules (Figure 5.8a). The light absorption and emission characteristics of GNPs can be exploited in colorimetric detection of analytes by measuring changes in the refractive index of the environment of the GNPs caused by absorption of target analytes. The wavelength of the light absorbed depends on whether the GNPs are separate or aggregated. A GNP suspension will thus appear red to the eye, which corresponds to the wavelength of light that is not absorbed. However, upon aggregation, the peak plasmon resonance of these particles shifts to blue-violet.

This change in optical properties can be exploited for both diagnostic and therapeutic purposes and can be seen easily with the naked eye. Colloidal gold conjugated with antibody or antigen has been used in development of lateral flow immunoassays for fish pathogens (see earlier). Nucleic acid probes conjugated with nanoparticles have been designed for rapid identification of aetiological agents. Oligonucleotide probes based on GNPs and detection of fish pathogens by their agglomeration were developed by Saleh *et al.* (2012), who detected SVCV RNA after only ~1 hour of hybridization. The samples were denatured at 95 °C for 30 seconds, annealed at 58 °C for 30 seconds and then cooled at room temperature for 10 minutes. A GNP solution (10 μL) was added and results were observed within one minute. Cyprinid herpesvirus-3 has also been detected successfully using GNP-based assays (Saleh *et al.*, 2013). Therefore, GNP-based methods facilitate rapid, easy assays of fish diseases with a high level of accuracy and low cost.

Magnetic nanoparticle-based assays enable rapid detection of pathogens. The method makes use of magnetic nanoparticles carrying antibodies directed against the target immobilized on a mylar film, based on a high-transition temperature DC superconducting quantum interference device (SQUID) (Chemla *et al.*, 2000). Unbound nanoparticles quickly relax by Brownian rotation and do not affect the signal. After binding to the target, the nanoparticles undergo Néel relaxation, resulting in a gradually dispersing magnetic flux that can be detected by the SQUID (Chemla *et al.*, 2000). Recently, Chung *et al.* (2013) reported a magneto-DNA method using magnetic nanoparticles (MNPs) and oligonucleotide probes to specifically detect target nucleic acids. This assay is based on a sandwich hybridization technique wherein two oligonucleotide probes bind to each end of the target nucleic acid (Figure 5.8b,c). The bead–MNP complexes were washed several times to remove unbound nucleic acids and signal was then read using a miniaturized micro-NMR (μNMR) system.

This new technology may have potential for development of highly sensitive and rapid pathogen detection tools or point-of-care testing devices for aquaculture. However, at present these methods do not provide information on the metabolic state of the infecting micro-organisms, and thus would not assist selection of appropriate antimicrobial agents.

MALDI-TOF Mass Spectrometry for Microbial Identification

Matrix-assisted laser desorption/ionization time-of-flight mass spectrometry (MALDI-TOF MS) can be used to differentiate bacterial species based on the mass profile of molecular

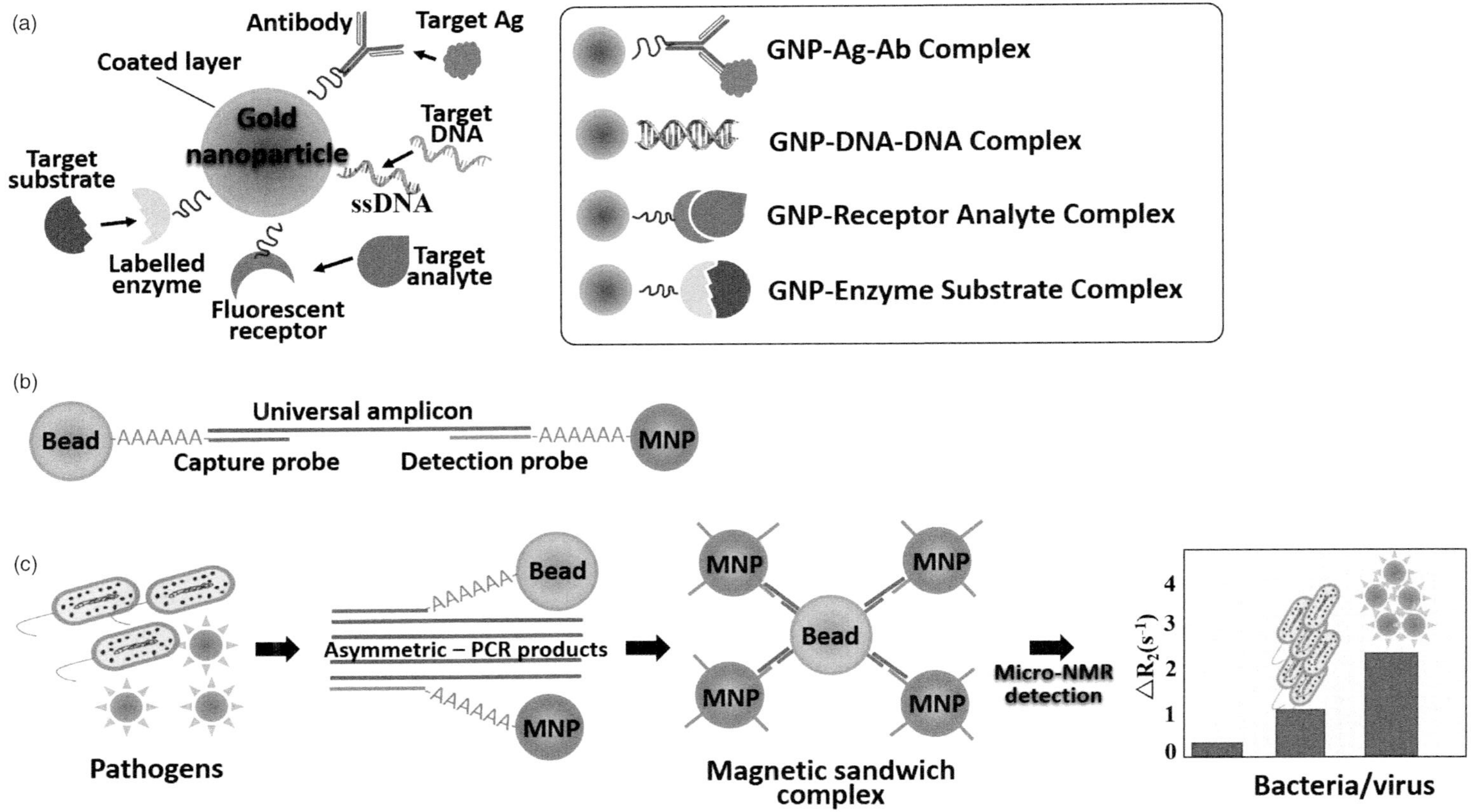

Figure 5.8 Potential detection of pathogens using nanoparticles. (a) Functionalization of gold nanoparticles in biomedical applications. (b) Schematic universal probes targeting a conserved region of bacterial 16S rRNA and conjugated to bead and magnetic nanoparticles (MNPs) at the end of each probe in the magneto-DNA assay. (c) Main steps of the assay procedure including amplification of target 16S rRNA; the binding of target DNA to capture probes conjugated to beads; hybridization of target DNA-capture probe with magnetic nanoparticles (MNPs) to form a magnetic sandwich complex. The results are then analysed by using a micronuclear magnetic resonance (μNMR) system. (*See plate section for the color representation of this figure.*)

analytes with low mass (<20 kDa) (Böhme *et al.*, 2010). This method is based on highly conserved proteins with housekeeping functions of bacteria and, to a lesser extent, fungi. Detected biomolecules correspond mostly to ribosomal proteins that are abundant, basic and of medium hydrophobicity; these biochemical traits favour ionization. Proteins ionized during the MALDI process include structural proteins, DNA- or RNA-binding proteins, ribosome modulation factors, carbon storage regulators, cold shock proteins and translation initiation factors. These biomarkers generate spectral fingerprints that vary among genera, species and subspecies of microorganisms (De Carolis *et al.*, 2014).

MALDI-TOF MS is used for identification of bacteria in research and in diagnostic laboratories (Clark *et al.*, 2013). The identification of bacteria using this technology is simple and reliable. Briefly, the sample to be analysed, which may be composed of whole bacterial cells, is mixed with a matrix solution (2,5-dihydrobenzoic acid to expand the mass range to 100 000 Da or hydroxyl cinnamonnic acid, the most common matrix in commercial systems), applied onto a metal plate target slide and irradiated with a laser. The matrix along with the sample analytes absorbs the laser light and vaporizes. Following ionization, proteins are accelerated by electrical fields into the time-of-flight mass spectrometer, where they are divided according to their mass-to-charge ratio. Their abundance is measured and a characteristic spectrum generated (Figure 5.9). Comparison of the mass peaks in the sample spectrum with reference spectra in commercially available databases results in a numerical value for evaluation of pattern matching. Values in the threshold range defined by the instrument manufacturer facilitate accurate and rapid identification of micro-organisms to the species level.

In addition, this technique may be applied to the detection of antibiotic resistance (Griffin *et al.*, 2012), although the findings are conflicting. Indeed, Jansson *et al.* (2015) successfully applied MALDI-TOF MS to the identification of fish pathogenic bacteria, including *F. columnare*, *F. psychrophilum*, *V. anguillarum*, *V. vulnificus* and *Y. ruckeri*, but not for differentiating subspecies of *A. salmonicida* as they were not accurately distinguished in the database. They suggested that the system has considerable potential for identifying other bacterial pathogens as reference data are updated.

However, the critical challenge of application of MALDI-TOF MS to micro-organism identification is the limited coverage of the available libraries. It is not possible to search an unknown spectrum directly against the library, and only species present in the database can be identified. The system is expensive to run, and the accuracy of detection can be affected by the cultivation duration; this also requires pure or well-isolated colonies. Furthermore, some micro-organisms require protein extraction prior to analysis. As accurate identification depends on the contents of the database, application of this technique to fish and shellfish pathogens is a considerable challenge.

High-throughput Sequencing Technologies

Whole-genome Sequencing of Bacterial Pathogens

Next-generation sequencing (NGS) is also referred to as high-throughput or massively parallel sequencing. This technique enables production of an enormous amount of sequence data rapidly and at lower cost compared with conventional Sanger sequencing. NGS generates hundreds of gigabases of short reads, 50–500 base pairs (Glenn, 2011; Zhang *et al.*, 2011). NGS platforms with different sequencing principles are commercially available, and vary in read length, read number, amplification methods and run time (Glenn, 2011; Metzker, 2010). Whole-genome sequencing (WGS), using NGS technologies, of several bacterial

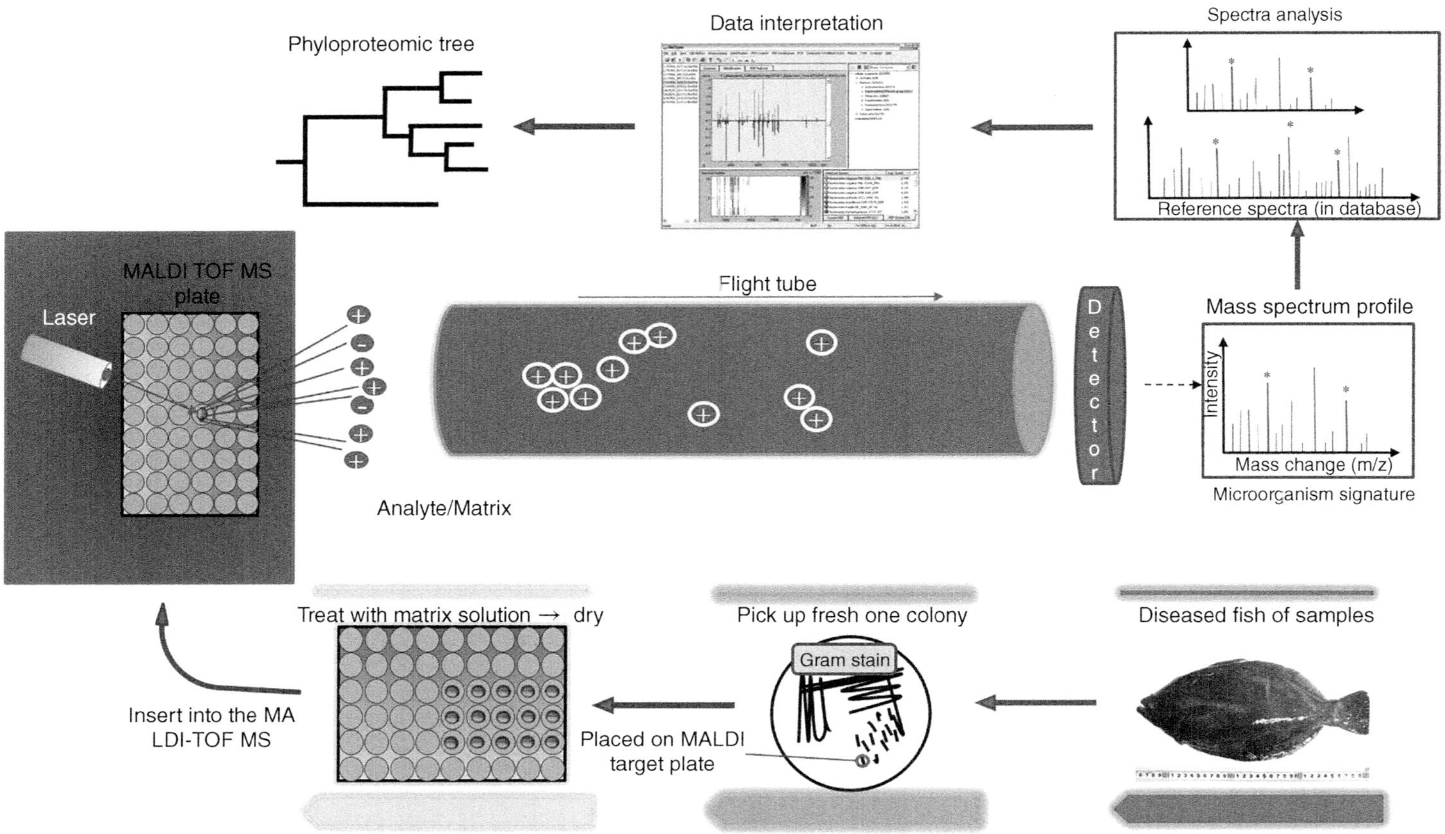

Figure 5.9 Principle of MALDI-TOF MS for bacterial identification. Microbial samples are deposited on a conductive metallic target plate and overlaid with a matrix solution composed of an organic acid. Once placed in the instrument, the samples are ionized by short laser followed by acceleration of variably charged particles through an electric field. (*See plate section for the color representation of this figure.*)

fish pathogens – *Aeromonas salmonicida* subsp. *salmonicida* (Reith *et al.*, 2008), *Edwardsiella tarda* (Wang *et al.*, 2009) and *Vibrio anguillarum* (Naka *et al.*, 2011) – has been conducted, and the sequence data provided not only rapid and accurate identification of pathogens but also insight into evolutionary and host adaptation pathways.

Indeed, the pragmatic species concept for bacteria is ultimately based on DNA-DNA hybridization (DDH), which is the traditional 'gold standard' used to distinguish a bacterial species (Auch *et al.*, 2010). However, it is known that DDH has several drawbacks in terms of the complex and time-consuming nature of the technique, and the impossibility of building cumulative databases based on DDH results (Auch *et al.*, 2010; Gevers *et al.*, 2005). There have been many attempts to find an alternative to the traditional standard, and the advent of WGS allowed the development of new methods for bacterial identification and taxonomic classification at a genome level. One of these is *in silico* or digital DNA-DNA hybridization (*is*DDH or dDDH), which is a molecular biological technique that allows for the direct experimental comparison of two genomes based on digitally derived genome-to-genome distances (Auch *et al.*, 2010). Another powerful genome-based method is the average nucleotide identity (ANI) based on pairwise genome comparison of all shared orthologous protein coding genes (Konstantinidis and Tiedje, 2005). This seems to be one of the best alternatives for a gold standard (Richter and Rosselló-Mora, 2009). In addition, interestingly, WGS can provide information on similarities and dissimilarities between bacterial strains isolated from different origins at an infra-subspecies level (Chaudhry and Prabhu, 2016). These new bioinformatics tools will greatly improve microbial identification and taxonomic classification, particularly for *Aeromonas* and *Vibrio*, taxonomically challenging genera with many aquatic pathogens (Colston *et al.*, 2014; Vincent *et al.*, 2016).

Although WGS has potential for the typing and characterization of bacterial pathogens, several studies have demonstrated examples of clinical use in humans. One diagnostic application of bacterial WGS is culture-independent *in silico* antimicrobial susceptibility testing, providing clinically relevant data within a time frame that can influence disease control (Köser *et al.*, 2012a,b; Torok and Peacock, 2012). Recently, Hasman *et al.* (2013) achieved rapid and precise identification of causative pathogens (bacteria) and their resistance genes, using direct WGS of clinical samples. In addition, future applications of bacterial WGS will include more accurate epidemiological maps of disease outbreaks (Eyre *et al.*, 2012; Gardy *et al.*, 2011). As an obvious application of WGS is epidemiological typing to reconstruct transmission pathways between healthcare centres, hospital wards or patients in the same ward (Köser *et al.*, 2012a,b), this technique will facilitate monitoring of disease outbreaks in real time in nearby fish farms and epidemiological studies at the global and national level, which is increasingly important as international trade expands. However, the most important barrier to use of rapid WGS in routine practice is the lack of automated interpretation software that can provide clinically meaningful information to microbiologists (rather than bioinformaticians) (Torok and Peacock, 2012). Moreover, although WGS is currently too expensive for routine use in most clinical laboratories, the price and turnaround time will most likely fall (Köser *et al.*, 2012a). Therefore, WGS will in the not too distant future become a standard diagnostic tool for infectious diseases in aquaculture.

Metagenomics Approaches for Pathogen Detection

Metagenomics based on NGS is a novel technique for culture-independent sequence-based microbial detection and identification as well as characterization of the entire microbiota of a sample. Two metagenomics approaches can be used for pathogen detection: deep amplicon sequencing and shotgun metagenomics (Miller *et al.*, 2013). The first is a targeted strategy involving a PCR amplification step prior to NGS to selectively amplify a taxonomic marker, such as the 16S rRNA gene. The latter is a broader strategy, in which the total nucleic acid extracted from a sample is sequenced either directly or following an enrichment step. As indicated by Pallen (2014), the term metagenomics is often used indiscriminately to cover deep amplicon sequencing approaches; thus, in the strict sense, shotgun metagenomics is a general approach to the discovery and detection of microbial pathogens in clinical samples. Indeed, shotgun metagenomics has marked potential in clinical diagnostics, public health monitoring and pathogen discovery (Bibby, 2013; Miller *et al.*, 2013). In conventional molecular techniques (see earlier), sequence information and the target pathogen must be known, while NGS can be unbiased and has the potential to detect and identify the full spectrum of not only fastidious bacteria and viruses but emerging and unknown pathogens (Cheval *et al.*, 2011; Lipkin, 2010). Application of this technique to viral detection would be useful as, in cases of infections with rare or novel viruses, routine culturing and diagnostic tests are often insufficient and inconclusive (Bibby, 2013). This method can also be applied to detect bacterial and parasitic pathogens, although it is little used for parasite detection (Griffing *et al.*, 2011; Nakamura *et al.*, 2008). Since shotgun metagenomics enables postmortem diagnosis of infection (Schuenemann *et al.*, 2013), this technique can be used for metagenomic diagnosis of infectious disease in long-dead animals, especially for samples stored in a freezer or stabilization reagent for a prolonged period. Shotgun metagenomics can be applied to any specimen to detect bacteria, viruses, fungi and parasites.

Although this new approach has tremendous potential in aquaculture, few studies have been performed to date (Alavandi and Poornima, 2012). However, it has a number of drawbacks that must be addressed before its routine use in clinical laboratories. The high cost of the equipment or sequencing is a major disadvantage. Also, skilled personnel with appropriate bioinformatics expertise are needed to access the computational power required to analyse very large sequence datasets (Capobianchi *et al.*, 2013). Moreover, DNA contamination is problematic, and nucleic acid of a target pathogen may be present at a very low level, as the pathogenic species is not always the most abundant (Pallen, 2014). Diagnostic metagenomics will become a key approach to the detection and characterization of pathogens in aquaculture in the near future.

Conclusion

Effective strategies for infectious diseases in aquatic animals require principally rapid and accurate diagnosis, which facilitates prompt and appropriate implementation of control measures and so a sustainable future for aquaculture. Diverse methods of conventional and modern diagnostics are addressed in this chapter (Figure 5.10), and the latter have generally many advantages in terms of higher specificity and sensitivity for rapid detection and identification of pathogens at reasonable cost, although each technique has its own strong and weak points. In particular, rapid and accurate molecular-based methods have become important diagnostic tools for aquatic animals, are increasingly applicable to aquaculture and should be continuously developed. Lateral-flow immunoassays, for example, based on nanoparticles could be applied to aquaculture as a point-of-care detection tool. Like DNA microarray, proteins or glycans can also be immobilized on a solid surface of microarray to probe different target molecules (nucleic acids, proteins, glycans) labelled with fluorescence,

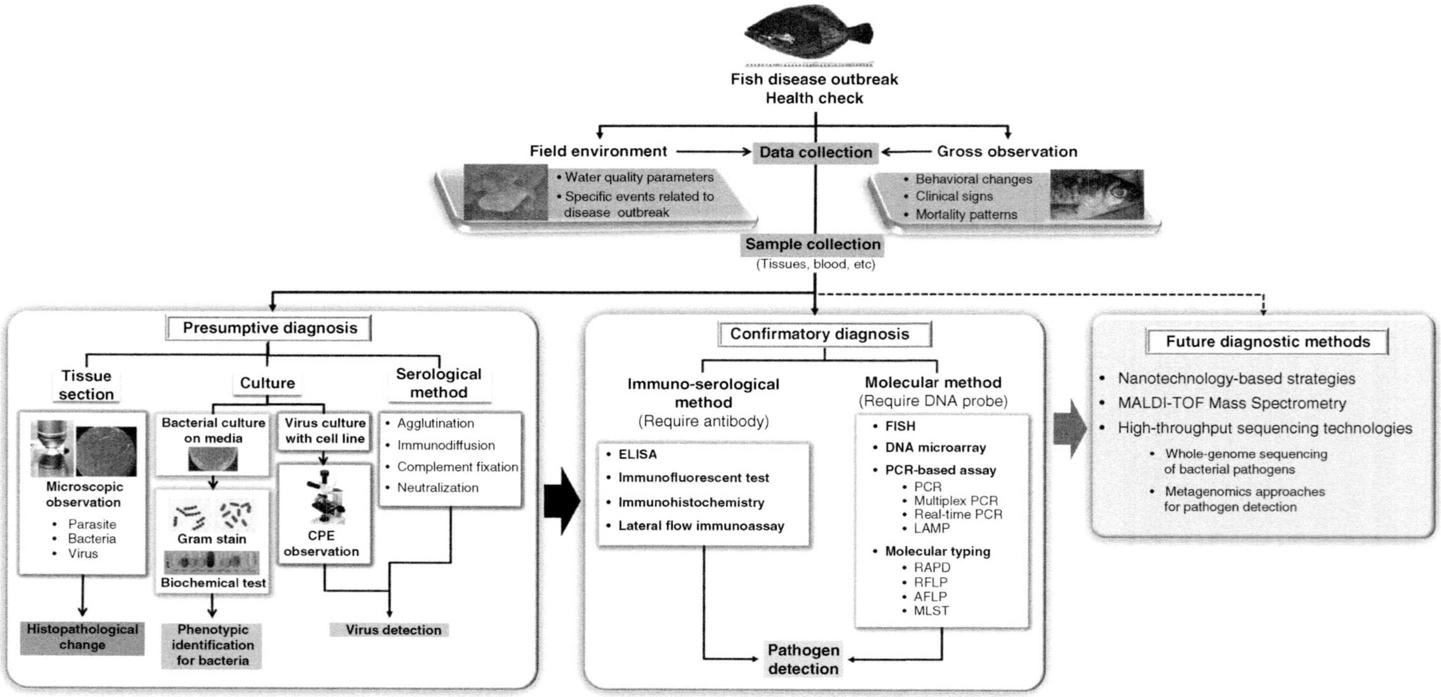

Figure 5.10 Conventional and modern diagnostic methods that can be used in aquatic animal health laboratories. (*See plate section for the color representation of this figure.*)

indicating there will be diverse applications of microarray tools for the study of pathogen detection and ecology (Santos *et al.*, 2014). In addition, use of NGS in aquatic animal health laboratories has increased for integrated investigation of the aetiology and epidemiology of diseases and host–pathogen interactions without previous knowledge. This advanced technique will provide insight into the diagnosis, prevention and control of diseases, enabling use of effective prophylactic strategies. Moreover, it is important to understand that the diagnostic process covers not only the sensitivity and specificity of each technique but also everything from sample collection (from eggs to adult animals) in the field through to processing in the diagnostic laboratory. In recent years, modern molecular diagnostic methods have influenced the practice of clinical medicine, and will soon be routine tools in aquatic animal health laboratories.

However, basic observations such as gross signs of disease, behavioural anomalies and mortality patterns and record keeping on the farm or production site are of great value as they lead to more accurate interpretation of the results of modern tests performed by the diagnostic laboratory. Although these basic practices were not addressed in this chapter, it should be remembered that clinicians, including fish health professionals and veterinarians, are required to understand the situations at a diseased farm or site before the causative agent is identified using the results of diagnostic tests. More importantly, precise interpretation of diagnostic test results together with field observations will enable development of short- and long-term control strategies, including antimicrobial and preventive (e.g. vaccines) measures.

References

Adams, A. and Thompson, K.D. (2008) Recent applications of biotechnology to novel diagnostics for aquatic animals. *Revue Scientifique et Technique (International Office of Epizootics)*, **27**(1), 197–209.

Adams, A., Burnell, G. and Allan, G. (2009) *Advances in disease diagnosis, vaccine development and other emerging methods to control pathogens in aquaculture. New Technologies in Aquaculture:* Improving Production Efficiency, Quality and Environmental Management, 197–214.

Adzitey, F., Huda, N. and Ali, G.R.R. (2013) Molecular techniques for detecting and typing of bacteria, advantages and application to foodborne pathogens isolated from ducks. *3 Biotech*, **3**(2), 97–107.

Alavandi, S.V. and Poornima, M. (2012) Viral metagenomics: a tool for virus discovery and diversity in aquaculture. *Indian Journal of Virology*, **23**, 88–98.

Altinok, I., Capkin, E. and Kayis, S. (2008) Development of multiplex PCR assay for simultaneous detection of five bacterial fish pathogens. *Veterinary Microbiology*, **131**(3), 332–338.

Ashrafi, R., Pulkkinen, K., Sundberg, L.R., Pekkala, N. and Ketola, T. (2015) A multilocus sequence analysis scheme for characterization of *Flavobacterium columnare* isolates. *BMC Microbiology*, **15**(1), 243.

Auch, A.F., Jan, M., Klenk, H.P., and Göker, M. (2010) Digital DNA-DNA hybridization for microbial species delineation by means of genome-to-genome sequence comparison. *Standards in Genomic Sciences*, **2**(1), 117–134.

Austin, B. (2011) Taxonomy of bacterial fish pathogens. *Veterinary Research*, **42**(1), 20.

Avendaño-Herrera, R., Rodríguez, J., Magariños, B., Romalde, J.L. and Toranzo, A.E. (2004) Intraspecific diversity of the marine fish pathogen *Tenacibaculum maritimum* as determined by randomly amplified polymorphic DNA-PCR. *Journal of Applied Microbiology*, **96**(4), 871–877.

Aznar, R., Ludwig, W. and Schleifer, K.H. (1993) Ribotyping and randomly amplified polymorphic DNA analysis of *Vibrio vulnificus* biotypes. *Systematic and Applied Microbiology*, **16**(2), 303–309.

Balcázar, J.L., Vendrell, I., de Blas, I. Ruiz Zarzuela, I., Gironés, O. and Múzquiz, J.L. (2007) Quantitative detection of *Aeromonas salmonicida* in fish tissue by real-time PCR using self-quenched, fluorogenic primers. *Journal of Medical Microbiology*, **56**(3), 323–328.

Baliarda, A., Faure , D. and Urdaci, M C. (2002) Development and application of a nested PCR to monitor brood stock salmonid ovarian fluid and spleen for detection of the fish pathogen *Flavobacterium psychrophilum*. *Microbiology*, **92**(3), 510–516.

Beaz-Hidalgo, R., Alperi, A., Buján, N., Romalde, J.L. and Figueras, M.J. (2010) Comparison of phenotypical and genetic identification of *Aeromonas* strains isolated from diseased fish. *Systematic and Applied Microbiology*, **33**(3), 149–153.

Behura, B.B., Samantray, B.R., Samal, S.K., Mukherjee, S.C. and Das, B.K. (2015) Use of randomly amplified polymorphic DNA analysis to differentiate *Vibrio anguillarum* and *Vibrio parahaemolyticus*. *International Journal of Current Microbiology and Applied Sciences*, **4**(10), 816–828.

Bibby, K. (2013) Metagenomic identification of viral pathogens. *Trends in Biotechnology*, **31**(5), 275– 279.

Biering, E. and Bergh, O. (1996) Experimental infection of Atlantic halibut, *Hippoglossus hippoglossus* L., yolk-sac larvae with infectious pancreatic necrosis virus: detection of virus by immunohistochemistry and in situ hybridization. *Journal of Fish Diseases*, **19**(4), 261–269.

Biswas, G. and Sakai, M. (2014) Loop-mediated isothermal amplification (LAMP) assays for detection and identification of aquaculture pathogens: current state and perspectives. *Applied Microbiology and Biotechnology*, **98**(7), 2881–2895.

Böhme, K., Fernández-No, I.C., Barros-Velázquez, J., Gallardo, J.M., Calo-Mata, P. and Canas, B. (2010) Species differentiation of seafood spoilage and pathogenic gram-negative bacteria by MALDI-TOF mass fingerprinting. *Journal of Proteome Research*, **9**(6), 3169–3183.

Bondad-Reantaso, M.G., McGladdery, S.E., East, L. and Subasinghe, R. (2001) *Asia Diagnostic Guide to Aquatic Animal Diseases*, Food and Agriculture Organization, Rome.

Botella, S., Pujalte, M.J., Macián, M.C., Ferrús, M.A., Hernandez, J. and Garay, E. (2002) Amplified fragment length polymorphism (AFLP) and biochemical typing of *Photobacterium damselae* subsp. *damselae*. *Journal of Applied Microbiology*, **93**(4), 681–688.

Cai, H.Y., Caswell, J.L. and Prescott, J.F. (2014) Nonculture molecular techniques for diagnosis of bacterial disease in animals a diagnostic laboratory perspective. *Veterinary Pathology*, **51**(2), 341–350.

Cai, X. Q., Xu, M.J., Wang, Y.H., *et al.* (2010) Sensitive and rapid detection of Clonorchis sinensis infection in fish by loop–mediated isothermal amplification (LAMP). *Parasitology Research*, **106**(6), 1379–1383.

Caipang, C.M.A., Sibonga, M.F.J., Geduspan, J.S. and Amar, M.J.A. (2012) An optimized loop-mediated isothermal amplification (LAMP) assay for the detection of white spot syndrome virus (WSSV) among cultured shrimps in the Philippines. *Journal of Animal and Plant Sciences*, **22**, 927–932.

Calvez, S., Fournel, C., Douet, D.G. and Daniel, P. (2015) Pulsed-field gel electrophoresis and multi locus sequence typing for characterizing genotype variability of *Yersinia ruckeri* isolated from farmed fish in France. *Veterinary Research*, **46**(1), 1–13.

Capobianchi, M.R., Giombini, E. and Rozera, G. (2013) Next-generation sequencing technology in clinical virology. *Clinical Microbiology and Infection*, **19**(1), 15–22.

Chakroun, C., Urdaci, M.C., Faure, D., Grimont, F. and Bernardet, J.F. (1997) Random amplified polymorphic DNA analysis provides rapid differentiation among isolates of the fish pathogen *Flavobacterium psychrophilum* and among *Flavobacterium* species. *Diseases of Aquatic Organisms*, **31**(3), 187–196.

Chang, C.I., Hung, P.H., Wu, C.C., *et al.* (2012) Simultaneous detection of multiple fish pathogens using a naked-eye readable DNA microarray. *Sensors (Basel)*, **12**(3), 2710–2728.

Chaudhry, V. and Prabhu, B. P. (2016) Genomic investigation reveals evolution and lifestyle adaptation of endophytic *Staphylococcus epidermidis. Scientific Reports*, **6**, 19263 10.1038/srep19263.

Chemla, Y.R., Grossman, H.L., Poon, Y., *et al.* (2000) Ultrasensitive magnetic biosensor for homogeneous immunoassay. *Proceedings of the National Academy of Sciences USA*, **97**(26), 14268–14272.

Chen, Y., Zhang, W. and Knabel, S.J. (2007) Multi-virulence-locus sequence typing identifies single nucleotide polymorphisms which differentiate epidemic clones and outbreak strains of *Listeria monocytogenes. Journal of Clinical Microbiology*, **45**(3), 835–846.

Cheval, J., Sauvage, V., Frangeul, L. *et al.* (2011) Evaluation of high-throughput sequencing for identifying known and unknown viruses in biological samples. *Journal of Clinical Microbiology*, **49**(9), 3268–3275.

Chico, V., Gomez, N. Estepa, A. and Perez, L. (2006) Rapid detection and quantitation of viral hemorrhagic septicemia virus in experimentally challenged rainbow trout by real-time RT-PCR. *Journal of Virological Methods*, **132**(1), 154–159.

Chung, H.J., Castro, C.M., Im, H., Lee, H. and Weissleder, R. (2013) A magneto-DNA nanoparticle system for rapid detection and phenotyping of bacteria. *Nature Nanotechnology*, **8**(5), 369–375.

Clark, A.E., Kaleta, E.J., Arora, A. and Wolk, D.M. (2013) Matrix-assisted laser desorption ionization-time of flight mass spectrometry: a fundamental shift in the routine practice of clinical microbiology. *Clinical Microbiology Reviews*, **26**(3), 547–603.

Colston, S.M., Fullmer, M.S., Beka, L., Lamy, B., Gogarten, J.P. and Graf, J. (2014) Bioinformatic genome comparisons for taxonomic and phylogenetic assignments using *Aeromonas* as a test case. *MBio*, **5**(6), e02136-14.

Crockford, M., Jones, J.B., McColl, K. and Whittington, R.J. (2008) Comparison of three molecular methods for the detection of Pilchard herpesvirus in archived paraffin-embedded tissue and frozen tissue. *Diseases of Aquatic Organisms*, **82**(1), 37–44.

Crumlish, M., Diab, A.M., George, S. and Ferguson, H.W. (2007) Detection of the bacterium *Flavobacterium psychrophilum* from a natural infection in rainbow trout, *Oncorhynchus mykiss* (Walbaum), using formalin-fixed, wax-embedded fish tissues. *Journal of Fish Diseases*, **30**(1), 37–41.

Dabbs, D.J. (2013) *Diagnostic Immunohistochemistry*, 4th edn, Elsevier Health Sciences, Philadelphia.

De Carolis, E., Vella, A., Vaccaro, L., *et al.* (2014) Application of MALDI-TOF mass spectrometry in clinical diagnostic microbiology. *Journal of Infection in Developing Countries*, **8**(09), 1081–1088.

Ding, Z.F., Xia, S.Y., Xue, H., *et al.* (2015) Direct visualization of the novel pathogen, *Spiroplasma eriocheiris*, in the freshwater crayfish *Procambarus clarkii* (Girard) using fluorescence *in situ* hybridization. *Journal of Fish Diseases*, **38**(9), 787–794.

Dixon, P.F. and Hill, B.J. (1984) Rapid detection of fish rhabdoviruses by the enzyme-linked immunosorbent assay (ELISA). *Aquaculture*, **42**(1), 1–12.

Duan, Y.B., Ge, C.Y., Zhang, X.K., Wang, J.X. and Zhou, M.G. (2014) Development and evaluation of a novel and rapid detection assay for *Botrytis cinerea* based on loop-mediated isothermal amplification. *PLoS One*, **9**(10), e111094.

El-Ansary, A. and Al-Daihan, S. (2009) On the toxicity of therapeutically used nanoparticles: an overview. *Journal of Toxicology* **2009**, 745810.

Eyre, D.W., Golubchik, T., Gordon, N.C., *et al.* (2012) A pilot study of rapid benchtop sequencing of *Staphylococcus aureus* and *Clostridium difficile* for outbreak detection and surveillance. *BMJ Open*, **2**(3), e001124.

Feist, S.W. and Longshaw, M. (2008) Histopathology of fish parasite infections – importance for populations. *Journal of Fish Biology*, **73**(9), 2143–2160.

Figueras, M.J., Beaz-Hidalgo, R., Collado, L. and Martínez-Murcia, A.J. (2011) Point of view on the recomendations for new bacterial species description and their impact on the genus *Aeromonas* and *Arcobacter*. *Bulletin of Bergeys International Society for Microbial Systematics*, **2**, 1–16.

Fukushima, M., Kakinuma, K., Hayashi, H., Nagai, H., Ito, K. and Kawaguchi, R. (2003) Detection and identification of *Mycobacterium* species isolates by DNA microarray. *Journal of Clinical Microbiology*, **41**(6), 2605–2615.

Gardy, J.L., Johnston, J.C., Sui, S.J.H., *et al.* (2011) Whole-genome sequencing and social-network analysis of a tuberculosis outbreak. *New England Journal of Medicine*, **364**, 730–739.

Genten, F., Terwinghe, E. and Danguy, A. (2009) *Atlas of Fish Histology*, CRC Press, Boca Raton.

Gevers, D., Cohan, F.M., Lawrence, J.G., *et al.* (2005) Re-evaluating prokaryotic species. *Nature Reviews Microbiology*, **3**, 733–739.

Glenn, T.C. (2011) Field guide to next-generation DNA sequencers. *Molecular Ecology Resources*, **11**, 759–769.

González, S.F., Krug, M.J., Nielsen, M E., Santos, Y. and Call, D.R. (2004) Simultaneous detection of marine fish pathogens by using multiplex PCR and a DNA microarray. *Journal of Clinical Microbiology*, **42**(4), 1414–1419.

Goodwin, A E., Merry, G.E. and Sadler, J. (2006) Detection of the herpesviral hematopoietic necrosis disease agent (Cyprinid herpesvirus 2) in moribund and healthy goldfish: validation of a quantitative PCR diagnostic method. *Diseases of Aquatic Organisms*, **69**(2/3), 137.

Graham, D.A., Taylor, C., Rodgers, D., *et al.* (2006) Development and evaluation of a one-step real-time reverse transcription polymerase chain reaction assay for the detection of salmonid alphaviruses in serum and tissues. *Diseases of Aquatic Organisms*, **70**(1/2), 47.

Gregory, A. (2002) Detection of infectious salmon anaemia virus (ISAV) by *in situ* hybridisation. *Diseases of Aquatic Organisms*, **50**(2), 105–110.

Griffin, P.M., Price, G.R., Schooneveldt, J.M., *et al.* (2012) Use of matrix-assisted laser desorption ionization-time of flight mass spectrometry to identify vancomycin-resistant enterococci and investigate the epidemiology of an outbreak. *Journal of Clinical Microbiology*, **50**(9), 2918–2931.

Griffing, S.M., Mixson-Hayden, T., Sridaran, S., *et al.* (2011) South American *Plasmodium falciparum* after the malaria eradication era: clonal population expansion and survival of the fittest hybrids. *PLoS One*, **6**, e23486.

Gunimaladevi, I., Kono, T., Lapatra, S.E. and Sakai, M. (2005) A loop mediated isothermal amplification (LAMP) method for detection of infectious hematopoietic necrosis virus (IHNV) in rainbow trout (Oncorhynchus mykiss) *Archives of Virology*, **150**(5), 899–909.

Haines, D.M. and Clark, E.G. (1991) Enzyme immunohistochemical staining of formalin-fixed tissues for diagnosis in veterinary pathology. *Canadian Veterinary Journal*, **32**(5), 295.
Han, H.J., Jung, S.J., Oh, M.J. and Kim, D.H. (2011) Rapid and sensitive detection of *Streptococcus iniae* by loop-mediated isothermal amplification (LAMP). *Journal of Fish Diseases*, **34**(5), 395–398.
Haridas, D.V., Pillai, D., Manojkumar, B., Nair, C.M. and Sherief, P.M. (2010) Optimisation of reverse transcriptase loop–mediated isothermal amplification assay for rapid detection of *Macrobrachium rosenbergii* noda virus and extra small virus in *Macrobrachium rosenbergii*. *Journal of Virological Methods*, **167**(1), 61–67.
Hasman, H., Saputra, D., Sicheritz-Ponten, T., *et al.* (2013) Rapid whole-genome sequencing for detection and characterization of microorganisms directly from clinical samples. *Journal of Clinical Microbiology*, **52**, 139–146.
Hodneland, K. and Endresen, C. (2006) Sensitive and specific detection of Salmonid alphavirus using real-time PCR (TaqMan®). *Journal of Virological Methods*, **131**(2), 184–192.
Huang, X., El-Sayed, I.H., Qian, W. and El-Sayed, M.A. (2007) Cancer cells assemble and align gold nanorods conjugated to antibodies to produce highly enhanced, sharp, and polarized surface Raman spectra: a potential cancer diagnostic marker. *Nano Letters*, **7**(6), 1591–1597.
Jansson, E., Eriksson, E., Säker, E., *et al.* (2015) Matrix-assisted laser desorption/ionization time of flight, MALDI-TOF, mass spectrometry for identification of fish pathogenic bacteria. Presented at the 17th International Conference on Diseases of Fish and Shellfish.
Kaittanis, C., Santra, S. and Perez, J.M. (2010) Emerging nanotechnology-based strategies for the identification of microbial pathogenesis. *Advanced Drug Delivery Reviews*, **62**(4), 408–423.
Kono, T., Savan, R., Sakai, M. and Itami, T. (2004) Detection of white spot syndrome virus in shrimp by loop-mediated isothermal amplification. *Journal of Virological Methods*, **115**(1), 59–65.
Konstantinidis, K. and Tiedje, J.M. (2005) Genomic insights that advance the species definition for prokaryotes. *Proceedings of the National Academy of Sciences USA*, **102**, 2567–2592.
Köser, C.U., Ellington, M.J., Cartwright, E.J.P., *et al.* (2012a) Routine use of microbial whole genome sequencing in diagnostic and public health microbiology. *PLoS Pathogens*, **8**(8), e1002824.
Köser, C.U., Holden, M.T.G., Ellington, M.J., *et al.* (2012b) Rapid whole-genome sequencing for investigation of a neonatal MRSA outbreak. *New England Journal of Medicine*, **366**, 2267–2275.
Koutna, M., Vesely, T., Psikal, I. and Hulova, J. (2003) Identification of spring viraemia of carp virus (SVCV) by combined RT-PCR and nested PCR. *Diseases of Aquatic Organisms*, **55**(3), 229–235.
Kozińska, A. (2007) Dominant pathogenic species of mesophilic aeromonads isolated from diseased and healthy fish cultured in Poland. *Journal of Fish Diseases*, **30**(5), 293–301.
Kulkarni, A., Caipang, C.M.A., Brinchmann, M.F., Korsnes, K. and Kiron, V. (2009) Use of loop-mediated isothermal amplification assay for the detection of *Vibrio anguillarum* O2β, the causative agent of vibriosis in Atlantic cod, *Gadus morhua*. *Journal of Rapid Methods & Automation in Microbiology*, **17**(4), 503–518.
LaFrentz, B.R., Waldbieser, G.C., Welch, T.J. and Shoemaker, C.A. (2014) Intragenomic heterogeneity in the 16S rRNA genes of *Flavobacterium columnare* and standard protocol for genomovar assignment. *Journal of Fish Diseases*, **37**(7), 657–669.
Law, J.W.F., Ab Mutalib, N.S., Chan, K.G. and Lee, L.H. (2015) Rapid methods for the detection of foodborne bacterial pathogens: principles, applications, advantages and limitations. *Frontiers in Microbiology*, **5**, 770.

Li, C., Shields, J.D., Small, H.J., *et al.* (2006) Detection of *Panulirus argus* Virus 1 (PaVI) in the Caribbean spiny lobster using fluorescence *in situ* hybridization (FISH). *Diseases of Aquatic Organisms*, **72**(3), 185–192.

Liao, H. and Hafner, J.H. (2005) Gold nanorod bioconjugates. *Chemistry of Materials*, **17**(18), 4636–4641.

Lievens, B., Frans, I., Heusdens, C., *et al.* (2011) Rapid detection and identification of viral and bacterial fish pathogens using a DNA array-based multiplex assay. *Journal of Fish Diseases*, **34**(11), 861–875.

Lipkin, W.I. (2010) Microbe hunting. *Microbiology and Molecular Biology Reviews*, **74**(3), 363–377.

Liu, H., Wang, Y., Xiao, J., Wang, Q., Liu, Q. and Zhang, Y. (2015) An immunochromatographic test strip for rapid detection of fish pathogen *Edwardsiella tarda*. *Bioresources and Bioprocessing*, **2**(1), 1–8.

Longshaw, M., Frear, P.A., Nunn, A.D., Cowx, I.G. and Feist, S.W. (2010) The influence of parasitism on fish population success. *Fisheries Management and Ecology*, **17**(5), 426–434.

Loy, A. and Bodrossy, L. (2006) Highly parallel microbial diagnostics using oligonucleotide microarrays. *Clinica Chimica Acta*, **363**(1), 106–119.

Lua, D.T., Yasuike, M., Hirono, I. and Aoki T. (2005) Transcription program of red sea bream iridovirus as revealed by DNA microarrays. *Journal of Virological Methods*, **79**(24), 15151–15164.

Magariños, B., Toranzo, A.E., Barja, J.L. and Romalde, J.L. (2000) Existence of two geographically–linked clonal lineages in the bacterial fish pathogen *Photobacterium damselae* subsp. *piscicida* evidenced by random amplified polymorphic DNA analysis. *Epidemiology and Infection*, **125**(01), 213–219.

McCarthy, U.M., Urquhart, K.L. and Bricknell, I.R. (2008) An improved *in situ* hybridization method for the detection of fish pathogens. *Journal of Fish Diseases*, **31**(9), 669–677.

Metzker, M.L. (2010) Sequencing technologies – the next generation. *Nature Reviews Genetics*, **11**(1), 31–46.

Miller, R.R., Montoya, V., Gardy, J.L., Patrick, D.M. and Tang, P. (2013) Metagenomics for pathogen detection in public health. *Genome Medicine*, **5**(9), 81.

Mori, Y., Nagamine, K., Tomita, N. and Notomi, T. (2001) Detection of loop-mediated isothermal amplification reaction by turbidity derived from magnesium pyrophosphate formation. *Biochemical and Biophysical Research Communications*, **289**(1), 150–154.

Morris, D.J., Adams, A. and Richards, R.H. (1999) In situ hybridization of DNA probes to PKX, the causative organism of proliferative kidney disease (PKD). *Journal of Fish Diseases*, **22**(2), 161–163.

Nagamine, K., Watanabe, K., Ohtsuka, K., Hase, T. and Notomi, T. (2001) Loop-mediated isothermal amplification reaction using a nondenatured template. *Clinical Chemistry*, **47**(9), 1742–1743.

Naka, H., Dias, G.M., Thompson, C.C., Dubay, C., Thompson, F.L. and Crosa, J.H. (2011) Complete genome sequence of the marine fish pathogen *Vibrio anguillarum* harboring the pJM1 virulence plasmid and genomic comparison with other virulent strains of *V. anguillarum* and *V. ordalii*. *Infection and Immunity*, **79**(7), 2889–2900.

Nakamura, S., Maeda, N., Mrion, I.M., *et al.* (2008) Metagenomic diagnosis of bacterial infections. *Emerging Infectious Diseases*, **14**(11), 1784–1786.

Nguyen, T.L., Lim, Y.J., Kim, D.H. and Austin, B. (2016) Development of real-time PCR for detection and quantitation of *Streptococcus parauberis*. *Journal of Fish Diseases*, **39**(1), 31–39.

Nilsen, H., Sundell, K., Duchaud, E., *et al.* (2014) Multilocus sequence typing (MLST) identifies epidemic clones of *Flavobacterium psychrophilum* in Nordic countries. *Applied and Environmental Microbiology*, **80**(9), 2728–2736.

Odell, I. and Cook, D. (2013) Immunofluorescence techniques. *Journal of Investigative Dermatology*, **133**(1), 34.

Olesen, N.J. and Jørgensen, P.E.V. (1991) Rapid detection of viral haemorrhagic septicaemia virus in fish by ELISA. *Journal of Applied Ichthyology*, **7**(3), 183–186.

Oreshkova, S.F., Shchelkunov, I.S., Tikunova, N.V., Shchelkunova, T.I., Puzyrev, A.T. and Ilyichev, A.A. (1999) Detection of spring viremia of carp virus isolates by hybridization with non-radioactive probes and amplification by polymerase chain reaction. *Virus Research*, **63**(1), 3–10.

Pallen, M.J. (2014) Diagnostic metagenomics: potential applications to bacterial, viral and parasitic infections. *Parasitology*, **141**(14), 1856–1862.

Panangala, V.S., van Shoemaker, C.A., Santen, V.L., Dybvig, K. and Klesius, P.H. (2007a) Multiplex-PCR for simultaneous detection of 3 bacterial fish pathogens, *Flavobacterium columnare, Edwardsiella ictaluri,* and *Aeromonas hydrophila. Diseases of Aquatic Organisms*, **74**(3), 199–208.

Panangala, V.S., Shoemaker, C.A. and Klesius, P.H. (2007b) Taq Man real-time polymerase chain reaction assay for rapid detection of *Flavobacterium columnare. Aquaculture Research*, **38**(5), 508–517.

Posthuma-Trumpie, G.A., Korf, J. and van Amerongen, A. (2009) Lateral flow (immuno) assay: its strengths, weaknesses, opportunities and threats. A literature survey. *Analytical and Bioanalytical Chemistry*, **393**(2), 569–582.

Ramos-Vara, J.A. (2005) Technical aspects of immunohistochemistry. *Veterinary Pathology*, **42**, 405–426.

Reith, M.E., Singh, R.K., Curtis, B., *et al.* (2008) The genome of *Aeromonas salmonicida* subsp. *salmonicida* A449: insights into the evolution of a fish pathogen. *BMC Genomics*, **9**, 427.

Richter, M. and Rosselló-Móra, R. (2009) Shifting the genomic gold standard for the prokaryotic species definition. *Proceedings of the National Academy of Sciences USA*, **106**, 19126–19131.

Rodnick, K J., St-Hilaire, S., Battiprolu, P.K., *et al.* (2008) Evidence for sex and or habitat differences in swimming performance, parasite infestation, tissue biochemistry, and morphology of juvenile coho salmon in Oregon's West Fork Smith River. *Transactions of the American Fisheries Society*, **137**, 1571–1590.

Romalde, J.L., Magariños, B., Villar, C., Barja, J.L. and Toranzo, A.E. (1999) Genetic analysis of turbot pathogenic *Streptococcus parauberis* strains by ribotyping and random amplified polymorphic DNA. *FEMS Microbiology Letters*, **179**(2), 297–304.

Sajid, M., Kawde, A.N. and Daud, M. (2014) Designs, formats and applications of lateral flow assay: a literature review. *Journal of Saudi Chemical Society*, **19**(6), 689–705.

Sakai, M., Baxa, D.V., Kurobe, T., Kono, T., Shivappa, R.B. and Hedrick, R.P. (2009) Detection of *Nucleospora salmonis* in cutthroat trout (*Oncorhynchus clarki*) and rainbow trout (*Oncorhynchus mykiss*) by loop-mediated isothermal amplification. *Aquaculture*, **288**(1), 27–31.

Saksida, S.M., Marty, G.D., Jones, S.R.M., *et al.* (2012) Parasites and hepatic lesions among pink salmon, *Oncorhynchus gorbuscha* (Walbaum), during early seawater residence. *Journal of Fish Diseases*, **35**(2), 137–151.

Saleh, M., Soliman, H., Haenen, O. and El-Matbouli, M. (2011) Antibody-coated gold nanoparticles immunoassay for direct detection of *Aeromonas salmonicida* in fish tissues. *Journal of Fish Diseases*, **34**(11), 845–852.

Saleh, M., Soliman, H., Schachner, O. and El-Matbouli, M. (2012) Direct detection of unamplified spring viraemia of carp virus RNA using unmodified gold nanoparticles. *Marine Ecology Progress Series*, **100**(1), 3–10.

Saleh, M., Gotesman, M. and El-Matbouli, M. (2013) Going for gold in the detection of Cyprinid herpesvirus-3. Presented at the 16th International Conference on Diseases of Fish and Shellfish, European Association of Fish Pathologists, September 2–6, Tampere, Finland.

Sanders, G.E., Batts, W.N. and Winton, J.R. (2003) Susceptibility of zebrafish (*Danio rerio*) to a model pathogen, spring viremia of carp virus. *Comparative Medicine*, **53**(5), 514–521.

Santos, F., Martinez-Garcia, M., Parro, V. and Anton, J. (2014) Microarray tools to unveil viral-microbe interactions in nature. *Frontiers in Ecology and Evolution*, **2**, article 31.

Savan, R., Igarashi, A., Matsuoka, S. and Sakai, M. (2004) Sensitive and rapid detection of edwardsiellosis in fish by a loop-mediated isothermal amplification method. *Applied and Environmental Microbiology*, **70**(1), 621–624.

Schacht, V. and Kern, J.S. (2015) Basics of immunohistochemistry. *Journal of Investigative Dermatology*, **135**(3), e30.

Schuenemann, V.J., Singh, P., Mendum, T.A., *et al.* (2013) Genome-wide comparison of medieval and modern *Mycobacterium leprae*. *Science*, **341**, 179–183.

Sithigorngul, W., Rukpratanporn, S., Sittidilokratna, N., *et al.* (2007) A convenient immunochromatographic test strip for rapid diagnosis of yellow head virus infection in shrimp. *Journal of Virological Methods*, **140**(1), 193–199.

Soliman, H. and El-Matbouli, M. (2006) Reverse transcription loop-mediated isothermal amplification (RT-LAMP) for rapid detection of viral hemorrhagic septicaemia virus (VHS). *Veterinary Microbiology*, **114**(3), 205–213.

Sritunyalucksana, K., Apisawetakan, S., Boon-nat, A., Withyachumnarnkul, B. and Flegel, T. W. (2006) A new RNA virus found in black tiger shrimp *Penaeus monodon* from Thailand. *Virus Research*, **118**, 31–38.

Stentiford, G.D., Longshaw, M., Lyons, B.P., Jones, G., Green, M. and Feist, S.W. (2003) Histopathological biomarkers in estuarine fish species for the assessment of biological effects of contaminants. *Marine Environmental Research*, **55**(2), 137–159.

Strepparava, N., Wahli, T., Segner, H., Polli, B. and Petrini, O. (2012) Fluorescent *in situ* hybridization: a new tool for the direct identification and detection of *F. psychrophilum*. *PLoS One*, **7**(11), e49280.

Tanner, M., Gancberg, D., Di Leo, A., *et al.* (2000) Chromogenic in situ hybridization: a practical alternative for fluorescence *in situ* hybridization to detect HER-2/neu oncogene amplification in archival breast cancer samples. *American Journal of Pathology*, **157**(5), 1467–1472.

Tao, Z., Larsen, A.M., Bullard, S.A., Wright, A.C. and Arias, C.R. (2012) Prevalence and population structure of *Vibrio vulnificus* on fishes from the northern Gulf of Mexico. *Applied and Environmental Microbiology*, **78**(21), 7611–7618.

Tomita, N., Mori, Y., Kanda, H. and Notomi, T. (2008) Loop-mediated isothermal amplification (LAMP) of gene sequences and simple visual detection of products. *Nature Protocols*, **3**(5), 877–882.

Topić Popović, N., Čož-Rakovac, R. and Strunjak-Perović, I. (2007) Commercial phenotypic tests (API 20E) in diagnosis of fish bacteria. *Veterinarni Medicina*, **52**(2), 49–53.

Torok, M.E. and Peacock, S.J. (2012) Rapid whole-genome sequencing of bacterial pathogens in the clinical microbiology laboratory– pipe dream or reality? *Journal of Antimicrobial Chemotherapy*, **67**, 2307–2308.

Uttamchandani, M., Neo, J.L., Zhung Ong, B.N. and Moochhala, S. (2009) Applications of microarrays in pathogen detection and biodefence. *Trends in Biotechnology*, **27**(1), 53–61.

Vincent, A.T., Trudel, M.V., Freschi, L., *et al.* (2016) Increasing genomic diversity and evidence of constrained lifestyle evolution due to insertion sequences in *Aeromonas salmonicida*. *BMC Genomics*, **17**, 1.

Wang, Q., Yang, M., Xiao, J., *et al.* (2009) Genome sequence of the versatile fish pathogen *Edwardsiella tarda* provides insights into its adaptation to broad host ranges and intracellular niches. *PLoS One*, **4**(10), e7646.

Warsen, A.E., Krug, M.J., LaFrentz, S., Stanek, D.R., Loge, F.J. and Call, D.R. (2004) Simultaneous discrimination between 15 fish pathogens by using 16S ribosomal DNA PCR and DNA microarrays. *Applied Environmental Microbiology*, **70**(7), 4216–4221.

Wassenaar, T.M. and Newell, D.G. (2000) Genotyping of *Campylobacter* spp. *Applied and Environmental Microbiology*, **66**(1), 1–9.

Whittington, R.J. and Steiner, K.A. (1993) Epizootic haematopoietic necrosis virus (EHNV): improved ELISA for detection in fish tissues and cell cultures and an efficient method for release of antigen from tissues. *Journal of Virological Methods*, **43**(2), 205–220.

World Organization for Animal Health (2015) *Manual of Diagnostic Tests for Aquatic Animals*. World Organization for Animal Health (OIE), Paris.

Yu, L.P., Hu, Y.H., Zhang, X.H. and Sun, B.G. (2013) Development of a triplex loop-mediated isothermal amplification method for rapid on-site detection of three *Vibrio* species associated with fish diseases. *Aquaculture*, **414**, 267–273.

Yue, Z., Teng, Y., Liang, C., *et al.* (2008) Development of a sensitive and quantitative assay for spring viremia of carp virus based on real-time RT-PCR. *Journal of Virological Methods*, **152**(1), 43–48.

Zhang, D.F., Zhang, Q.Q. and Li, A.H. (2014) Development of a multiplex PCR assay for rapid and simultaneous detection of four genera of fish pathogenic bacteria. *Letters in Applied Microbiology*, **59**(5), 471–478.

Zhang, J., Chiodini, R., Badr, A. and Zhang, G. (2011) The impact of next-generation sequencing on genomics. *Journal of Genetics and Genomics*, **38**(3), 95–109.

Zhao, P., Wu, Y., Zhu, Y., *et al.* (2014) Upconversion fluorescent strip sensor for rapid determination of *Vibrio anguillarum*. *Nanoscale*, **6**(7), 3804–3809.

6

Immunostimulant Diets and Oral Vaccination In Fish

Eva Vallejos-Vidal[1], *Felipe Reyes-López*[2] *and Simon MacKenzie*[3]

[1] Institut de Biotecnologia i Biomedicina, Universitat Autonoma de Barcelona, Bellaterra, Spain
[2] Department of Cell Biology, Physiology and Immunology, Universitat Autonoma de Barcelona, Bellaterra, Spain
[3] Institute of Aquaculture, University of Stirling, Stirling, Scotland, UK

Introduction

An immunostimulant (IS) is a natural or chemical substance that stimulates the immune system by specific (vaccines or antigens) or non-specific (irrespective of antigenic specificity) routes. In aquaculture, non-specific immunostimulants have been widely used, probably due to the limited knowledge of the immune response in fish and the ease of their application. Although fish are indeed the most diverse group of vertebrates, there are well-conserved mechanisms across the immune system. These systems, often innate immunity, are the most commonly used to measure the response of the fish to the dietary supplement in question. This, in part, is due to the relative simplicity of such measurements that are often based upon straightforward biochemical tests in leucocytes. This cell group in particular is useful due to the ease of their purification from fish in culture.

Our aim in this chapter is not to provide a review of fish immunity, which has been extensively covered in many excellent reviews throughout the pertinent literature, but rather to provide some insight into the target tissue of many IS diets; the fish mucosa. As stated, many studies have focused upon the innate immune response at a cellular and humoral level due to the ease of access to blood. However, the mucosal immune systems that are in direct contact with the pathogens are in fact the target tissues for evaluation, that is, the surfaces in contact with the external environment: gills, nose, gastrointestinal tract and skin. These tissue–environment interfaces are also commonly named as the portals of entry when described in a pathogen context.

The mucosal tissues contain a significant diversity of pathogen recognition receptors (PRRs) and are capable of mounting a robust immune response against pathogens (Gomez *et al.*, 2013; Salinas *et al.*, 2011). In fish, four mucosal-associated lymphoid tissues (MALT) have been described; nose-associated lymphoid tissue (NALT), skin-associated lymphoid tissue (SALT), gill-associated lymphoid tissue (GIALT), and gut-associated lymphoid tissue (GALT), each responsible for the immune response at a specific site (Salinas, 2015). The described cellular environment within each of these MALTs lacks organized lymphoid structures, such as lymphoid nodes or germinal centres in a mammalian sense, and therefore leucocyte populations are dispersed within the tissues. Each tissue has been shown to have secretory Igs

Diagnosis and Control of Diseases of Fish and Shellfish, First Edition. Edited by Brian Austin and Aweeda Newaj-Fyzul.

in the mucus that are transported into the lumen through a polymeric Ig receptor (pIgR) and the presence of a specialized mucosal Ig class, IgT/Z, is a defining factor. Furthermore, there are commensal bacteria across the tissues and in some cases they are coated by Igs (Parra *et al.*, 2015).

However, understanding of the individual properties of each of these MALTs and their overall impact upon immunity and survival is still in its infancy. GALT, a major player in immunostimulant diet design as this is the targeted interface, is a complex tissue containing resident granulocytes, macrophages, lymphocytes and plasma cells (lamina propria leucocytes, LPLs), and T- and B-cells among epithelial cells (intraepithelial lymphocytes, IELs). Additionally, there are significant populations of epithelial, neuroendocrine and goblet cells that are able to produce cell activity mediators and regulate gut immune responses (Parra *et al.*, 2015).

Surprisingly, given the central role of the gastrointestinal (GI) tract in diet design for aquaculture, there is little information available concerning GALT regulation. The skin (SALT) and gill (GIALT) mucosal surfaces represent the largest surface areas in contact with the external environment and therefore exposure to pathogens. The skin is the outermost organ of the body and the first line of defence from external insult (Xu *et al.*, 2013). SALT has mucus-secreting cells in the epidermis and this characteristic defines it as a mucosal tissue. Tissue responses have been reported based upon lysozyme, complement, lectins and proteolytic enzymes (Nigam *et al.*, 2012), while secreted IgM and IgT have also been detected (Maki *et al.*, 2003; Xu *et al.*, 2013). From a total surface area point of view, the GIALT has the largest of all tissues in contact with the external environment. Furthermore, the intimate contact with the bloodstream places this MALT as a particularly important line of defence. Lymphocyte cell aggregation in the interbranchial lymphoid tissue (ILT) (Haugarvoll *et al.*, 2008), mainly T-cells and some scattered B-cells (Koppang *et al.*, 2010), has been reported in salmonids. However, several microbiological studies have shown that bacterial penetration of GIALT and subsequent colonization of internal organs of the fish take place in a matter of hours (Callol *et al.*, 2015a,b).

Therefore, there exists an urgency to generate knowledge that allows a more profound understanding of the function of these tissues before the effect of IS diets can be functionally assessed with a view to reinforcing MALTs through diet.

Commonly Measured Immunological Parameters

The immunostimulant effect of dietary supplements in fish has been focused mainly on the evaluation of non-specific immune parameters and, therefore, on the consequences of these treatments on the innate immune system. The innate immune system has both cellular and humoral components by which it carries out its protective function. The major components of the innate immune system at the cellular level are leucocytes, mainly monocytes, macrophages and granulocytes (Magnadóttir, 2006; Secombes and Fletcher, 1992). Among the granulocytes, neutrophils are the most abundant cell type and their presence has been described in Salmoniformes, Cypriniformes and Perciformes (Flerova and Balabanova, 2013). Neutrophils and macrophages are responsible for the production of bioactive molecules for pathogen recognition and destruction, cellular communication and activation, initiation of an adaptive immune response and later, resolution of an inflammatory response and tissue repair. Furthermore, these cell types are responsible in the majority for phagocytosis (Silva and Correia-Neves, 2012), one of the main mediators of innate immunity to remove pathogens such as bacteria, viruses and parasites. For this reason, these immune cell types are also called phagocytes. This microbe/killing mechanism triggers diverse antimicrobial processes that use a wide variety of mechanisms including cellular activation, production of oxidative radicals and the production of cytokines driving the inflammatory response, amongst others.

Two of the most important antimicrobial systems of phagocytic cells are the NADPH phagocyte oxidase and inducible nitric oxide synthase (iNOS) pathways, which are responsible for the generation of superoxide (O_2^-) and nitric oxide (NO) radicals, respectively. NADPH oxidase, a multi-subunit complex, catalyses a one-electron reduction of molecular oxygen into superoxide anion (O_2^-), also referred to as reactive oxygen species (ROS), which is converted either spontaneously to H_2O_2 or enzymatically by superoxide dismutase (SOD). In comparison to neutrophils, the size of the respiratory burst is much reduced in macrophages (Iles and Forman, 2002). Since O_2^- is the first product to be released from the respiratory burst, the measurement of O_2^- has been accepted as a direct and accurate way of measuring respiratory burst activity (Secombes and Olivier, 1997): the reduction of ferricytochrome c to determine extracellular O_2^-, and the reduction of the nitroblue tetrazolium (NBT) redox dye to determine intracellular O_2^- (Dügenci *et al.*, 2003). On the other hand, iNOS is responsible for NO production and its derivatives, which are collectively known as reactive nitrogen species (RNS). Unlike ROS, macrophages generally produce considerably more RNS than neutrophils (Nathan and Shiloh, 2000). iNOS is activated by interferon (IFN) gamma or tumour necrosis factor (TNF) (Green *et al.*, 1993). Also, NO has been demonstrated to activate nuclear factor (NF)-kappaB in peripheral blood mononuclear cells, an important transcription factor in iNOS gene expression in response to inflammation (Kaibori *et al.*, 1999). The ROS and RNS antibacterial activities have been widely discussed (Fang, 2004).

Although less studied, myeloperoxidase (MPO) is a lysosomal protein stored in azurophilic granules also involved in antimicrobial mechanisms and is also produced by phagocytes. It is most abundantly expressed in neutrophils although is also present in circulating mammalian monocytes but is lost as these mature into macrophages (Locksley *et al.*, 1987). It possesses antimicrobial activity via hypohalous acid production (Klebanoff, 2005) and is released into the extracellular space during degranulation (Spitznagel *et al.*, 1983).

Among the immune cell parameters, red blood cell (RBC) count is frequently used to evaluate possible undesired collateral effects (anaemia) provoked by immunostimulants administered in supplemented feed. Interestingly, RBCs have received increased attention over the last few years due to the reported participation of these cells in the rainbow trout immune response (Morera *et al.*, 2011).

In addition to the cellular response, humoral elements also participate in the innate immune response, including lysozyme or the complement system (Magnadóttir 2006; Secombes and Fletcher, 1992). IgM is the most common immunoglobulin in serum and mucus and is the key player in systemic immune responses (Parra *et al.*, 2015). For this reason, the total immunoglobulin and total protein level (an indirect antibody level measurement) are frequently evaluated in immunostimulant supplemented diets. IgM also participates in the opsonization of pathogens, facilitating their phagocytosis. In this ambit, complement is a vital component of innate immunity and represents one of the major effector mechanisms of the innate immune system (Dunkelberger and Song, 2010). It starts with the identification of pathogenic surfaces and leads to the generation of potent proinflammatory mediators (anaphylatoxins), opsonization (coating) of the pathogenic surface through various complement opsonins (such as C3b), and targeted lysis of the pathogenic surface through the assembly of membrane-penetrating pores known as the membrane attack complex (MAC). The complement system can be activated through three major pathways: classical (antigen: antibody immune complexes), lectin (PAMP recognition by lectins) and the alternative pathway (spontaneous hydrolysis/pathogenic surfaces) (Dunkelberger and Song, 2010).

Various lytic enzymes, acting alone or in cascade, are also important in the defence against pathogens. Lysozyme is one of the most analysed lytic enzyme activities used to evaluate immunostimulant-enhanced improvement of innate immunity. Lysozyme is bactericidal, hydrolyzing β-[1,4] linked glycoside bonds of both Gram-positive and -negative bacterial cell wall peptidoglycans resulting in lysis (Magnadóttir, 2006). As with the innate components described above, it is also present in fish mucosa (Parra *et al.*, 2015).

Finally, at the gene expression level, proinflammatory (interleukin (IL)-1, IL-6, TNF-alpha) and anti-inflammatory or immunosuppressive (IL-10, transforming growth factor (TGF)-beta) cytokines have been evaluated in fish fed with immunostimulant-supplemented diets. Thus, the limited available information addressing gene expression modulation does not allow a direct understanding of the possible pathways and immunological functions stimulated by the administration of immunostimulants in a global context.

The cortisol and glucose response to immunostimulant administration has not been extensively explored. Based on changing dietary composition over recent years (i.e. vegetable protein source instead of animal protein), using cortisol and glucose measurements to evaluate the effects of dietary administration of new immunostimulants could be important not only for the effect on the stress response but also for the consequences upon the host–pathogen response as intimate regulation between endocrine and immune system is a central requirement for effective responses (Tort, 2011).

The evaluation of changes in the modulation of genes associated with the immune system has not been routine practice in evaluating the immunostimulant effects in diets. Moreover, three recent studies have evaluated the gene expression profile in fish fed with immunostimulant diets, making an effort to complement the general and systemic information provided in these types of studies such as growth, non-specific humoral and cellular innate immune parameters, and cumulative mortality against pathogens. Based on the limited existing information, upregulation of IL-1-beta and TNF-alpha (Giri *et al.*, 2015; Wang *et al.*, 2015; Yang *et al.*, 2015) and downregulation of IL-10 and TGF-beta (Giri *et al.*, 2015; Wang *et al.*, 2015) have been observed, suggesting the expression of these genes as potential candidates contributing to the observed immunomodulation in fish fed with different immunostimulant diets. Further studies evaluating the transcriptomic response of fish fed with immunostimulant diets are needed to confirm this hypothesis.

Plant, Herbal and Algal Extracts

Diverse efforts, using many different experimental systems, have been made in order to evaluate the immunostimulant effects of algae, herbs and plant extracts in various fish species. The immunostimulants covered in this chapter that are composed of plant, herb or algal extracts (Table 6.1) are presented below. This details the different dietary supplements used, where they have been tested and upon which fish species.

Table 6.1 Plant, Herb And Algae Extracts Used in Fish

Plant		Herbal	Algae/Fungi
Achyranthes aspera	*Echinacea*	*Andrographis paniculata*	*Ascophyllum nodosum*
Aegle marmelos	*Eclipta alba*	*Angelicae Sinensis*	*Durvillaea antarctica*
Allium sativum	*Ficus carica*	*Astagalus radix*	*Haematococcus pluvialis*
Aloe vera	*Nigella sativa*	*Ocimum sanctum*	*Laminaria digitata*
Avicennia marina	*Psidium guajava*	*Rehmannia glutinosa*	*Navicula spp*
Azadirachta indica	*Rauvolfia tetraphylla*		*Porphyridium cruentum*
Camellia sinensis	*Rhizophora apiculata*		*Spirulina platensis*
Cedrus deodara	*Urtica dioica*		
Citrus sinensis	*Viscum album Coloratum*		*Ganoderma lucidum*
Coffea arabica	*Zingiber officinale*		*Lentinula edodes*
Cotinus coggyria			

Plant and Herb Extracts

Andrographis paniculata

The dietary administration of andrographolide, the main medicinal compound of *Andrographis paniculata*, native to India and Sri Lanka with antimicrobial, antioxidant, anti-inflammatory and immunomodulator properties (Chao *et al.*, 2010; Gao *et al.*, 2009; Levita *et al.*, 2010; Xu *et al.*, 2006), had a stimulatory effect on non-specific immune parameters in *Labeo rohita* (Basha *et al.*, 2013), a similar effect to that observed in fish infected with *Aphanomyces invadans* fed with *Rauvolfia tetraphylla*-supplemented diets (Yogeshwari *et al.*, 2015), a plant of the family *Apocynaceae* distributed in tropical countries including India.

Aloe barbadensis

Aloe barbadensis, also called *Aloe vera* (family Xanthorrhoeaceae), is a plant frequently used in traditional medicine with multiple properties including antiviral and immunomodulatory activity (Kim *et al.*, 1999; Vázquez *et al.*, 1996). In a study in Nile tilapia, *O.nilotocus*, fed an *Aloe vera*-supplemented diet and propolis, no significant differences were found in any measured parameters (Dotta *et al.*, 2014). However, in another strain of Nile tilapia (GIFT) after challenge with *Streptococcus iniae*, an increase in growth performance was observed with slight changes in RBC and white blood cell (WBC) counts, haemoglobin and haematocrit and no changes in glucose and cortisol (Gabriel *et al.*, 2015). These differences may be related to differences in the *A. vera* concentration used: in both studies, fish were fed with 0.5%, 1% and 2% of the supplemented diet but in the case of Nile tilapia, the *A. vera* was mixed equally with propolis. Overall, no significant favourable health status changes were observed in tilapia (GIFT) fed with the *A. vera*-supplemented diet. Similarly, no differences were observed in Nile tilapia fed with a propolis-supplemented diet, although 1% propolis-ethanolic-extract increased the monocyte count and decreased neutrophils 28 days after treatment (Abd-El-Rhman, 2009).

In steelhead rainbow trout (*Oncorhynchus mykiss*, Walbaum), dietary *Aloe vera* inclusion had no effect on growth, non-specific immune parameters, the expression of several immune-related genes and the immune response to formalin-killed atypical *Aeromonas salmonicida* (Zanuzzo *et al.*, 2015). The authors suggest that prolonged feeding with *A. vera* may cause an undesirable effect but no significant differences were found in Nile tilapia fed for two weeks (Dotta *et al.*, 2014) and few changes were observed in haemato-immune parameters (RBC, WBC) in tilapia (GIFT) challenged with *S. iniae* that were fed for eight weeks prior to challenge (Gabriel *et al.*, 2015). Thus, further studies are needed to evaluate the effective impact of *A. vera* as an immunostimulant in fish. Of course, one has to be wary of making comparisons between such phylogenetically distinct species with different life histories and dietary requirements.

Chinese Herbs

The immunostimulant effects of several Chinese herbs have been evaluated in different cyriniform species. The *Astragalus* root (*Astragalus radix*, AR), a plant that contains polysaccharides, alkaloids and volatile oils, has been shown to modulate the function of immune system-relevant cell populations, including T-cells, B-cells, natural killer (NK) cells and macrophages (Kong *et al.*, 2003; Liu, 2002). Polysaccharides extracted from angelica root (*Angelica sinensis*, AS) possess biological properties, including haematopoietic, immunomodulation, antitumour, antioxidant, radioprotective and hypoglycaemic activity (Jin *et al.*, 2012). In the large yellow croaker (*Pseudosciaena crocea*), the effect of combined *Astragalus* and *Angelica* roots was evaluated and a significant enhancement of respiratory burst activity of phagocytic cells, phagocytosis and lysozyme activities in plasma was recorded (Jian and W,u 2003). Similar effects were reported in common carp fed with *Astragalus* and *Ganoderma lucidum* (GL) (Yin *et al.*, 2009). A range of non-specific immune parameters were found to be enhanced, including SOD and peroxidase (POD) activity, in tilapia (*Oreochromis niloticus*) supplemented with a Chinese herbal mixture composed of *Astragalus*, *Angelica*, hawthorn, licorice root and honeysuckle (Tang *et al.*, 2014). This was accompanied by reduced mortality following *A. hydrophila* challenge. Furthermore, upregulation of IL-1 and TNF-alpha was reported (Tang *et al.*, 2014), confirming these mRNAs as potential biomarker candidates. In our opinion, this highlights the need to further identify the underpinning molecular mechanisms contributing to the observable impact of immunostimulants.

Azadirachta indica

The effect of azadirachtin, a high-value carotenoid from the Indian plant (*Azadirachta indica*) responsible for its antibacterial property (Mistry *et al.*, 2014), has been evaluated in goldfish (*Carassius auratus*), resulting in high nitroblue tetrazolium (NBT) activity, serum lysozyme, erythrocyte and leucocyte counts (Kumar *et al.*, 2013). Further studies are warranted in view of these positive results.

Camellia sinensis

Green tea (*Camellia sinensis* L.) (GT) is a medicinal herb with non-oxidized and unfermented leaves, which have anti-inflammatory, antioxidative, antiproliferative, antibacterial and antiviral properties (Crespy and Williamson 2004; Isogai *et al.*, 2001; Weber *et al.*, 2003). In Nile tilapia fed a GT experimental diet for 12 weeks, a higher growth performance, haematoimmune parameters and cumulative survival against *A. hydrophila* were observed

(Abdel-Tawwab *et al.*, 2010), while in yellowtail (*Seriola quinqueradiata*) fed with GT polyphenols, no significant differences were observed (Ishihara *et al.*, 2002).

Green tea extracts have also been evaluated in rainbow trout and a decaffeinated GT extract showed a higher lysozyme and peroxidase content (Sheikhzadeh *et al.*, 2011). However, when rainbow trout were fed with epigallocatechin-3-gallate (EGCG), a very potent antioxidant derived from GT, no significant differences were observed (Thawonsuwan *et al.*, 2010). These results are consistent with those observed in Nile tilapia fed with GT with changes in immune parameters (Abdel-Tawwab *et al.*, 2010) but no significant differences were observed with a GT polyphenol-supplemented diet (Ishihara *et al.*, 2002).

Cedrus deodara

Dihydroquercetin obtained from deodar (*Cedrus deodara,* family Pinaceae), a traditional plant used in Hindu medicine native to the Indian subcontinent with a broad spectrum of action (Chandur *et al.*, 2011), was evaluated in gilthead seabream (*Sparus aurata*). These studies detected an increase in cellular (phagocytosis and respiratory burst activities) and humoral (serum complement activity, antiprotease, total protein, peroxidase, bactericidal activity and IgM levels) activities, with the highest increases related to the lowest doses (Awad *et al.*, 2015).

Citrus sinensis

Another tree mainly cultivated in subtropical regions with antimicrobial and antifungal properties is the sweet orange (*Citrus sinensis*), a member of the Citrus family (Chee *et al.*, 2009; Sharma and Tripathi, 2008). In tilapia (*Oreochromis mossambicus*) fed with essential oil, an increase in weight gain, specific growth rate (SGR), serum biochemical and haematoimmunological parameters and survival against *S. iniae* infection was reported with a concomitant decrease in feed conversion rate (FCR), albumin and mean cell haemoglobin (MCH) (Acar *et al.*, 2015).

Coffea arabica

Coffee is one of the most popular drinks in the world, with *Coffea arabica* (coffee bean, Rubiaceae family) representing 75–80% of the world coffee production. Caffeine has been reported to improve defence against different stressors (Lacorte *et al.*, 2013). In carp, dietary administration of roasted coffee beans (RCB) did not improve fish growth (Abdel-Tawwab *et al.*, 2015). Along the same lines, RCB in Nile tilapia did not improve growth performance (Abdel-Tawwab *et al.*, 2015) and there was an adverse effect at a concentration higher than 1 g/kg reported in seabream (Chatzifotis *et al.*, 2008). However, RCB were reported to improve some immune parameters in carp (Abdel-Tawwab *et al.*, 2015), suggesting the possibility of using non-conventional immunostimulants in fish diets.

Echinacea

The historical and traditional use of *Echinacea purpurea*, a flowering plant in the Asteraceae family, has been subject to a few studies based upon tilapia. Echinacea activates macrophages and stimulates phagocytic function in humans (See *et al.*, 1997). The dietary effect of echinacea extract was evaluated in Nile tilapia (*Oreochromis niloticus*) where a positive impact upon weight gain, SGR, monocyte activity, neutrophil adherence and survival rate against *A. hydrophila* was recorded (Aly and Mohamed, 2010).

Eclipta alba

The immunostimulant effect of the Indian medicinal plant *Eclipta alba* (L.), a herb also belonging to the Asteraceae, has been reported to confer anti-inflammatory and antimicrobial properties (Leal *et al.*, 2000; Wiart *et al.*, 2004). In tilapia, *E. alba* stimulated an increase of the non-specific humoral response (lysozyme, antiprotease and complement) and the cellular response (myeloperoxidase content, production of reactive oxygen and nitrogen species), with improved survival against *A. hydrophila* (Christybapita *et al.*, 2007).

Mentha piperita

Mentha piperita (also known as peppermint) is a traditional medicinal herb and one of the most widely used in both Eastern and Western traditions. This perennial herb belongs to the Lamiaceae family and has reported antioxidant, antiviral and antibacterial properties (McKay and Blumberg, 2006). Although increases in haematological, mucosal and systemic immune system parameters were reported, a decrease in the number of lymphocytes was observed in fry of the Caspian white fish (*Rutilus frisii kutum*) fed with peppermint-supplemented diets (Adel *et al.*, 2015).

Ocimum sanctum (Tulsi, Queen of Plants)

Ocimum sanctum fed to *Labeo rohita* increased protection against *A. hydrophila* infection. This was accompanied with enhanced non-specific immune (superoxide anion production, lysozyme activity, total protein, Ig) and haematoimmune parameters (total RBC/WBC counts, haemoglobin content) (Das *et al.*, 2013).

Psidium guajava L

Guava (*Psidium guajava L.*) leaves, colloquially known as the 'poor man's apple of the tropics' and widely distributed throughout Asia, including India, have been reported to have antimicrobial and antioxidant activities (Chen and Yen, 2007; Metwally *et al.*, 2010). This treatment has shown not only better growth and immune parameters in immunostimulated groups of *Labeo rohita* but also changes in the mRNA abundance of genes related to the inflammatory response: upregulation of IL-1-beta and TNF-alpha and downregulation of IL-10, TGF-beta, inducible nitric oxide synthase (iNOS), cyclo-oxygenase-2 (COX-2) and nuclear factor (NF)-kappa-B (Giri *et al.*, 2015). Furthermore, increased resistance against *A. hydrophila* (Basha *et al.*, 2013; Giri *et al.*, 2015; Kumar *et al.*, 2013) and *Aphanomyces invadans* (Yogeshwari *et al.*, 2015) infections was reported.

Rehmannia glutinosa

Rehmannia glutinosa (RG) (also known as di-huang in China), which belongs to the family of Scrophulariaceae, and *Ficus carica* polysaccharide (FCP), obtained from a plant which belongs to the largest genus of the Moraceae family with anti-inflammatory, antitumour and antioxidant properties (Baek *et al.*, 2012; Chao *et al.*, 2006; Yu *et al.*, 2006), were tested in carp (*Cyprinus carpio*), showing increases in plasma lysozyme activity and leucocyte phagocytic activity (Wang *et al.*, 2015; Yin *et al.*, 2009). This was also reported in the Chinese sucker (*Myxocyprinus asiaticus*) (Zhang *et al.*, 2009). In Jian carp (*Cyprinus carpio* var. Jian) fed with AS, the number of NBT-positive cells (blood), and lysozyme and complement activity (serum) was also registered (Jian and Wu, 2004). At the gene expression level, upregulation of IL-1-beta, TNF-alpha and iNOS and downregulation of IL-10 and TGF-beta were detected in carp (Wang *et al.*, 2015) while in FCP-fed grass carp (*Ctenopharyngodon idella*), upregulation of IL-1 and TNF-alpha with HSP70 downregulation was registered (Yang *et al.*, 2015). An increase in respiratory burst activity and in phagocytic activity of isolated blood cells and plasma lysozyme activity was observed when fish were immunostimulated with AR + GL and vaccinated against *A. hydrophila*/*A. salmonicida* (Yin *et al.*, 2009). A high survival rate in RG-treated carp challenged with *A. hydrophila* (Wang *et al.*, 2015) and high resistance to *Flavobacterium columnare* in grass carp fed with FCP (Yang *et al.*, 2015) were observed, indicating a potential value of the immune response for these immunostimulants in aquaculture.

Rhizophora apiculata

Rhizophora apiculata (family *Rhizophoraceae*) is one of the widely distributed mangrove tree species in tropical countries, with reported antimicrobial and antiviral activity (Bandaranayake, 2002; Premanathan *et al.*, 1999). Survival rates were higher in clownfish (*Amphiprion sebae*) infected with *Vibrio alginolyticus* (Dhayanithi *et al.*, 2015a) and, interestingly, the same survival rate (although with different immunostimulant doses) was observed when diets were supplemented with *Avicennia marina* (Dhayanithi *et al.*, 2015b), another mangrove tree widely distributed along tropical and subtropical coastlines with antioxidant, antibacterial and antiviral activity (Abeysinghe 2010; Khafagi *et al.*, 2008; Lincy *et al.*, 2013).

Cotinus coggyria

Cotinus coggyria (tetra) is a medicinal plant with antimicrobial and antibacterial effects (Dülger *et al.*, 2009). In rainbow trout fed with a 1% dose, it increased extracellular and intracellular respiratory burst activity, phagocytic and lysozyme activity and total protein level (Bilen *et al.*, 2011).

Urtica dioica

Urtica dioica, the stinging nettle, has been used as an immunostimulant in fish diet. This herbaceous perennial flowering plant is native to Europe, Asia, northern Africa and western North America and has been reported to have immunostimulatory, anti-inflammatory, antioxidant, antiviral, antibacterial and antifungal activities (Gülçin *et al.*, 2004; Hadizadeh *et al.*, 2009; Uncini Manganelli *et al.*, 2005). Together with an increase in haematological and immunological parameters, it was noted that plasma cortisol and glucose decreased with increasing doses in the diet of juvenile and adult *Labeo victorianus* after challenge with *A. hydrophila* (Ngugi *et al.*, 2015).

Black cumin seed oil (*Nigella sativa*) has also been evaluated in the rainbow trout, *O.mykiss*. While black cumin has antibacterial, antioxidant and anti-inflammatory effects (El-Saleh *et al.*, 2004; Hanafy and Hatem, 1991; Zedlitz *et al.*, 2002), stinging nettle has antimicrobial activity with effectiveness against a wide range of micro-organisms (Gülçin *et al.*, 2004). These supplements induced an increase in lysozyme, myeloperoxidase and antiprotease activities, and total serum protein and IgM levels (Awad *et al.*, 2013).

Viscum album coloratum

Viscum album coloratum (Korean mistletoe) fed to Japanese eel had an immunostimulant effect. Korean mistletoe is a semi-parasitic woody perennial commonly found growing in deciduous trees which possesses activity as an immunoadjuvant that has been suggested to be derived from lectins (Yoon *et al.*, 1999, 2003). Extract activity was evaluated by measuring the induction of cytokines and stimulation of NK cell activity (Hajto 1986; Kuttan *et al.*, 1992; Männel *et al.*, 1991; Metzner *et al.*, 1985; Mueller and Anderer, 1990). An increase in lysozyme and phagocytic activity in doses of 0.1%, 0.5% and 1% and also a dose-dependent increase in the total survival rate in eels challenged with *A. hydrophila* were reported (Choi *et al.*, 2008), thus implicating *V. album* in potentiating defence against bacterial infection in the eel.

Zingiber officinale

The majority of reported studies have evaluated immunostimulant effects in the rainbow trout (*O. mykiss*). In rainbow trout fed a diet containing a 1% aqueous extract of powdered ginger roots for three weeks, a significant non-specific immune response increase was recorded, including extracellular respiratory burst activity and phagocytosis of blood leucocytes. These processes, considered to be one of the most important mechanisms involved in the bactericidal activity of macrophages and an increase in plasma protein levels (Dügenci *et al.*, 2003), indicate that humoral factors may enhance phagocytosis in fish (Chung and Secombes, 1987). Also, a proliferation in the number of neutrophils, macrophages and lymphocytes, and enhanced phagocytic, respiratory burst, lysozyme, bactericidal, antiprotease activities, and an augmented relative survival in fish challenged with *A. hydrophila* were observed in rainbow trout fed with ginger (Nya and Austin, 2009). Ginger has anti-inflammatory and antioxidative activity and its effect upon a range of bacterial, fungal and parasitic conditions has been reported (Agarwal *et al.*, 2001; Chrubasik *et al.*, 2005; Endo *et al.*, 1990; Grzanna *et al.*, 2005; Kim *et al.*, 2007). A higher survival rate was also observed in rainbow trout supplemented with garlic (*Allium sativum*) (Nya and Austin, 2011).

Algae and Fungi Extracts

Algae-derived supplements as potential immunostimulants have received increasing attention in recent years. In the spotted wolffish (*Anarhichas minor*), the effect of alginate, a polysaccharide found in brown algae cell walls composed of M- and G-blocks, was evaluated (Haug *et al.*, 1967). An increase in SGR was reported with a 0.01% alginate feeding group but similar results were not observed in either of the other dietary groups (0.06% and 0.1%) (Vollstad *et al.*, 2006). Despite the differences observed in SGR, no significant differences were found in mortality between any of the groups when infected with atypical *A. salmonicida* (Vollstad *et al.*, 2006). In Atlantic cod (*Gadus morhua*) fed with 0.01%, 0.06% and 0.1% of alginate, an increase in the SGR was observed in all groups compared to fish fed a control diet (Vollstad *et al.*, 2006). These contrasting observations suggest a species specificity in response to alginate extracts in the diet.

Astaxanthin

This is another algae-derived compound evaluated as an immunostimulant in fish. It is a high-value carotenoid produced from microalgae with anti-inflammatory activity and antioxidant benefits, and enhances the release of the proinflammatory cytokines IL-1-β and TNF-α (Guerin *et al.*, 2003; Higuera-Ciapara *et al.*, 2006; Lorenz and Cysewski, 2000). In carp fed with an astaxanthin-supplemented diet, an increase in RBC and WBC, haemoglobin, haematocrit, and a better survival curve was registered against *A. hydrophila* (Jagruthi *et al.*, 2014).

Navicula

Another immunostimulant used as an additive is the marine diatom *Navicula* sp., a boat-shaped alga belonging to the family Naviculaceae rich in antioxidant carotenoids and vitamins (Patil *et al.*, 2007). Silage microalgae *Navicula* enriched with *Lactobacillus sakei* enhanced immunity in gilthead seabream (Reyes-Becerril *et al.*, 2013). This effect was evaluated in separate diets in a different fish species, Pacific red snapper (*Lutjanus peru*), showing increased growth rate, humoral immune response and antioxidant capabilities in fish supplemented with *Navicula* + *L. sakei* (a probiotic) or *L. sakei* alone (Reyes-Becerril *et al.*, 2014).

Porphyridium cruentum

For *Porphyridium cruentum* extracts, efforts have focused on the evaluation of derivatives mainly administered to fish through artemia and rotifers enriched with this algae (Conceição *et al.*, 2001; Makridis *et al.*, 2009; Skjermo and Bergh, 2004; Skjermo *et al.*, 1995). In fish, the only reported study whose administration strategy was via artemia and rotifers was in Senegalese sole (*Solea senegalensis*) using lyophilized red algae as an immunostimulant (*Porphyridium cruentum*). Using a commercial diet routinely employed on farms, no statistical differences were found for the respiratory burst activity of phagocytes (Díaz-Rosales *et al.*, 2008). A similar result was observed when fish larvae were immunostimulated with high-M alginate-enriched artemia in halibut (Skjermo and Bergh, 2004) and turbot (Skjermo *et al.*, 1995). However, Conceição *et al.* (2001) reported that turbot larvae fed with rotifers enriched with alginate capsules containing 86% mannuronic acid polymers (FMI) had a threefold higher protein turnover compared to the control group. The authors suggested this may contribute to higher larval viability and survival in case of environmental/disease stress (Conceição *et al.*, 2001). The rich alginate compounds contributed to an improved survival rate against *Vibrio anguillarum* both in juvenile turbot (Skjermo *et al.*, 1995) and halibut larvae (Skjermo and Bergh, 2004). The high-M alginate has a stimulatory effect on human monocytes, inducing the expression of TNF-alpha (Espevik *et al.*, 1993; Otterlei *et al.*, 1991). TNF-alpha production was induced by TLR2 and TLR4/MD-2 receptor complexes and membrane CD14 in humans and mice (Flo *et al.*, 2002) with response intensity correlating to the molecular weight of high-M alginate (Otterlei *et al.*, 1993). Thus, alginate-dependent TNF-alpha production may be involved in the observed increase in survival of halibut and turbot larvae against *V. anguillarum*.

Spirulina platensis

Spirulina platensis, which belongs to the Cyanobacteria (blue-green algae) family, can upregulate IL-1-beta and TNF-alpha mRNAs, increase phagocytic activity and superoxide anion production in carp leucocytes (Watanuki *et al.*, 2006) while in rainbow trout, increases in haematoimmune parameters (RBC, WBC, total protein) and decreases in plasma cortisol and glucose were observed (Yeganeh *et al.*, 2015). The decreases in the latter have been previously reported (Ngugi *et al.*, 2015), confirming the need to further investigate the effects and mechanisms of immunostimulants on the stress response.

Spirulina platensis does not have a cellulose cell wall and therefore fish can digest it (Karkos *et al.*, 2008); however, some non-digestible components such as dietary fibre have been introduced as diet supplements. Vitacel, a pure raw fibre composed of cellulose and hemicelluloses, has shown in rainbow trout fed with 10 g/kg an increase in serum lysozyme, ACH50, bactericidal activity. The increase in plasma lysozyme was also reported in sturgeon, although with a greater amount administrated (13 g/kg) (Heidarieh *et al.*, 2011). Also, feeding with Vitacel decreased cumulative mortality after challenge with *A. hydrophila* (Yarahmadi *et al.*, 2014). Importantly, HSP70 gene expression was downregulated (Yarahmadi *et al.*, 2014). The downregulation of HSP70 has been reported in fish fed a supplemented diet (Yang *et al.*, 2015), so the effect of immunostimulant diets on the expression of stress-related genes may be an interesting area for study. The effects of Vitacel have also been evaluated in the giant sturgeon (*Huso huso*) fed with 1.3% Vitacel per kg of food. The results showed an increase in plasma lysozyme activity after 15 and 90 days, and also an increase in number of neutrophil and eosinophil cells after 90 days (Heidarieh *et al.*, 2011). Thus, the administration of Vitacel may enhance the innate immune system and growth performance in juvenile sturgeon.

Ganoderma lucidum

Ganoderma lucidum (GL) is a mushroom whose polysaccharides have been reported to be effective in modulating immune responses, inhibiting tumour growth, preventing oxidative damage and activating B lymphocytes (Yin *et al.*, 2009; You and Lin 2002; Zhang *et al.*, 2002).

Lentinula edodes

The medicinal mushroom *Lentinula edodes* as a supplement in trout diets induced an increase in the number of total leucocytes (percentage of monocytes and neutrophils was higher but lymphocytes were lower), phagocytic and lysozyme activity and serum IgM levels. When fish were challenged against *Lactococcus garvieae*, higher survival was observed in fish fed with the *L. edodes* extract (Baba *et al.*, 2015).

Diets Containing Pathogen-Associated Molecular Patterns

Activation of the immune response in the presence of pathogens requires that the host recognizes specific and structurally conserved components that are produced by the pathogen. These conserved components are called pathogen-associated molecular patterns (PAMPs) and are typically lipopolysaccharide (LPS), peptidoglycan (PGN), lipoproteins, flagellin, CpG DNA and muramyl dipeptide (MDP) from bacteria, fungal beta-glucans and zymosan, and double-stranded RNA (dsRNA) from virus. PAMP recognition is mediated by pathogen recognition receptors (PRRs) that are structurally and functionally conserved between vertebrates, invertebrates and plants, and allow the host to distinguish among different classes of pathogen in order to mount an appropriate immune response. This immune response is mediated through the induction of inflammatory cytokines, chemokines and co-stimulatory molecules that facilitate leucocyte recruitment to the site of the infection, activation of adaptive immunity and activation of antimicrobial effectors (Boltaña *et al.*, 2011a; Janeway and Medzhitov, 2002).

Throughout the last 15 years, the use of PAMPs as immunostimulants has been reported for several different species. Beta-glucans are commonly used in immunostimulant diets for aquaculture. This major structural component of yeast and fungal cell walls is widely used in fish diets as an additive in commercial supplements such as Biosaf, DVAQUA, Ecoactiva, Ergosan, Fibosel, MacroGard and VitaStim. We have also included commentaries on chitin, lipolysaccharides , mannan-oligosaccharides (MOS), peptidoglycans and yeast extracts.

Beta-Glucan

The PAMP most commonly used in dietary immunostimulants is beta-glucan, which has been directly studied as an extract from *S. cerevisiae* or in one of its commercial forms (MacroGard, Sigma). The effect of MacroGard dietary immunostimulation upon the expression of selected inflammatory genes in carp has been studied (TNF-1-alpha, TNF-2-alpha-, IL-1-beta, IL-6 family and IL-10) in gut and head kidney after 14 days of feeding. TNF-2-alpha was significantly downregulated in gut and head kidney, IL-10 was downregulated in gut, and a posterior challenge with *A. salmonicida* stimulated the production of TNF-1-alpha and TNF-2-alpha at 6 hpi in the head kidney (Falco *et al.*, 2012). Also, in carp fed with MacroGard for 25 days, it was observed that most of the selected cytokines analysed (IL-1-beta, IL-10, TNF-1-alpha, TNF-2-alpha and CXCa) were downregulated although expression of Mx mRNA transcripts was increased in liver, head kidney, spleen and mid-gut after challenge with dsRNA (Falco *et al.*, 2014). In another study in carp fed with MacroGard, an increase in alternative complement activity was reported after 25 days of feeding and this was detected in conjuncton with regulation of several complement-related mRNA transcripts at seven and 25 days in the liver and head kidney. The fish also had high serum CRP levels after seven days (Pionnier *et al.*, 2014). In the mid-gut after seven days, Bf/C2, C3 and MAP2 were upregulated, and CRP2 and C3 were also upregulated at 25 days of feeding. A follow-on PAMP challenge using LPS or poly (I:C) as immunostimulants reported regulation of CRP and complement-related gene expression profiles, with a significant effect in fish fed with beta-glucan; however, for CRP levels, and serum complement activity, the effect was lower than in control fish. The authors suggested that beta-glucan immunostimulation was sufficient enough to reduce the effects of a PAMP challenge (Pionnier *et al.*, 2014).

The use of beta-glucan (Sigma) in a basal diet for one week reported no significant differences for orally administered beta-glucan compared to control diets for bacterial killing, O_2^- production/NBT or survival to *A. hydrophila* infection (Selvaraj *et al.*, 2005). In contrast, in Rohu (*Labeo rohita*) fingerlings fed four different diets containing 100, 250 or 500 mg of Sigma beta-glucan/kg over 56 days, immune parameters including leucocyte count, phagocytic ratio, phagocytic index, lysozyme activity, complement activity and serum bactericidal activity were affected. Highest levels were reported 42 days after feeding with the 250 mg beta-glucan/kg diet in parallel with a significant reduction in mortality compared to control during *A. hydrophila* and *E. tarda* infection (Misra *et al.*, 2006). Sahoo and Mukherjee (2001) described that fish fed for one week with beta-glucan at a dose of 0.1% showed an increase in bacterial agglutination, haemagglutination and haemolysin titre, bactericidal activity, serum phagocytic ratio, serum phagocytic index and serum leucocrit compared with control; an increase in survival to *A. hydrophila* challenge was also reported. These data suggest that in Rohu, administration of beta-glucan has a protective effect against bacterial pathogens. The effect of a combined diet of beta-glucan and LPS (0.1% beta-glucan + 0.025% LPS, 0.5% beta-glucan + 0.125% LPS, 1% beta-glucan + 0.25% LPS) administered for one, seven and 14 days and analysed after 16 days was an increase in bactericidal activity compared to control fish. An increase in survival against *A. hydrophila* was observed in the fish fed with the highest dose; 1% beta-glucan + 0.25% LPS (Selvaraj *et al.*, 2006). Interestingly, administration of a LPS-only diet at doses of 1, 2.5 and 5 mg did not show any protective effect or increased antibody titre to an *A. hydrophila* challenge (Selvaraj *et al.*, 2009).

Beta-glucan extracts in the diet of the large yellow croaker, *Larimichthys crocea*, at doses of 0.09% and 0.18% over eight weeks produced an increase in serum lysozyme content and phagocytic and respiratory burst activity in head kidney macrophages at the lower doses. In addition, a reduction in mortality rate was reported after *V. harveyi* challenge (Ai *et al.*, 2007). In the Nile tilapia, *Oreochromis niloticus*, fed with 0.1% beta-glucan, an increase in the above mentioned parameters was also reported in addition to increases in serum bactericidal activity, serum NO and lymphocyte transformation index after 21 days of diet (El-Boshy *et al.*, 2010). In tilapia fed with 10 g/kg of Biosaf (commercial extract) an increase in the same immunological parameters was reported, except the lymphocyte transformation index had no significant differences (El-Boshy *et al.*, 2010). Again after challenge with *A. hydrophila*, a reduction in the mortality rate was reported (El-Boshy *et al.*, 2010). These data suggest that beta-glucans are effective in this group of fish species.

The effect of EcoActiva, another commercial beta-glucan, in snapper diets at 0.1% in winter and summer seasons during 84 days was reported by Cook *et al.* (2003). During the winter season, an increase in respiratory burst activity of head kidney macrophages was observable even at 56 days post diet administration but when administrated in the summer season, this parameter increased only at day 28, suggesting important temperature-related effects upon diet efficacy (Cook *et al.*, 2003).

The commercial extracts Fibosel and VitaStim (1 g/kg of feed, 10 g/kg of feed) were tested in the gilthead sea bream, *Sparus aurata*, and the study highlighted an increase in spleen macrophage respiratory burst activity at lower doses with both supplements and also at higher doses using Fibosel. Importantly, both immunostimulants caused a significant reduction in mortality rate after *P. damselae subsp. piscicida* bath challenge (Couso *et al.*, 2003). European sea bass, *Dicentrachus labrax*, fed with 2% MacroGard for two weeks every three months showed increased serum complement activity and plasma lysozyme activity at the end of three cycles (Bagni *et al.*, 2000). Further studies have shown that MacroGard at 0.1% for 15 days also increased serum complement activity, serum lysozyme activity and gill HSP70 content at 30 days from the end of the treatment period. In contrast, when the diet was administered over a longer term (four cycles of 15 days every 60 days), no effect was found (Bagni *et al.*, 2005).

In salmonid fish, many reports have focused on evaluating the immunostimulant effect of beta-glucan but the capacity of dietary beta-glucan to stimulate the immune system remains unclear. In 1994, Siwicki *et al.* described the effect of different beta-glucan-containing feeds including MacroGard 0.2 g/100 g, *C. utilis* 2.7 g/100 g, *S. cerevisiae* 2.7 g/100 g and a deacylated chitin 0.5 g/100 g formulation in rainbow trout over sevem days. In all diets the respiratory burst activity in blood, phagocytic index, MPO activity, serum total Ig and blood bactericidal killing activities increased after one week (Siwicki *et al.*, 1994). However, Kunttu *et al.* (2009) administered MacroGard at doses of 0.2%, 0.6% and 1.8%, and were only able to report an increase in blood respiratory burst activity at the two higher doses after 21 days. In another parallel study in rainbow trout, MacroGard at a dose of 4.5 g/kg of feed and a beta-glucan extracted from *H. vulgare* at 12.2, 16.7 and 26.4 g/kg of diet were compared for nine weeks. None of these treatments was able to immunostimulate any of the measured parameters (Sealey *et al.*, 2008).

An interesting study was carried out by Ghaedi *et al.* (2015) in which they fed 4 kg female rainbow trout broodstock for three months prior to spawning with 0.1% and 0.2% of MacroGard and a control diet. Their fry were then fed the same doses of the immunostimulant diet for two months (Ghaedi *et al.*, 2015). Broodstock fish fed with 0.2% beta-glucan diet had the highest levels of ACH50 and lysozyme activity. The total serum Ig and IgM content was significantly higher for both doses in comparison to controls. The descendent fry fed with the immunostimulant diets showed increases in ACH50, lysozyme, total Ig and IgM and also a significant increase in survival, but the fry descended from the IS diet fed broodstock did not show any transgenerational gain in immunity (Ghaedi *et al.*, 2015). The effects of beta-glucan diets in trout have been difficult to pin down, with contrasting results published. The response of salmonid fish to beta-glucan clearly requires further study.

Finally, in the Asian catfish (*Clarias batrachus*), diets containing beta-glucan and synthetic levamisole (Sigma) were evaluated. Interestingly, increased respiratory burst activity in blood was reported in conjunction with an increase in leucocyte myeloperoxidase content 31 days post diet for both treatments (Kumari and Sahoo, 2006).

Overall, it appears that beta-glucans have a strong effect upon measured blood parameters such as respiratory burst across all fish species, suggesting that a direct impact upon blood leucocyte populations is a generic response to this PAMP. However, the underpinning mechanisms of this activity remain unknown.

Saccharomyces cerevisiae

The effect of baker's yeast extract (*S. cerevisiae*), a supplement containing both nucleotides and beta-glucan, upon immune parameters in carp after 10 days of feeding demonstrated immunostimulation (Biswas *et al.*, 2012). The expression of proinflammatory cytokines, including IL-1-beta, TNF-alpha, IL-12p35, IL-12p40 and IFN-gamma-2, was significantly increased in the head kidney after one day and the expression of CXC-chemokines was increased after one, five and seven days of feeding. Interestingly, a concurrent reduction of IL-10 gene expression was reported, suggesting an inflammatory response to the diet. O_2^- production and phagocytic activity in head kidney leucocytes increased at three days in fish fed with the IS diet and phagocytic activity increased both at one and three days. A parallel increase in resistance to bacterial infection was observed at six hours post injection of *A. hydrophila* in IS diet-fed fish (Biswas *et al.*, 2012). A longer trial, 60 days, was reported using microbial levan at 0.25%, 0.5%, 0.75%, 1.0% and 1.25% in juvenile Rohu. Within the treatment groups, albumin/globulin ratios globally decreased in a dose-dependent manner whereas haemoglobin content, total leucocyte count and serum total protein increased with supplementation at 1% or more. A gradual concomitant increase in serum lysozyme activity and respiratory burst activity was observed, with the highest activity in the 0.75% and 1.0% levan groups. A reduction of mortality rate for all levan diet-fed fish was reported in challenges with *A. hydrophila* (Gupta *et al.*, 2008).

In sea bream and sea bass, the most frequently studied dietary additives have been derived from yeast cultures, by adding the whole yeast (Cuesta *et al.*, 2004; He *et al.*, 2009; Ortuño *et al.*, 2002; Rodríguez *et al.*, 2003), the yeast cell walls (Yu *et al.*, 2014) and also extracts such as MOS (Torrecillas *et al.*, 2007), chitin (Cuesta *et al.*, 2004; Esteban *et al.*, 2001) and beta-glucan, either extracted directly (Ai *et al.*, 2007; El-Boshy *et al.*, 2010) or using commercially available additives such as Biosaf (El-Boshy *et al.*, 2010), VitaStim (Couso *et al.*, 2003), Sanictum (Kirchhoff *et al.*, 2011), EcoActiva (Cook *et al.*, 2003), Fibosel (Couso *et al.*, 2003) and MacroGard (Bagni *et al.*, 2000, 2005; Couso *et al.*, 2003).

Whole yeast preparations at doses of 1, 5 and 10 g/kg were fed for four weeks to gilthead sea bream and significant effects increased respiratory burst activity, phagocytic ability, natural cytotoxic activity and MPO content in the head kidney of sea bream leucocytes in a dose-dependent manner (Ortuño *et al.*, 2002). Increases in serum IgM content two weeks after treatment were also reported (Cuesta *et al.*, 2004). Rodriguez *et al.* (2003) evaluated the effect of a modified strain of *S. cerevisiae* (fsk-1) which has a lower glucan and higher chitin composition in the cell wall and reported that at doses of 10 g/kg of feed, serum lysozyme, phagocytic ability and capacity were increased whereas serum complement activity and peroxidase content decreased after six weeks of the diet (Rodríguez *et al.*, 2003). In Japanese sea bass, *Lateolabrax japonicas*, yeast cell wall (YCW) supplementation at doses of 250, 500, 1000,

2000 and 20 000 mg/kg was examined in a 72-day trial. No significant effect was observed for C3 activity, IgM levels, myeloperoxidase content, respiratory burst or anti-O_2^- content but 500 mg/kg of YCW did increase cumulative survival of sea bass challenged with *A. veronii* (Yu *et al.*, 2014).

The commercial product DVAQUA (product of fermentation of *S. cerevisiae*) was used in doses of 0.125, 0.25, 0.50, 1.0 and 2.0 g/kg of feed in hybrid tilapia (*Oreochromis niloticus* ♀ *x O. aureus* ♂) for eight weeks. An increase in serum lysozyme activity, serum C3 and C4 content and macrophage phagocytic activity isolated from head kidney at the end of the eight weeks was reported for all dosages whereas an increase in head kidney macrophage respiratory burst activity was evident at 0.125, 0.25 and 1.0 g/kg of DVAQUA (He *et al.*, 2009).

Chitin

Chitin (poly [1→4]-β-N-acetyl-D-glucosamine) is an insoluble polysaccharide present in the exoskeleton of shellfish and insects and in the cell walls of fungi. The synthetic compound was used to test immunostimulatory ability in gilthead sea bream with doses of 25, 50 and 100 mg/kg of feed over six weeks. All doses induced an increase in natural haemolytic complement activity and head kidney-leucocyte natural cytotoxic activity after two weeks. Furthermore, increased head kidney-leucocyte respiratory burst activity was also reported after four weeks (Esteban *et al.*, 2001). Interestingly, at a concentration of 25 mg/kg, an increase in the total content of serum IgM was identified after six weeks (Cuesta *et al.*, 2004).

Other derivatives of yeast have also been used, including MOS (extracted from *S. cerevisiae*) which when administered at 4% in the diet over a nine-week period caused an increase in phagocytic macrophage HK-activity in European sea bass. This same diet when tested in a *V. alginolyticus* co-habitation challenge model produced a significant reduction in infected fish at doses of 2% and no infected fish were found at 4% of MOS (Torrecillas *et al.*, 2007).

In rainbow trout, diets enriched with peptidoglycan (PGN), a key component of the bacterial cell wall, have been evaluated. The expression of antimicrobial peptides (AMP) was analysed in fish fed with PG for 14 days and at higher PG doses a scaled expression pattern was induced over time where defensins were typically expressed early and cathelicidins and LEAPs later on in the course of the experiment (Casadei *et al.*, 2013). A withdrawal of PG diets at day 14 resulted in a fall in expression level of AMPs that was particularly apparent with cathelicidins and LEAP expression whereas defensins remained at high levels (Casadei *et al.*, 2015). In rainbow trout fed with 20 μg/kg/day of bacterial LPS (extracted from *P. agglomerans*) for 93 days, bactericidal activity, lysozyme activity, blood haemolytic activity and respiratory burst were found to increase in comparison to controls (Skalli *et al.*, 2013). In contrast, previous studies in Atlantic salmon fry fed LPS extracted from *A. salmonicida* at a concentration of 0.1% for 62 days did not reveal changes in plasma immunoglobulin levels (Guttvik *et al.*, 2002).

Receptors Mediating Immunostimulation Via PAMPs

In the last decade there has been growing interest in the use of plant, herb and algae extracts as immunostimulant dietary supplements in fish. However, in most cases the mechanisms responsible for the underpinning physiological response in fish are still unknown (Reverter *et al.*, 2014). The Toll-like receptors (TLRs) are an archetypal group of pathogen recognition receptors (PRRs) that are type I transmembrane proteins associated with the innate immune response involved in the sensing of microbial-specific molecular structures (PAMPs). This is probably the most studied group of PRRs in all vertebrates, including fish. PAMP recognition may occur in various cellular compartments, including the plasma membrane, endosomes, lysosomes and endolysosomes (Akira *et al.*, 2006). TLRs activate pathways through a variety of TIR-domain-containing adaptor proteins responsible for cell signalling cascade activation, such as MyD88 and TRIF, which activate transcription factors (NF-kappa-B, IRFs) and mitogen-activated protein kinases (MAPKs) to promote a proinflammatory response (Kawai and Akira, 2010), thus modulating innate and adaptive immune response. In teleosts, there are more than 17 TLRs identified (Tanekhy, 2016) with evolutionary conservation of key components of the TLR-signalling pathway (Purcell *et al.*, 2007). However, fish TLRs also exhibit very distinct features and significant diversity (Palti, 2011).

Although many civilizations have used natural extracts for centuries, several studies in mammals have shown that plants extracts modulate TLRs (Chahal *et al.*, 2013). Thus, some plants and algae compounds can downregulate mRNA expression (Arora *et al.*, 2016; Robertson *et al.*, 2015; Zhong *et al.*, 2014) and induction (Granica *et al.*, 2015; Nguyen *et al.*, 2015) of TLRs, suppressing the TLR/NF-kappa-B signalling pathway (Kim *et al.*, 2014). Conversely, other extracts promote the proinflammatory response (Ghochikyan *et al.*, 2014) and enhance TLR9 and IRF7 activation, inducing interferon (IFN)-beta protein expression (Lin *et al.*, 2015). These extracts also elicit the M1 and M2 macrophage response through the TLR/NF-kappa-B signalling pathway (Ryu *et al.*, 2015). In fish, the effects of plant, herbal and algal extracts have been poorly described. Only one study using a zebrafish model suggests an anti-inflammatory effect of leuropein (primary phenolic compound present in olive leaf) by inhibiting TLR and MAPK signalling (Ryu *et al.*, 2015).

In general, the phytochemical subcomponents of plant-derived extracts are diverse, including phenolics, terpenoids, polysaccharides and proteins. Thus, the extraction solvent is important in determining the final composition of the extract. In this respect, it has been demonstrated while aqueous extracts reduce TLR activation, ethanolic extracts from the same plant increased activation of the same TLRs (Ahn *et al.*, 2006a,b; Nakaya *et al.*, 2004; Pannacci *et al.*, 2006; Rhule *et al.*, 2008). Therefore, it seems that not only the nature of the plant-derived extract is important to determine the immunomodulatory effect, but also the extraction method employed. In conclusion, it appears that it is essential to address the implications of the extraction method for plant-derived compounds. The nature of the potential regulatory ligands also requires further study in order to understand the linkage between the extracts and functional TLR outputs, whether stimulatory or inhibitory. This area has significant potential, reaching beyond fish to a possible impact upon human health.

One of the most commonly used strategies to stimulate the immune system in fish is the administration of purified immunostimulants in the diet. This strategy follows the premise of recognition, identification and response to PAMPs which can be used to modulate immunological activity. To date, the most commonly used PAMPs in fish immunostimulant diets are lipopolysaccharide (LPS), peptidoglycan (PGN) and beta-glucans. In mammals, LPS, a component of the outer membrane of Gram-negative bacteria, recognized by TLR4, forms a complex with co-receptors lymphocyte antigen 96 (MD2) and CD14 on the cell surface that serves as the main LPS-binding component leading to activation of multiple signalling components and the subsequent production of proinflammatory cytokines (Park and Lee, 2013). The utilization of LPS as an immunostimulant for fish seems to be contradictory as fish, and most non-mammalian vertebrates, are highly resistant to the toxic effects of LPS (Swain *et al.*,

2008), due to the significant evolutionary differences observed between these two groups in terms of TLR4. The vast majority of fish do not express TLR4 and neither CD14 nor MD2 has been isolated (Tanekhy, 2016).

Thus, it has been proposed for fish that (1) LPS interacts with alternative factors such as beta-2-integrins which are abundantly expressed on rainbow trout mononuclear phagocytes after stimulation with high concentrations of LPS (Iliev *et al.*, 2005); and (2) TLR4 negatively regulates the MyD88-dependent TLR pathway (Sepulcre *et al.*, 2009). PGN is the basic component of the bacterial cell wall. In mammals, PGN activates both the TLR2 and NOD pathways but does not activate TLR4-mediated signal transduction (Girardin *et al.*, 2003; Schwandner *et al.*, 1999). In rainbow trout macrophages, PGN stimulation induced the expression of MyD88, IRAK and TNF activated factor (TRAF6), suggesting TLR involvement in PGN-mediated inflammatory response in trout (Boltaña *et al.*, 2011b). Interestingly, both compounds are likely to be present in most PAMP preparations unless ultra-pure compounds are used. This is unlikely and not economical for IS diet production for aquaculture so a mixture of potentially antagonist effects is probably occurring as each signalling pathway is activated, influencing the final response outcome.

The most commonly used PAMPs included in immunostimulant diets are the beta-glucans, the major structural components of yeast and fungal cell walls. Beta-glucans consist of a heterogeneous group of glucose polymers also named beta-1,3/1,6-glucans. In mammals, although various receptors such as complement receptor C3 and TLR1/6 have been described (Dalmo and Bøgwald, 2008), dectin-1 is considered to be the main beta-glucan receptor (Brown and Gordon, 2003). However, dectin-1 has not been identified in fish and it has been suggested that beta-glucan could be detected by TLRs although the actual target receptor is unknown (Pietretti *et al.*, 2013).

Despite growing knowledge of the mechanisms involved in the TLR-mediated fish innate immune response, more efforts are needed to determine the underlying effects upon the recognition and activation of the fish immune response by PAMP-associated immunostimulants. The complex composition of immunostimulant extracts from plant, algal and microbial sources makes the identification of specific activation/suppression pathways and receptor-ligand relationships particularly difficult. When economic constraints are also taken into consideration for the application of a complex IS diet, understanding the underlying immune response is a significant challenge.

Oral Vaccination

Vaccines are available for several aquaculture fish species; most target bacterial pathogens and only a few have been raised against viruses (Embregts and Forlenza, 2016). Commercially available vaccines are administered orally (by mixing with the feed), by immersion (dip or bath) or injection through the intraperitoneal or intramuscular route. Recently, a new strategy using nasal-associated lymphoid tissue has been reported, resulting in a reportedly high protection in trout (Salinas *et al.*, 2015). While protection is generally highest with injection-based vaccination, this approach is also associated with intensive handling and by consequence increased stress for the fish. There is also a size element in that fish that are too small to be injected are usually vaccinated orally or by immersion. The oral administration of vaccines is a very attractive route for antigen delivery for aquaculture as it offers a simple route to deliver antigen with almost no human manipulation. This method is considered less stressful, therefore resulting in increased fish welfare and no side effects have been reported so far. On the other hand, the low efficacy and short protection reported are significant disadvantages of this vaccination method. For these reasons, a combination of oral, immersion and injection vaccination during the life cycle of the fish is suggested to ensure protection (Embregts and Forlenza, 2016). Taking into account the total number of commercially available fish vaccines, a small portion are orally administered (Brudeseth *et al.*, 2013; Dhar *et al.*, 2014; Sommerset *et al.*, 2005) and have been deployed in a few countries, mainly those involved in Atlantic salmon aquaculture (Chile, Norway and Scotland). These vaccine preparations only provide short-term protection and are mostly used as a primer or booster vaccination (Brudeseth *et al.*, 2013)

The low efficacy observed in oral vaccines is probably due to antigen degradation during passage through the stomach, reducing structural integrity and absorption in the second segment of the intestine that has being identified as the main site for antigen uptake (Fujino *et al.*, 1987; Georgopoulou *et al.*, 1986; Iida and Yamamoto 1985; Noaillac-Depeyre and Gas, 1973; Rombout and Berg, 1989; Stroband and Kroon, 1981). Furthermore, it is very difficult to determine individual dosage as the only possible quantifier is to calculate the amount of feed on average consumed by the population. In this context, the quantity of antigen per pellet is also difficult to address as the distribution of the antigen in the feed may be uneven (for top-coating in powder or liquid), or when the antigen is mixed with the feed the impact of the high temperatures in the extrusion process may impact upon antigen integrity. Thus, the combination of several parameters that are difficult to control probably contributes to the compromised outcome of oral immunizations that is often reported.

Current licensed oral vaccines for fish are all formulated on heat-killed or formalin-killed pathogens and the majority are enteric pathogens or those affecting mucosal organs. Orally administered antigens are taken up and transported via the end-gut, and if an adequate amount of antigen reaches this segment, local as well as systemic antibody responses are induced in fish (Rombout *et al.*, 1986). These vaccines incorporate an antigen-protecting vehicle or the MicroMatrix delivery system. These vehicles aim to protect the antigens from gastric degradation and promote antigen uptake by enhancing adhesion to mucosal surfaces (Embregts and Forlenza, 2016). Tobar *et al.* (2015) reported prolonged protection against *P. salmonis* and the ISA virus upon oral administration of MicroMatrix-encapsulated vaccines at repeated intervals over 10 days. This protection was correlated to a high serum IgM and when serum IgM decreased, a window of susceptibility to infection was reported, suggesting an association between antibody levels and fish protective status (Tobar *et al.*, 2015).

Gut Immunity

In teleost fish, a layer of mucus containing antimicrobial peptides, complement factors, immunoglobulins and other surface host defence proteins such as the defensins covers the mucosal surface of the gut. Gut-associated lymphoid tissue (GALT) containing resident monocytes and macrophages and intraepithelial B- and T-lymphocytes is present where teleost B-cells have phagocytic properties (Li *et al.*, 2006; Zhang *et al.*, 2010). The immunoglobin IgT in the gut has been shown to coat commensal gut bacteria (Zhang *et al.*, 2010) and mucosal antigen uptake is linked to the expression of both proinflammatory cytokines, including IL-1-beta, TNF-alpha and IL-8, in the gut (Buchmann 1999; Chettri *et al.*, 2014; Kai *et al.*, 2014), and chemokines such as CCR6, CCR9B, CXCL10 and CK12 that are expressed in response to antigen delivery through the gut mucosa (Baoprasertkul *et al.*, 2004; Dixon *et al.*, 2013; Montero *et al.*, 2011). These data collectively suggest that gut vaccination may develop the same response as parental vaccination.

In respect of immunoglobulins in the gut, IgM, IgD and IgT (or IgZ) have been detected in teleost fish. IgT is specialized at mucosal surfaces and can account for the largest proportion of the B-cell population found in the gut (Chen *et al.*, 2015). Several studies have also shown that CD8-alpha (marker for activated cytotoxic T-lymphocytes (CTLs) in fish) accounts for the largest proportion of T-lymphocytes in the gut of fish (Chen *et al.*, 2014; Min *et al.*, 2012; Plant and LaPatra, 2011) and its activation may correspond to the elimination of cells infected with intracellular pathogens. As for CD4 responses in fish, transcription factors for their specification into Th1 and Th2 subtypes have been characterized: T-bet, GATA-3 and FoxP3 (Kumari *et al.*, 2009; Mitra *et al.*, 2010; Munang'andu *et al.*, 2013; Takizawa *et al.*, 2014; Wang *et al.*, 2010a,b; Zhang *et al.*, 2011). These data suggest that the gut mucosa of finfish is endowed with a cellular-mediated immune response orchestrated by CD4 and CD8 proteins expressed in response to mucosal vaccination. However, the major caveat that impedes the development of this methodology remains the effective delivery of intact antigen to the target cell population. In order to achieve this, significant research activity has been devoted to developing and testing different delivery systems.

Non-encapsulated Vaccines

Many efforts have been reported for the development of oral vaccines of non-encapsulated antigens such as inactivated bacteria, yeast, plants or commensal bacteria expressing antigens. However, only very short-term protection has been achieved, 2–3 months after vaccination, and consecutive administrations did not demonstrate any significant difference in protection observed from a single application (Choi *et al.*, 2011; Huang *et al.*, 2014; Kondo *et al.*, 2003; Li *et al.*, 2015; Tu *et al.*, 2010). Several methods using enteric pathogens that do not affect fish or commensal microbes as vaccine vehicles have showed promising levels of protection (Anuradha *et al.*, 2010; Cui *et al.*, 2015; Lu *et al.*, 2011; Nur-Nazifah *et al.*, 2014). Live commensals might retain their ability to colonize the gut and persist long enough to deliver antigen to mucosal surfaces but in contrast, due to host tolerance the response to antigen may not be sufficient to trigger strong local responses and promote long-term protection (Embregts and Forlenza, 2016). Yeasts are a well-characterized system to express antigens where the yeast wall can protect the antigen from degradation in the stomach, and also may act as an adjuvant as it is rich in beta-glucans. Recently, high efficacy was reported against rock bream iridovirus (RBIV) using a feed containing lyophilized rice callus expressing the major capsid protein of RBIV (Shin *et al.*, 2013), highlighting the potential utility of using antigens produced in plants.

Encapsulated Oral Vaccines

In contrast with the whole bacteria, yeast- or plant-derived vaccines based upon purified proteins, plasmid DNA and recombinant protein subunits need protection to avoid breakdown in the stomach. This is essential for proper delivery and uptake in the second segment of the intestine and the main driver to develop different methods for antigen encapsulation. In fish, specifically in the Atlantic salmon, cells that are equivalent in function to the mammalian microfold cells (M cells) that are able to uptake gold-BSA particles have been identified (Fuglem *et al.*, 2010). This cellular characteristic further strengthens the case for microencapsulation as a promising field for oral vaccine delivery. Microencapsulation for oral vaccines has been addressed using alginate particles, nanoparticles of poly D,L-lactic-co-glycolic acid (PGLA), chitosan, liposomes, MicroMatrix and biofilms or artemia (Mutoloki *et* al., 2015; Plant and LaPatra, 2011; Tafalla *et al.*, 2013). Alginate-encapsulated vaccines have been the most successful, probably due to the ability of alginate to protect the antigen from degradation in the stomach, and also the ability to diffuse through the gut mucus layer where it might be actively taken up by M cells, thus mimicking a natural route of infection.

In summary, oral vaccines have huge potential that needs to be exploited as this method of delivering protection is highly desirable within aquaculture production systems. The development of new methods for the production and encapsulation of antigen that improve delivery, therefore creating a long-term response, is essential. Underlying these efforts are the continuing research that will provide a better understanding of the immune response following oral vaccination and therefore be able to drive and direct formulation strategies.

Future Perspectives

There has been a significant amount of information generated from research on immunostimulants in fish. Research has investigated many different species that cover the entire range of finfish aquaculture and represent many different and distinct environments, each with advantages and limitations. Furthermore, each has a different set of potential threats although on the whole, most IS diet studies have focused upon response to bacterial disease. For the immunostimulants themselves, a diverse range of compounds and extracts have been tested, many of them in very different formulations that reflect intensive to semi-intensive aquaculture systems. In view of the actual dosage of immunostimulant and extract contents, that is the active ingredients that experimental fish are exposed to and the difficulty in measuring the IS compounds, it is difficult to reconcile realistic doses with observed responses. However, in some cases clear dose–response thresholds have been described. Overall, few studies have been able to record a clear dose-dependent effect that translates to increased immune response although increased survival to challenges after IS diet treatment has been regularly observed. The design of robust experiments, with detailed analyses, that seek to clarify these points will be of great advantage in understanding the impact of IS compounds upon the immune system in different species.

Interestingly the majority of studies report upon increasing values of haematological parameters including superoxide production, respiratory burst and myeloperoxidase activity, and often these are supported by PCR-based observation of gene expression in distinct tissues. Many studies have also directly measured both head kidney and splenic responses but have not addressed gut immunity. This aspect of immunity has been poorly developed in most fish species, particularly in omnivorous species such as tilapia that are farmed globally and are exposed to hugely different sources of nutrition and are grown over a wide environmental spectrum. It would seem likely that the gut-associated response would be the driver for these responses and therefore it may be useful to concentrate more attention upon this tissue in the future in order to understand the sequence of events leading to a modified outcome. This itself will contribute to the evaluation of immunomodulation in fish and the efficacy of the compounds chosen, leading to a more informed translational research effort. It will be critical to understand how IS compounds achieve systemic activation of the immune response and whether this represents a positive response for the treated fish. Chronically activated immune responses that are often of an inflammatory nature incur a significant metabolic cost that may influence growth rate.

In conclusion, the use of immunostimulant-containing diets in aquaculture is widespread and encompasses a wide diversity of products that range from large feed producers using yeast extracts to more local custom production often using traditional remedies and extracts. Although the use of IS diets is generally accepted, there is little agreement across the scientific literature as to which IS extracts and compounds produce a reliable and robust response in fish that leads to increased protection and survival. In fact, there remains much contradictory evidence in published research. It is very positive that the body of knowledge addressing the actions of IS diets is steadily increasing as the global aquaculture industry expands and this increased activity will pave the way to a more profound understanding of immunomodulation in fish through diet.

References

Abd-El-Rhman, A. M. M. (2009) Antagonism of *Aeromonas hydrophila* by propolis and its effect on the performance of Nile tilapia, *Oreochromis niloticus*. *Fish & Shellfish Immunology*, **27**, 454–9. doi:10.1016/j.fsi.2009.06.015

Abdel-Tawwab, M., Ahmad, M. H., Seden, M. E., *et al.* (2010) Use of green tea, *Camellia sinensis* L., in practical diet for growth and protection of Nile tilapia, *Oreochromis niloticus* (L.), against *Aeromonas hydrophila* infection. *Journal of the World Aquaculture Society*, **41**, 203–213. doi:10.1111/j.1749-7345.2010.00360.x

Abdel-Tawwab, M., Sharafeldin, K. M., Mosaad, M. N. M., *et al.* (2015) Coffee bean in common carp, *Cyprinus carpio* L. diets: Effect on growth performance, biochemical status, and resistance to waterborne zinc toxicity. *Aquaculture*, **448**, 207–213. doi:10.1016/j.aquaculture.2015.06.010

Abeysinghe, P. (2010) Antibacterial activity of some medicinal mangroves against antibiotic resistant pathogenic bacteria. *Indian Journal of Pharmaceutical Sciences*, **72**, 167–172.

Acar, Ü., Kesbiç, O. S., Yılmaz, S., *et al.* (2015) Evaluation of the effects of essential oil extracted from sweet orange peel (*Citrus sinensis*) on growth rate of tilapia (*Oreochromis mossambicus*) and possible disease resistance against *Streptococcus iniae*. *Aquaculture*, **437**, 282–286. doi:10.1016/j.aquaculture.2014.12.015

Adel, M., Abedian Amiri, A., Zorriehzahra, J., *et al.* (2015) Effects of dietary peppermint (*Mentha piperita*) on growth performance, chemical body composition and hematological and immune parameters of fry Caspian white fish (*Rutilus frisii kutum*). *Fish & Shellfish Immunology*, **45**, 841–847. doi:10.1016/j.fsi.2015.06.010

Agarwal, M., Walia, S., Dhingra, S., *et al.* (2001) Insect growth inhibition, antifeedant and antifungal activity of compounds isolated/ derived from *Zingiber officinale* Roscoe (ginger) rhizomes. *Pest Management Science*, **57**, 289–300. doi:10.1002/ps.263

Ahn, J. Y., Choi, I. S., Shim, J. Y., *et al.* (2006) The immunomodulator ginsan induces resistance to experimental sepsis by inhibiting Toll-like receptor-mediated inflammatory signals. *European Journal of Immunology*, **36**, 37–45. doi:10.1002/eji.200535138

Ahn, J. Y., Song, J. Y., Yun, Y. S., *et al.* (2006) Protection of *Staphylococcus aureus*-infected septic mice by suppression of early acute inflammation and enhanced antimicrobial activity by ginsan. *FEMS Immunology and Medical Microbiology*, **46**, 187–197. doi:10.1111/j.1574-695X.2005.00021.x

Ai, Q., Mai, K., Zhang, L., *et al.* (2007) Effects of dietary beta-1, 3 glucan on innate immune response of large yellow croaker, *Pseudosciaena crocea*. *Fish & Shellfish Immunology*, **22**, 394–402. doi:10.1016/j.fsi.2006.06.011

Akira, S., Uematsu, S., & Takeuchi, O. (2006) Pathogen recognition and innate immunity. *Cell*, **124**, 783–801. doi:10.1016/j.cell.2006.02.015

Aly, S. M., & Mohamed, M. F. (2010) *Echinacea purpurea* and *Allium sativum* as immunostimulants in fish culture using Nile tilapia (*Oreochromis niloticus*). *Journal of Animal Physiology and Animal Nutrition*, **94**. doi:10.1111/j.1439-0396.2009.00971.x

Anuradha, K., Foo, H. L., Mariana, N. S., *et al.* (2010) Live recombinant *Lactococcus lactis* vaccine expressing aerolysin genes D1 and D4 for protection against *Aeromonas hydrophila* in tilapia (*Oreochromis niloticus*). *Journal of Applied Microbiology*, **109**, no-no. doi:10.1111/j.1365-2672.2010.04789.x

Arora, N., Shah, K., & Pandey-Rai, S. (2016) Inhibition of imiquimod-induced psoriasis-like dermatitis in mice by herbal extracts from some Indian medicinal plants. *Protoplasma*, **253**, 503–515. doi:10.1007/s00709-015-0829-y

Awad, E., Austin, D., & Lyndon, A. R. (2013) Effect of black cumin seed oil (*Nigella sativa*) and nettle extract (Quercetin) on enhancement of immunity in rainbow trout, *Oncorhynchus mykiss* (Walbaum). *Aquaculture*, **388–391**, 193–197. doi:10.1016/j.aquaculture.2013.01.008

Awad, E., Awaad, A. S., & Esteban, M. A. (2015) Effects of dihydroquercetin obtained from deodar (*Cedrus deodara*) on immune status of gilthead seabream (*Sparus aurata* L.). *Fish & Shellfish Immunology*, **43**, 43–50. doi:10.1016/j.fsi.2014.12.009

Baba, E., Uluköy, G., & Öntaş, C. (2015) Effects of feed supplemented with *Lentinula edodes* mushroom extract on the immune response of rainbow trout, *Oncorhynchus mykiss*, and disease resistance against *Lactococcus garvieae*. *Aquaculture*, **448**, 476–482. doi:10.1016/j.aquaculture.2015.04.031

Baek, G.-H., Jang, Y.-S., Jeong, S.-I., *et al.* (2012) *Rehmannia glutinosa* suppresses inflammatory responses elicited by advanced glycation end products. *Inflammation*, **35**, 1232–1241. doi:10.1007/s10753-012-9433-x

Bagni, M., Archetti, L., Amadori, M., *et al.* (2000) Effect of long-term oral administration of an immunostimulant diet on innate immunity in sea bass (*Dicentrarchus labrax*). *Journal of Veterinary Medicine. B, Infectious Diseases and Veterinary Public Health*, **47**, 745–51. Retrieved from http://www.ncbi.nlm.nih.gov/pubmed/11204129

Bagni, M., Romano, N., Finoia, M. G., *et al.* (2005) Short- and long-term effects of a dietary yeast beta-glucan (Macrogard) and alginic acid (Ergosan) preparation on immune response in sea bass (*Dicentrarchus labrax*). *Fish & Shellfish Immunology*, **18**, 311–25. doi:10.1016/j.fsi.2004.08.003

Bandaranayake, W. M. (2002) Bioactivities, bioactive compounds and chemical constituents of mangrove plants. *Wetlands Ecology and Management*, **10**, 421–452. doi:10.1023/A:1021397624349

Baoprasertkul, P., Peatman, E., Chen, L., *et al.* (2004) Sequence analysis and expression of a CXC chemokine in resistant and susceptible catfish after infection of *Edwardsiella ictaluri*. *Developmental & Comparative Immunology*, **28**, 769–780. doi:10.1016/j.dci.2003.12.002

Basha, K. A., Raman, R. P., Prasad, K. P., *et al.* (2013) Effect of dietary supplemented andrographolide on growth, non-specific immune parameters and resistance against *Aeromonas hydrophila* in *Labeo rohita* (Hamilton). *Fish & Shellfish Immunology*, **35**, 1433–41. doi:10.1016/j.fsi.2013.08.005

Bilen, S., Bulut, M., & Bilen, A. M. (2011) Immunostimulant effects of *Cotinus coggyria* on rainbow trout (*Oncorhynchus mykiss*). *Fish & Shellfish Immunology*, **30**, 451–5. doi:10.1016/j.fsi.2010.12.013

Biswas, G., Korenaga, H., Takayama, H., *et al.* (2012) Cytokine responses in the common carp, *Cyprinus carpio* L. treated with baker's yeast extract. *Aquaculture*, **356–357**, 169–175. doi:10.1016/j.aquaculture.2012.05.019

Boltaña, S., Reyes-Lopez, F., Morera, D., *et al.* (2011a) Divergent responses to peptidoglycans derived from different *E. coli* serotypes influence inflammatory outcome in trout, *Oncorhynchus mykiss*, macrophages. *BMC Genomics*, **12**, 34. doi:10.1186/1471-2164-12-34

Boltaña, S., Roher, N., Goetz, F. W., *et al.* (2011b) PAMPs, PRRs and the genomics of gram negative bacterial recognition in fish. *Developmental & Comparative Immunology*, **35**, 1195–203. doi:10.1016/j.dci.2011.02.010

Brown, G. D., & Gordon, S. (2003) Fungal beta-glucans and mammalian immunity. *Immunity*, **19**, 311–315. doi:10.1016/S1074-7613(03)00233-4

Brudeseth, B. E., Wiulsrød, R., Fredriksen, B. N., *et al.* (2013) Status and future perspectives of vaccines for industrialised fin-fish farming. *Fish and Shellfish Immunology*. doi:10.1016/j.fsi.2013.05.029

Buchmann, K. (1999) Immune mechanisms in fish skin against monogeneans - A model. *Folia Parasitologica*, **46**, 1–9.

Callol, A., Pajuelo, D., Ebbesson, L., *et al.* (2015) Early steps in the European eel *(Anguilla anguilla)-Vibrio vulnificus* interaction in the gills: role of the RtxA13 toxin. *Fish & Shellfish Immunology*, **43**, 502–9. doi:10.1016/j.fsi.2015.01.009

Callol, A., Reyes-López, F. E., Roig, F. J., *et al.* (2015) An enriched European eel transcriptome sheds light upon host-pathogen interactions with *Vibrio vulnificus*. *Plos One*, **10**, e0133328. doi:10.1371/journal.pone.0133328

Casadei, E., Bird, S., Vecino, J. L. G., *et al.* (2013) The effect of peptidoglycan enriched diets on antimicrobial peptide gene expression in rainbow trout (*Oncorhynchus mykiss*). *Fish & Shellfish Immunology*, **34**, 529–37. doi:10.1016/j.fsi.2012.11.027

Casadei, E., Bird, S., Wadsworth, S., *et al.* (2015) The longevity of the antimicrobial response in rainbow trout (*Oncorhynchus mykiss*) fed a peptidoglycan (PG) supplemented diet. *Fish & Shellfish Immunology*, **44**, 316–20. doi:10.1016/j.fsi.2015.02.039

Chahal, D. S., Sivamani, R. K., Rivkah Isseroff, R., *et al.* (2013) Plant-based modulation of toll-like receptors: An emerging therapeutic model. *Phytotherapy Research*, **27**, 1423–1438. doi:10.1002/ptr.4886

Chandur, U., Shashidhar, S., Chandrasekar, S., *et al.* (2011) Studies of preliminary phytochemical and anti-arthritic activity of heart wood of *Cedrus deodar* (Roxb.). *Research Journal of Pharmaceutical, Biological and Chemical Sciences*, **2**, 654–660.

Chao, J. C. J., Chiang, S. W., Wang, C. C., *et al.* (2006) Hot water-extracted *Lycium barbarum* and *Rehmannia glutinosa* inhibit proliferation and induce apoptosis of hepatocellular carcinoma cells. *World Journal of Gastroenterology*, **12**, 4478–4484.

Chao, W. W., Kuo, Y. H., & Lin, B. I. F. (2010) Anti-inflammatory activity of new compounds from *Andrographis paniculata* by NF-κB transactivation inhibition. *Journal of Agricultural and Food Chemistry*, **58**, 2505–2512. doi:10.1021/jf903629j

Chatzifotis, S., Kokou, F., Ampatzis, K., *et al.* (2008) Effects of dietary caffeine on growth, body composition, somatic indexes, and cerebral distribution of acetyl-cholinesterase and nitric oxide synthase in gilthead sea bream (*Sparus aurata*), reared in winter temperature. *Aquaculture Nutrition*, **14**, 405–415. doi:10.1111/j.1365-2095.2007.00541.x

Chee, H. Y., Kim, H., & Lee, M. H. (2009) *In vitro* antifungal activity of Limonene against *Trichophyton rubrum*. *Mycobiology*, **37**, 243–6. doi:10.4489/MYCO.2009.37.3.243

Chen, H. Y., & Yen, G. C. (2007) Antioxidant activity and free radical-scavenging capacity of extracts from guava (*Psidium guajava* L.) leaves. *Food Chemistry*, **101**, 686–694. doi:10.1016/j.foodchem.2006.02.047

Chen, L., Evensen, Ø., & Mutoloki, S. (2015) IPNV antigen uptake and distribution in Atlantic salmon following oral administration. *Viruses*, **7**, 2507–17. doi:10.3390/v7052507

Chen, L., Klaric, G., Wadsworth, S., *et al.* (2014) Augmentation of the antibody response of Atlantic salmon by oral administration of alginate-encapsulated IPNV antigens. *PLoS ONE*, 9. doi:10.1371/journal.pone.0109337

Chettri, J. K., Kuhn, J. A., Jaafar, R. M., *et al.* (2014) Epidermal response of rainbow trout to *Ichthyobodo necator* : immunohistochemical and gene expression studies indicate a Th1-/Th2-like switch. *Journal of Fish Diseases*, **37**, 771–783. doi:10.1111/jfd.12169

Choi, S. H., Kim, M. S., & Kim, K. H. (2011) Protection of olive flounder (*Paralichthys olivaceus*) against *Edwardsiella tarda* infection by oral administration of auxotrophic mutant *E. tarda* (Δalr Δasd E. tarda). *Aquaculture*, **317**, 48–52. doi:10.1016/j.aquaculture.2011.04.021

Choi, S.-H., Park, K.-H., Yoon, T.-J., *et al.* (2008) Dietary korean mistletoe enhances cellular non-specific immune responses and survival of Japanese eel (*Anguilla japonica*). *Fish & Shellfish Immunology*, **24**, 67–73. doi:10.1016/j.fsi.2007.08.007

Christybapita, D., Divyagnaneswari, M., & Dinakaran Michael, R. (2007) Oral administration of *Eclipta alba* leaf aqueous extract enhances the non-specific immune responses and disease resistance of *Oreochromis mossambicus*. *Fish & Shellfish Immunology*, **23**, 840–852. doi:10.1016/j.fsi.2007.03.010

Chrubasik, S., Pittler, M. H., & Roufogalis, B. D. (2005) Zingiberis rhizoma: A comprehensive review on the ginger effect and efficacy profiles. *Phytomedicine*, **12**, 684–701. doi:10.1016/j.phymed.2004.07.009

Chung, S., & Secombes, C. J. (1987) Activation of rainbow trout macrophages. *Journal of Fish Biology*, **31**, 51–56.

Conceição, L. E. C., Skjermo, J., Skjåk-Bræk, G., *et al.* (2001) Effect of an immunostimulating alginate on protein turnover of turbot (*Scophthalmus maximus* L.) larvae. *Fish Physiology and Biochemistry*, **24**, 207–212.

Cook, M. T., Hayball, P. J., Hutchinson, W., *et al.* (2003) Administration of a commercial immunostimulant preparation, EcoActiva (TM) as a feed supplement enhances macrophage respiratory burst and the growth rate of snapper (*Pagrus auratus*, Sparidae (Bloch and Schneider)) in winter. *Fish & Shellfish Immunology*, **14**, 333–345. doi:10.1006/fsim.2002.0441

Couso, N., Castro, R., Magariños, B., *et al.* (2003) Effect of oral administration of glucans on the resistance of gilthead seabream to pasteurellosis. *Aquaculture*, **219**, 99–109. doi:10.1016/S0044-8486(03)00019-X

Crespy, V., & Williamson, G. (2004) A review of the health effects of green tea catechins in *in vivo* animal models. *The Journal of Nutrition*, **134**, 3431S–3440S.

Cuesta, A., Meseguer, J., & Esteban, M. A. (2004) Total serum immunoglobulin M levels are affected by immunomodulators in seabream (*Sparus aurata* L.). *Veterinary Immunology and Immunopathology*, **101**, 203–10. doi:10.1016/j.vetimm.2004.04.021

Cui, L.-C., Guan, X.-T., Liu, Z.-M., *et al.* (2015) Recombinant lactobacillus expressing G protein of spring viremia of carp virus (SVCV) combined with ORF81 protein of koi herpesvirus (KHV): A promising way to induce protective immunity against SVCV and KHV infection in cyprinid fish via oral vaccination. *Vaccine*, **33**, 3092–3099. doi:10.1016/j.vaccine.2015.05.002

Dalmo, R. A., & Bøgwald, J. (2008) Beta-glucans as conductors of immune symphonies. *Fish & Shellfish Immunology*, **25**, 384–96. doi:10.1016/j.fsi.2008.04.008

Das, R., Prakash Raman, R., Saha, H., *et al.* (2013) Effect of *Ocimum sanctum* Linn. (Tulsi) extract on the immunity and survival of *Labeo rohita* (Hamilton) infected with *Aeromonas hydrophila. Aquaculture Research*, 1111–1121. doi:10.1111/are.12264

Dhar, A. K., Manna, S. K., & Thomas Allnutt, F. C. (2014) Viral vaccines for farmed finfish. *Indian Journal of Virology*, **25**, 1–17. doi:10.1007/s13337-013-0186-4

Dhayanithi, N., Ajithkumar, T., Arockiaraj, J., *et al.* (2015) Immune protection by *Rhizophora apiculata* in clownfish against *Vibrio alginolyticus. Aquaculture*, **446**, 1–6. doi:10.1016/j.aquaculture.2015.04.013

Díaz-Rosales, P., Chabrillón, M., Abdala, R. T., *et al.* (2008) Effect of dietary administration of *Porphyridium cruentum* on the respiratory burst activity of sole, *Solea senegalensis* (Kaup), phagocytes. *Journal of Fish Diseases*, **31**, 489–495. doi:10.1111/j.1365-2761.2008.00923.x

Dixon, B., Luque, A., Abós, B., *et al.* (2013) Molecular characterization of three novel chemokine receptors in rainbow trout (*Oncorhynchus mykiss*). *Fish & Shellfish Immunology*, **34**, 641–651. doi:10.1016/j.fsi.2012.12.003

Dotta, G., de Andrade, J. I. A., Tavares Gonçalves, E. L., *et al.* (2014) Leukocyte phagocytosis and lysozyme activity in Nile tilapia fed supplemented diet with natural extracts of propolis and *Aloe barbadensis. Fish & Shellfish Immunology*, **39**, 280–4. doi:10.1016/j.fsi.2014.05.020

Dügenci, S. K., Arda, N., & Candan, A. (2003) Some medicinal plants as immunostimulant for fish. *Journal of Ethnopharmacology*, **88**, 99–106. doi:10.1016/S0378-8741(03)00182-X

Dülger, B., Hacıoglu, N., & Bilen, S. (2009) Antimicrobial activity of *Cotinus coggyria* from Turkey. *Asian Journal of Chemistry*, **21**, 4139–4140.

Dunkelberger, J. R., & Song, W.-C. (2010) Complement and its role in innate and adaptive immune responses. *Cell Research*, **20**, 34–50. doi:10.1038/cr.2009.139

El-Boshy, M. E., El-Ashram, A. M., Abdelhamid, F. M., *et al.* (2010) Immunomodulatory effect of dietary *Saccharomyces cerevisiae*, beta-glucan and laminaran in mercuric chloride treated Nile tilapia (*Oreochromis niloticus*) and experimentally infected with *Aeromonas hydrophila. Fish & Shellfish Immunology*, **28**, 802–8. doi:10.1016/j.fsi.2010.01.017

El-Saleh, S. C., Al-Sagair, O. a., & Al-Khalaf, M. I. (2004) Thymoquinone and *Nigella sativa* oil protection against methionine-induced hyperhomocysteinemia in rats. *International Journal of Cardiology*, **93**, 19–23. doi:10.1016/S0167-5273(03)00108-6

Embregts, C. W. E., & Forlenza, M. (2016) Oral vaccination of fish: Lessons from humans and veterinary species. *Developmental & Comparative Immunology*, **64**, 118–137. doi:10.1016/j.dci.2016.03.024

Endo, K., Kanno, E., & Oshima, Y. (1990) Structures of antifungal diarylheptenones, gingerenones A, B, C and isogingerenone B, isolated from the rhizomes of *Zingiber officinale. Phytochemistry*, **29**, 797–799. doi:10.1016/0031-9422(90)80021-8

Espevik, T., Otterlei, M., Skjåk-Braek, G., *et al.* (1993) The involvement of CD14 in stimulation of cytokine production by uronic acid polymers. *European Journal of Immunology*, **23**, 255–261. article. doi:10.1002/eji.1830230140

Esteban, M. a, Cuesta, A., Ortuno, J., *et al.* (2001) Immunomodulatory effects of dietary intake of chitin on gilthead seabream (*Sparus aurata* L.) innate immune system. *Fish & Shellfish Immunology*, **11**, 303–315. doi:10.1006/fsim.2000.0315

Falco, A., Frost, P., Miest, J., *et al.* (2012) Reduced inflammatory response to *Aeromonas salmonicida* infection in common carp (*Cyprinus carpio* L.) fed with β-glucan supplements. *Fish & Shellfish Immunology*, **32**, 1051–7. doi:10.1016/j.fsi.2012.02.028

Falco, A., Miest, J. J., Pionnier, N., *et al.* (2014) β-Glucan-supplemented diets increase poly(I:C)-induced gene expression of Mx, possibly via Tlr3-mediated recognition mechanism in common carp (*Cyprinus carpio*). *Fish & Shellfish Immunology*, **36**, 494–502. doi:10.1016/j.fsi.2013.12.005

Fang, F. C. (2004) Antimicrobial reactive oxygen and nitrogen species: concepts and controversies. *Nature Reviews. Microbiology*, **2**, 820–832. doi:10.1038/nrmicro1004

Flerova, E. A., & Balabanova, L. V. (2013) Ultrastructure of granulocytes of teleost fish (Salmoniformes, Cypriniformes, Perciformes). *Journal of Evolutionary Biochemistry and Physiology*, **49**, 223–233. doi:10.1134/S0022093013020126

Flo, T. H., Ryan, L., Latz, E., *et al.* (2002) Involvement of Toll-like receptor (TLR) 2 and TLR4 in cell activation by mannuronic acid polymers. *Journal of Biological Chemistry*, **277**, 35489–35495. doi:10.1074/jbc.M201366200

Fuglem, B., Jirillo, E., Bjerkås, I., *et al.* (2010) Antigen-sampling cells in the salmonid intestinal epithelium. *Developmental and Comparative Immunology*, **34**, 768–774. doi:10.1016/j.dci.2010.02.007

Fujino, Y., Ono, S.-I., & Nagai, A. (1987) Studies on uptake of rabbit's immunoglobulin into the columnar epithelial cells in the gut of rainbow trout *Salmo gairdneri*. *Nippon Suisan Gakkaishi*, **53**, 367–370.

Gabriel, N. N., Qiang, J., He, J., *et al.* (2015) Dietary *Aloe vera* supplementation on growth performance, some haemato-biochemical parameters and disease resistance against *Streptococcus iniae* in tilapia (GIFT). *Fish & Shellfish Immunology*, **44**, 504–14. doi:10.1016/j.fsi.2015.03.002

Gao, X., Wang, W., Wei, S., *et al.* (2009) Antioxidant, antioedema and analgesic activities of *Andrographis paniculata* extracts and their active constituent andrographolide. *Phytotherapy Research*, **23**, 958–964. doi:10.1002/ptr

Georgopoulou, U., Sire, M. F., & Vernier, J. M. (1986) Immunological demonstration of intestinal absorption and digestion of protein macromolecules in the trout (*Salmo gairdneri*). *Cell and Tissue Research*, **245**. doi:10.1007/BF00213946

Ghaedi, G., Keyvanshokooh, S., Mohammadi Azarm, H., *et al.* (2015) Effects of dietary β-glucan on maternal immunity and fry quality of rainbow trout (*Oncorhynchus mykiss*). *Aquaculture*, **441**, 78–83. doi:10.1016/j.aquaculture.2015.02.023

Ghochikyan, A., Pichugin, A., Bagaev, A., *et al.* (2014) Targeting TLR-4 with a novel pharmaceutical grade plant derived agonist, Immunomax®, as a therapeutic strategy for metastatic breast cancer. *Journal of Translational Medicine*, **12**, 322. doi:10.1186/s12967-014-0322-y

Girardin, S. E., Boneca, I. G., Carneiro, L. a M., *et al.* (2003) Nod1 detects a unique muropeptide from gram-negative bacterial peptidoglycan. *Science*, **300**, 1584–1587. doi:10.1126/science.1084677

Giri, S. S., Sen, S. S., Chi, C., *et al.* (2015) Effect of guava leaves on the growth performance and cytokine gene expression of *Labeo rohita* and its susceptibility to *Aeromonas hydrophila* infection. *Fish & Shellfish Immunology*, **46**, 217–224. doi:10.1016/j.fsi.2015.05.051

Gomez, D., Sunyer, J. O., & Salinas, I. (2013) The mucosal immune system of fish: The evolution of tolerating commensals while fighting pathogens. *Fish & Shellfish Immunology*, **35**, 1729–1739. doi:10.1016/j.fsi.2013.09.032

Granica, S., Piwowarski, J. P., & Kiss, A. K. (2015) Ellagitannins modulate the inflammatory response of human neutrophils *ex vivo*. *Phytomedicine*, **22**, 1215–1222. doi:10.1016/j.phymed.2015.10.004

Green, S. J., Nacy, C. A., Schreiber, R. D., *et al.* (1993) Neutralization of gamma interferon and tumor necrosis factor alpha blocks in vivo synthesis of nitrogen oxides from L-arginine and protection against *Francisella tularensis* infection in *Mycobacterium bovis* BCG-treated mice. *Infection and Immunity*, **61**, 689–698.

Grzanna, R., Lindmark, L., & Frondoza, C. G. (2005) Ginger-an herbal medicinal product with broad anti-inflammatory actions. *Journal of Medicinal Food*, **8**, 125–132. doi:10.1089/jmf.2005.8.125

Guerin, M., Huntley, M. E., & Olaizola, M. (2003) *Haematococcus* astaxanthin: Applications for human health and nutrition. *Trends in Biotechnology*, **21**, 210–216. doi:10.1016/S0167-7799(03)00078-7

Gülçin, I., Küfrevioğlu, Ö. I., Oktay, M., *et al.* (2004) Antioxidant, antimicrobial, antiulcer and analgesic activities of nettle (*Urtica dioica* L.). *Journal of Ethnopharmacology*, **90**, 205–215. doi:10.1016/j.jep.2003.09.028

Gupta, S. K., Pal, a K., Sahu, N. P., *et al.* (2008) Microbial levan in the diet of *Labeo rohita* Hamilton juveniles: effect on non-specific immunity and histopathological changes after challenge with *Aeromonas hydrophila*. *Journal of Fish Diseases*, **31**, 649–57. doi:10.1111/j.1365-2761.2008.00939.x

Guttvik, A., Paulsen, B., Dalmo, R. A., *et al.* (2002) Oral administration of lipopolysaccharide to Atlantic salmon (*Salmo salar* L.) fry. Uptake, distribution, influence on growth and immune stimulation. *Aquaculture*, **214**, 35–53. doi:10.1016/S0044-8486(02)00358-7

Hadizadeh, I., Peivastegan, B., & Hamzehzarghani, H. (2009) Antifungal activity of essential oils from some medicinal plants of Iran against *Alternaria alternate*. *American Journal of Applied Sciences*, **6**, 857–861.

Hajto, T. (1986) Immunomodulatory effect of Iscador: a *Viscum album* preparation. *Oncology*, **43**, 51–61.

Hanafy, M. S., & Hatem, M. E. (1991) Studies on the antimicrobial activity of *Nigella sativa* seed (black cumin). *Journal of Ethnopharmacology*, **34**, 275–278.

Haug, A., Myklestad, S., Larsen, B., *et al.* (1967) Correlation between chemical structure and physical properties of alginates. *Acta Chemica Scandinavica*. doi:10.3891/acta.chem.scand.21-0768

Haugarvoll, E., Bjerkås, I., Nowak, B. F., *et al.* (2008) Identification and characterization of a novel intraepithelial lymphoid tissue in the gills of Atlantic salmon. *Journal of Anatomy*, **213**, 202–209. doi:10.1111/j.1469-7580.2008.00943.x

He, S., Zhou, Z., Liu, Y., *et al.* (2009) Effects of dietary *Saccharomyces cerevisiae* fermentation product (DVAQUA®) on growth performance, intestinal autochthonous bacterial community and non-specific immunity of hybrid tilapia (*Oreochromis niloticus* ♀×*O. aureus* ♂) cultured . *Aquaculture*, **294**, 99–107. doi:10.1016/j.aquaculture.2009.04.043

Heidarieh, M., Soltani, M., Tamimi, A., *et al.* (2011) Comparative effect of raw fiber (Vitacel) and alginic acid (Ergosan) on growth performance, immunocompe- tent cell population and plasma lysozyme content of giant sturgeon (*Huso huso*). *Turkish Journal of Fisheries and Aquatic Sciences*, **11**, 445–450. doi:10.4194/1303-2712-v11

Higuera-Ciapara, I., Félix-Valenzuela, L., & Goycoolea, F. M. (2006) Astaxanthin: a review of its chemistry and applications. *Critical Reviews in Food Science and Nutrition*, **46**, 185–196. doi:10.1080/10408690590957188

Huang, L. Y., Wang, K. Y., Xiao, D., *et al.* (2014) Safety and immunogenicity of an oral DNA vaccine encoding Sip of *Streptococcus agalactiae* from Nile tilapia *Oreochromis niloticus* delivered by live attenuated *Salmonella typhimurium*. *Fish & Shellfish Immunology*, **38**, 34–41. doi:10.1016/j.fsi.2014.02.017

Iida, H., & Yamamoto, T. (1985) Intracellular transport of horseradish peroxidase in the absorptive cells of goldfish hindgut in vitro, with special reference to the cytoplasmic tubules. *Cell and Tissue Research*, **240**, 553–560. doi:10.1007/BF00216344

Iles, K. E., & Forman, H. J. (2002) Macrophage signaling and respiratory burst. *Immunologic Research*, **26**, 95–105. doi:10.1385/IR:26:1-3:095

Iliev, D. B., Roach, J. C., Mackenzie, S., *et al.* (2005) Endotoxin recognition: In fish or not in fish? *FEBS Lett*, **579**, 6519–6528. doi:10.1016/j.surg.2006.10.010.Use

Ishihara, N., Araki, T., Tamaru, Y., *et al.* (2002) Influence of green tea polyphenols on feed performance, growth performance, and fish body component in yellowtail (*Seriola quinqueradiata*). *Japanese Journal of Food Chemistry*, **9**, 7–14.

Isogai, E., Isogai, H., Hirose, K., *et al.* (2001) *In vivo* synergy between green tea extract and levofloxacin against enterohemorrhagic *Escherichia coli* O157 infection. *Current Microbiology*, **42**, 248–251. doi:10.1007/s002840010212

Jagruthi, C., Yogeshwari, G., Anbazahan, S. M., *et al.* (2014) Effect of dietary astaxanthin against *Aeromonas hydrophila* infection in common carp, *Cyprinus carpio*. *Fish & Shellfish Immunology*, **41**, 674–80. doi:10.1016/j.fsi.2014.10.010

Janeway, C. A., & Medzhitov, R. (2002) Innate immune recognition. *Annual Review of Immunology*, **20**, 197–216. doi:10.1146/annurev.immunol.20.083001.084359

Jian, J., & Wu, Z. (2003) Effects of traditional Chinese medicine on nonspecific immunity and disease resistance of large yellow croaker, *Pseudosciaena crocea* (Richardson). *Aquaculture*, **218**, 1–9. doi:10.1016/S0044-8486(02)00192-8

Jian, J., & Wu, Z. (2004) Influences of traditional Chinese medicine on non-specific immunity of Jian Carp (*Cyprinus carpio* var. Jian). *Fish & Shellfish Immunology*, **16**, 185–191. doi:10.1016/S1050-4648(03)00062-7

Jin, M., Zhao, K., Huang, Q., *et al.* (2012) Isolation, structure and bioactivities of the polysaccharides from *Angelica sinensis* (Oliv.) Diels: A review. *Carbohydrate Polymers*, **89**, 713–722. doi:10.1016/j.carbpol.2012.04.049

Kai, Y. H., Wu, Y. C., & Chi, S. C. (2014) Immune gene expressions in grouper larvae (*Epinephelus coioides*) induced by bath and oral vaccinations with inactivated betanodavirus. *Fish & Shellfish Immunology*, **40**, 563–569. doi:10.1016/j.fsi.2014.08.005

Kaibori, M., Sakitani, K., Oda, M., *et al.* (1999) Immunosuppressant FK506 inhibits inducible nitric oxide synthase gene expression at a step of NF-kappaB activation in rat hepatocytes. *Journal of Hepatology*, **30**, 1138–1145.

Karkos, P. D., Leong, S. C., Karkos, C. D., *et al.* (2008) *Spirulina* in clinical practice: Evidence-based human applications. *Evidence-Based Complementary and Alternative Medicine*, **2011**, 27–31. doi:10.1093/ecam/nen058

Kawai, T., & Akira, S. (2010) The role of pattern-recognition receptors in innate immunity: update on Toll-like receptors. *Nature Immunology*, **11**, 373–84. doi:10.1038/ni.1863

Khafagi, I., Gab-Alla, A., & Waleed SalamaMoustafa Fouda3 (2008) Biological activities and phytochemical constituents of the gray mangrove *Avicennia marina* (Forssk.) Vierh. *Journal of Coastal Research*, **5**, 62–69.

Kim, J.-K., Kim, Y., Na, K.-M., *et al.* (2007) [6]-Gingerol prevents UVB-induced ROS production and COX-2 expression *in vitro* and *in vivo*. *Free Radical Research*, **41**, 603–614. doi:10.1080/10715760701209896

Kim, K. H., Hwang, Y. J., & Bai, S. C. (1999) Resistance to *Vibrio alginolyticus* in juvenile rockfish (*Sebastes schlegeli*) fed diets containing different doses of aloe. *Aquaculture*, **180**, 13–21. doi:10.1016/S0044-8486(99)00143-X

Kim, S. J., Yoon, S. J., Kim, Y. M., *et al.* (2014) HS-23, *Lonicera japonica* extract, attenuates septic injury by suppressing toll-like receptor 4 signaling. *Journal of Ethnopharmacology*, **155**, 256–266. doi:10.1016/j.jep.2014.05.021

Kirchhoff, N. T., D'Antignana, T., Leef, M. J., *et al.* (2011) Effects of immunostimulants on ranched southern bluefin tuna *Thunnus maccoyii*: immune response, health and performance. *Journal of Fish Biology*, **79**, 331–55. doi:10.1111/j.1095-8649.2011.03019.x

Klebanoff, S. J. (2005) Myeloperoxidase : friend and foe. *Journal of Leukocyte Biology*, **77**, 598–625. doi:10.1189/jlb.1204697.1

Kondo, M., Kawai, K., Okabe, M., *et al.* (2003) Efficacy of oral vaccine against bacterial coldwater disease in ayu *Plecoglossus altivelis*. *Diseases of Aquatic Organisms*, **55**, 261–264. doi:10.3354/dao055261

Kong, X., Hu, Y., & Song, D. (2003) Research progress of immunopharmacology of *Astragalus* polysaccharide. *Journal of the Chinese Society of Veterinary Science*, **3**, 34–37 [China].

Koppang, E. O., Fischer, U., Moore, L., *et al.* (2010) Salmonid T cells assemble in the thymus, spleen and in novel interbranchial lymphoid tissue. *Journal of Anatomy*, **217**, 728–739. doi:10.1111/j.1469-7580.2010.01305.x

Kumar, S., Raman, R. P., Pandey, P. K., *et al.* (2013) Effect of orally administered azadirachtin on non-specific immune parameters of goldfish *Carassius auratus* (Linn. 1758) and resistance against *Aeromonas hydrophila*. *Fish & Shellfish Immunology*, **34**, 564–73. doi:10.1016/j.fsi.2012.11.038

Kumari, J., Bogwald, J., & Dalmo, R. A. (2009) Transcription factor GATA-3 in Atlantic salmon (Salmo salar): Molecular characterization, promoter activity and expression analysis. *Molecular Immunology*, **46**, 3099–3107. doi:10.1016/j.molimm.2009.06.008

Kumari, J., & Sahoo, P. K. (2006) Non-specific immune response of healthy and immunocompromised Asian catfish (*Clarias batrachus*) to several immunostimulants. *Aquaculture*, **255**, 133–141. doi:10.1016/j.aquaculture.2005.12.012

Kunttu, H. M. T., Valtonen, E. T., Suomalainen, L.-R., *et al.* (2009) The efficacy of two immunostimulants against *Flavobacterium columnare* infection in juvenile rainbow trout (*Oncorhynchus mykiss*). *Fish & Shellfish Immunology*, **26**, 850–7. doi:10.1016/j.fsi.2009.03.013

Kuttan, G., Vasudevan, D. M., & Kuttan, R. (1992) Tumour reducing activity of an isolated active ingredient from mistletoe extract and its possible mechanism of action. *Journal of Experimental & Clinical Cancer Research*, **11**, 7–12.

Lacorte, L. M., Seiva, F. R. F., Rinaldi, J. C., *et al.* (2013) Caffeine reduces cadmium accumulation in the organism and enhances the levels of antioxidant protein expression in the epididymis. *Reproductive Toxicology*, **35**, 137–143. doi:10.1016/j.reprotox.2012.10.009

Leal, L. K. a M., Ferreira, a. a G., Bezerra, G. a., *et al.* (2000) Antinociceptive, anti-inflammatory and bronchodilator activities of Brazilian medicinal plants containing coumarin: A comparative study. *Journal of Ethnopharmacology*, **70**, 151–159. doi:10.1016/S0378-8741(99)00165-8

Levita, J., Nawawi, A., Mutholib, A., *et al.* (2010) Andrographolide inhibits COX-2 expression in human fibroblast cells due to its interaction with arginine and histidine in cyclooxygenase site. *Journal of Applied Sciences*, **10**, 1481–1484.

Li, J., Barreda, D. R., Zhang, Y.-A. A., *et al.* (2006) B lymphocytes from early vertebrates have potent phagocytic and microbicidal abilities. *Nature Immunology*, **7**, 1116–1124. doi:10.1038/ni1389

Li, L. P., Wang, R., Liang, W. W., *et al.* (2015) Development of live attenuated *Streptococcus agalactiae* vaccine for tilapia via continuous passage invitro. *Fish & Shellfish Immunology*, **45**, 955–963. doi:10.1016/j.fsi.2015.06.014

Lin, C. J., Lin, H. J., Chen, T. H., *et al.* (2015) *Polygonum cuspidatum* and its active components inhibit replication of the influenza virus through Toll-like receptor 9-induced interferon beta expression. *PLoS ONE*, **10**, 1–13. doi:10.1371/journal.pone.0117602

Lincy, M. P., Paulpriya, K., & Mohan, V. R. (2013) *In vitro* antioxidant activity of *Avicennia marina* (Forssk) Vierh pneumatophore (Avicenniaceae). *Science Research Reporter*, **3**, 106–114.

Liu, H. (2002) Research status of Chinese herbal immunostimulants and their application in aquaculture. *Journal of Fisheries*, **15**, 91–94 [China].

Locksley, R. M., Nelson, C. S., Fankhauser, J. E., *et al.* (1987) Loss of granulemyeloperoxidase during in vitro culture of human monocytes correlates with decay in antiprotozoa activity. *The American Journal of Tropical Medicine and Hygiene*, **36**, 541–548.

Lorenz, R. T., & Cysewski, G. R. (2000) Commercial potential for *Haematococcus* microalgae as a natural source of astaxanthin. *Trends in Biotechnology*, **18**, 160–167. doi:10.1016/S0167-7799(00)01433-5

Lu, L., Xu, H., He, Y., *et al.* (2011) Protection of grass carp, *Ctenopharyngon idellus* (Valenciennes), through oral administration of a subunit vaccine against reovirus. *Journal of Fish Diseases*, **34**, 939–942. doi:10.1111/j.1365-2761.2011.01310.x

Magnadóttir, B. (2006) Innate immunity of fish (overview). *Fish & Shellfish Immunology*, **20**, 137–51. doi:10.1016/j.fsi.2004.09.006

Maki, J. L., Dickerson, H. W., Maki, J. L., *et al.* (2003) Systemic and cutaneous mucus antibody responses of Channel catfish immunized against the protozoan parasite *Ichthyophthirius multifiliis*. *Clinical and Diagnostic Laboratory Immunology*, **10**, 876–881. doi:10.1128/CDLI.10.5.876

Makridis, P., Moreira, C., Alves Costa, R., *et al.* (2009) Use of microalgae bioencapsulated in Artemia during the weaning of Senegalese sole (*Solea senegalensis* Kaup). *Aquaculture*, **292**, 153–157. doi:10.1016/j.aquaculture.2009.04.016

Männel, D. N., Becken, H., Gundt, A., *et al.* (1991) Induction of tumor necrosis factor expression by a lectin from *Viscum album*. *Cancer Immunology Immunotherapy*, **33**, 177–182.

McKay, D. L., & Blumberg, J. B. (2006) A review of the bioactivity and potential health benefits of peppermint tea (*Mentha piperita* L.). *Phytotherapy Research*, **20**, 619–633. doi:10.1002/ptr

Metwally, A. M., Omar, A. A., Harraz, F. M., *et al.* (2010) Phytochemical investigation and antimicrobial activity of *Psidium guajava* L. leaves. *Pharmacognosy Magazine*, **6**, 212–218. doi:10.4103/0973-1296.66939

Metzner, G., Franz, H., Kindt, A., *et al.* (1985) The in vitro activity of lectin I from mistletoe (ML I) and its isolated A and B chains on functions ofmacrophages and polymorphonuclear cells. *Immunobiology*, **169**, 461–71. article. doi:10.1016/S0171-2985(85)80002-4

Min, L., Li-Li, Z., Jun-Wei, G., *et al.* (2012) Immunogenicity of Lactobacillus-expressing VP2 and VP3 of the infectious pancreatic necrosis virus (IPNV) in rainbow trout. *Fish & Shellfish Immunology*, **32**, 196–203. doi:10.1016/j.fsi.2011.11.015

Misra, C., Das, B., Mukherjee, S., *et al.* (2006) Effect of long term administration of dietary beta-glucan on immunity, growth and survival of *Labeo rohita* fingerlings. *Aquaculture*, **255**, 82–94. Retrieved from http://www.sciencedirect.com/science/article/pii/S0044848605007696

Mistry, K. S., Sanghvi, Z., Parmar, G., *et al.* (2014) The antimicrobial activity of *Azadirachta indica, Mimusops elengi, Tinospora cardifolia, Ocimum sanctum* and 2% chlorhexidine gluconate on common endodontic pathogens: An *in vitro* study. *European Journal of Dentistry*, **8**, 172–177. doi:10.4103/1305-7456.130591

Mitra, S., Alnabulsi, A., Secombes, C. J., *et al.* (2010) Identification and characterization of the transcription factors involved in T-cell development, t-bet, stat6 and foxp3, within the zebrafish, Danio rerio. *FEBS Journal*, **277**, 128–147. doi:10.1111/j.1742-4658.2009.07460.x

Montero, J., Ordas, M. C., Alejo, A., *et al.* (2011) CK12, a rainbow trout chemokine with lymphocyte chemo-attractant capacity associated to mucosal tissues. *Molecular Immunology*, **48**, 1102–1113. doi:10.1016/j.molimm.2011.02.005

Morera, D., Roher, N., Ribas, L., *et al.* (2011) RNA-Seq reveals an integrated immune response in nucleated erythrocytes. *PLoS One*, **6**, e26998. Journal Article.

Mueller, E. A., & Anderer, F. A. (1990) Synergistic action of a plant rhamnogalacturonan enhancing antitumor cytotoxicity of human natural killer and lymphokine-activated killer cells: chemical specificity of target cell recognition. *Cancer Research*, **50**, 3646–51.

Munang'andu, H. M., Fredriksen, B. N., Mutoloki, S., *et al.* (2013) The kinetics of CD4+ and CD8+ T-cell gene expression correlate with protection in Atlantic salmon (*Salmo salar* L) vaccinated against infectious pancreatic necrosis. *Vaccine*, **31**, 1956–1963. doi:10.1016/j.vaccine.2013.02.008

Mutoloki, S., Munang'andu, H. M., & Evensen, Ø. (2015) Oral vaccination of fish - antigen preparations, uptake, and immune induction. *Frontiers in Immunology*, **6**, 1–10. doi:10.3389/fimmu.2015.00519

Nakaya, T. A., Kita, M., Kuriyama, H., *et al.* (2004) *Panax ginseng* induces production of proinflammatory cytokines via toll-like receptor. *Journal of Interferon and Cytokine Research*, **24**, 93–100. doi:10.1089/107999004322813336

Nathan, C., & Shiloh, M. U. (2000) Reactive oxygen and nitrogen intermediates in the relationship between mammalian hosts and microbial pathogens. *Proceedings of the National Academy of Sciences of the United States of America*, **97**, 8841–8848. doi:10.1073/pnas.97.16.8841

Ngugi, C. C., Oyoo-Okoth, E., Mugo-Bundi, J., *et al.* (2015) Effects of dietary administration of stinging nettle (*Urtica dioica*) on the growth performance, biochemical, hematological and immunological parameters in juvenile and adult Victoria Labeo (*Labeo victorianus*) challenged with *Aeromonas hydrophila*. *Fish & Shellfish Immunology*, **44**, 533–41. doi:10.1016/j.fsi.2015.03.025

Nguyen, C. T., Luong, T. T., Lee, S. Y., *et al.* (2015) *Panax ginseng* aqueous extract prevents pneumococcal sepsis *in vivo* by potentiating cell survival and diminishing inflammation. *Phytomedicine*, **22**, 1055–1061. doi:10.1016/j.phymed.2015.07.005

Nigam, A. K., Kumari, U., Mittal, S., *et al.* (2012) Comparative analysis of innate immune parameters of the skin mucous secretions from certain freshwater teleosts, inhabiting different ecological niches. *Fish Physiology and Biochemistry*, **38**, 1245–1256. doi:10.1007/s10695-012-9613-5

Noaillac-Depeyre, J., & Gas, N. (1973) Absorption of protein macromolecules by the enterocytes of the carp (*Cyprinus carpio* L.) - Ultrastructural and cytochemical study. *Zeitschrift fur Zellforschung und Mikroskopische Anatomie*, **146**, 525–541. doi:10.1007/BF02347181

Nur-Nazifah, M., Sabri, M. Y., & Siti-Zahrah, A. (2014) Development and efficacy of feed-based recombinant vaccine encoding the cell wall surface anchor family protein of *Streptococcus agalactiae* against streptococcosis in *Oreochromis* sp. *Fish & Shellfish Immunology*, **37**, 193–200. doi:10.1016/j.fsi.2014.01.011

Nya, E. J., & Austin, B. (2009) Use of dietary ginger, *Zingiber officinale* Roscoe, as an immunostimulant to control *Aeromonas hydrophila* infections in rainbow trout, *Oncorhynchus mykiss* (Walbaum). *Journal of Fish Diseases*, **32**, 971–977. doi:10.1111/j.1365-2761.2009.01101.x

Nya, E. J., & Austin, B. (2011) Development of immunity in rainbow trout (*Oncorhynchus mykiss*, Walbaum) to *Aeromonas hydrophila* after the dietary application of garlic. *Fish & Shellfish Immunology*, **30**, 845–850. doi:10.1016/j.fsi.2011.01.008

Ortuño, J., Cuesta, A., Rodríguez, A., *et al.* (2002) Oral administration of yeast, *Saccharomyces cerevisiae*, enhances the cellular innate immune response of gilthead seabream (*Sparus aurata* L.). *Veterinary Immunology and Immunopathology*, **85**, 41–50. Retrieved from http://www.ncbi.nlm.nih.gov/pubmed/11867166

Otterlei, M., Ostgaard, K., Skjåk-Braek, G., *et al.* (1991) Induction of cytokine production from human monocytes stimulated with alginate. *Journal of Immunotherapy*, **10**, 286–291. doi:10.1097/00002371-199108000-00007

Otterlei, M., Sundan, a., Skjak-Braek, G., *et al.* (1993) Similar mechanisms of action of defined polysaccharides and lipopolysaccharides: Characterization of binding and tumor necrosis factor alpha induction. *Infection and Immunity*, **61**, 1917–1925.

Palti, Y. (2011) Toll-like receptors in bony fish: From genomics to function. *Developmental & Comparative Immunology*, **35**, 1263–1272. doi:10.1016/j.dci.2011.03.006

Pannacci, M., Lucini, V., Colleoni, F., *et al.* (2006) *Panax ginseng* C.A. Mayer G115 modulates pro-inflammatory cytokine production in mice throughout the increase of macrophage toll-like receptor 4 expression during physical stress. *Brain, Behavior, and Immunity*, **20**, 546–551. doi:10.1016/j.bbi.2005.11.007

Park, B. S., & Lee, J.-O. (2013) Recognition of lipopolysaccharide pattern by TLR4 complexes. *Experimental & Molecular Medicine*, **45**, e66. doi:10.1038/emm.2013.97

Parra, D., Reyes-Lopez, F. E., & Tort, L. (2015) Mucosal immunity and B cells in teleosts: Effect of vaccination and stress. *Frontiers in Immunology*, **6**, 1–12. doi:10.3389/fimmu.2015.00354

Patil, V., Källqvist, T., Olsen, E., *et al.* (2007) Fatty acid composition of 12 microalgae for possible use in aquaculture feed. *Aquaculture International*, **15**, 1–9. doi:10.1007/s10499-006-9060-3

Pietretti, D., Vera-Jimenez, N. I., Hoole, D., *et al.* (2013) Oxidative burst and nitric oxide responses in carp macrophages induced by zymosan, MacroGard and selective dectin-1 agonists suggest recognition by multiple pattern recognition receptors. *Fish & Shellfish Immunology*, **35**, 847–857. doi:10.1016/j.fsi.2013.06.022

Pionnier, N., Falco, A., Miest, J. J., *et al.* (2014) Feeding common carp *Cyprinus carpio* with β-glucan supplemented diet stimulates C-reactive protein and complement immune acute phase responses following PAMPs injection. *Fish & Shellfish Immunology*, **39**, 285–95. doi:10.1016/j.fsi.2014.05.008

Plant, K. P., & LaPatra, S. E. (2011) Advances in fish vaccine delivery. *Developmental and Comparative Immunology*, **35**, 1256–62. doi:10.1016/j.dci.2011.03.007

Premanathan, M., Arakaki, R., Izumi, H., *et al.* (1999) Antiviral properties of a mangrove plant, *Rhizophora apiculata* Blume, against human immunodeficiency virus. *Antiviral Research*, **44**, 113–122. doi:10.1016/S0166-3542(99)00058-3

Purcell, M. K. M. M. K., Smith, K. D. K. D. K., Hood, L., *et al.* (2007) Conservation of toll-like receptor signaling pathways in teleost fish. *Comparative Biochemistry and Physiology Part D Genomics Proteomics*, **1**, 77–88. doi:10.1016/j.cbd.2005.07.003

Reverter, M., Bontemps, N., Lecchini, D., *et al.* (2014) Use of plant extracts in fish aquaculture as an alternative to chemotherapy: Current status and future perspectives. *Aquaculture*, **433**, 50–61. doi:10.1016/j.aquaculture.2014.05.048

Reyes-Becerril, M., Angulo, C., Estrada, N., *et al.* (2014) Dietary administration of microalgae alone or supplemented with *Lactobacillus sakei* affects immune response and intestinal morphology of Pacific red snapper (*Lutjanus peru*). *Fish & Shellfish Immunology*, **40**, 208–16. doi:10.1016/j.fsi.2014.06.032

Reyes-Becerril, M., Guardiola, F., Rojas, M., *et al.* (2013) Dietary administration of microalgae *Navicula* sp. affects immune status and gene expression of gilthead seabream (*Sparus aurata*). *Fish & Shellfish Immunology*, **35**, 883–9. doi:10.1016/j.fsi.2013.06.026

Rhule, A., Rase, B., Smith, J. R., *et al.* (2008) Toll-like receptor ligand-induced activation of murine DC2.4 cells is attenuated by *Panax notoginseng*. *Journal of Ethnopharmacology*, **116**, 179–186. doi:10.1016/j.jep.2007.11.019

Robertson, R. C., Guihéneuf, F., Bahar, B., *et al.* (2015) The anti-inflammatory effect of algae-derived lipid extracts on lipopolysaccharide (LPS)-stimulated human THP-1 macrophages. *Marine Drugs*, **13**, 5402–5424. doi:10.3390/md13085402

Rodríguez, A., Cuesta, A., Ortuño, J., *et al.* (2003) Immunostimulant properties of a cell wall-modified whole *Saccharomyces cerevisiae* strain administered by diet to seabream (*Sparus aurata* L.). *Veterinary Immunology and Immunopathology*, **96**, 183–192. doi:10.1016/S0165-2427(03)00164-8

Rombout, J. H. W. M., & Berg, A. A. (1989) Immunological importance of the second gut segment of carp. I. Uptake and processing of antigens by epithelial cells and macrophages. *Journal of Fish Biology*, **35**, 13–22. doi:10.1111/j.1095-8649.1989.tb03388.x

Rombout, J. W. H. M., Blok, L. J., Lamers, C. H. J., *et al.* (1986) Immunization of carp (*Cyprinus carpio*) with a *Vibrio anguillarum* bacterin: Indications for a common mucosal immune system. *Developmental and Comparative Immunology*, **10**, 341–351. doi:10.1016/0145-305X(86)90024-8

Ryu, S. J., Choi, H. S., Yoon, K. Y., *et al.* (2015) Oleuropein suppresses LPS-induced inflammatory responses in RAW 264.7 Cell and zebrafish. *Journal of Agricultural and Food Chemistry*, **63**, 2098–2105. doi:10.1021/jf505894b

Sahoo, P. K., & Mukherjee, S. C. (2001) Effect of dietary beta-1,3 glucan on immune responses and disease resistance of healthy and aflatoxin B1-induced immunocompromised rohu (*Labeo rohita* Hamilton). *Fish & Shellfish Immunology*, **11**, 683–95. doi:10.1006/fsim.2001.0345

Salinas, I. (2015) The mucosal immune system of teleost fish. *Biology*, **4**, 525–539. doi:10.3390/biology4030525

Salinas, I., LaPatra, S. E., & Erhardt, E. B. (2015) Nasal vaccination of young rainbow trout (Oncorhynchus mykiss) against infectious hematopoietic necrosis and enteric red mouth disease. *Developmental and Comparative Immunology*, **53**, 105–111. doi:10.1016/j.dci.2015.05.015

Salinas, I., Zhang, Y.-A., & Sunyer, J. O. (2011) Mucosal immunoglobulins and B cells of teleost fish. *Developmental & Comparative Immunology*, **35**, 1346–65. doi:10.1016/j.dci.2011.11.009

Schwandner, R., Roman, D., Holger, W., *et al.* (1999) Peptidoglycan-and lipoteichoic acid-induced cell activation is mediated by toll-like receptor 2. *Journal of Biological Chemistry*, **274**, 17406–17409. doi:10.1074/jbc.274.25.17406

Sealey, W. M., Barrows, F. T., Hang, A., *et al.* (2008) Evaluation of the ability of barley genotypes containing different amounts of β-glucan to alter growth and disease resistance of rainbow trout *Oncorhynchus mykiss*. *Animal Feed Science and Technology*, **141**, 115–128. doi:10.1016/j.anifeedsci.2007.05.022

Secombes, C. J., & Fletcher, T. C. (1992) The role of phagocytes in the protective mechanisms of fish. *Annual Review of Fish Diseases*, **2**, 53–71. doi:10.1016/0959-8030(92)90056-4

Secombes, C. J., & Olivier, G. (1997) *Host—Pathogen Interactions in Salmonids. Furunculosis. doi:DOI*: 10.1016/B978-012093040-1/50014-2

See, D., Broumand, N., Sahl, L., *et al.* (1997) *In vitro* effects of echinacea and ginseng on natural killer and antibody-dependent cell cytotoxicity in healthy subjects and chronic fatigue syndrome or acquired immunodeficiency syndrome patients. *Immunopharmacology*, **35**, 229–235.

Selvaraj, V., Sampath, K., & Sekar, V. (2005) Administration of yeast glucan enhances survival and some non-specific and specific immune parameters in carp (*Cyprinus carpio*) infected with *Aeromonas hydrophila*. *Fish & Shellfish Immunology*, **19**, 293–306. doi:10.1016/j.fsi.2005.01.001

Selvaraj, V., Sampath, K., & Sekar, V. (2006) Adjuvant and immunostimulatory effects of beta-glucan administration in combination with lipopolysaccharide enhances survival and some immune parameters in carp challenged with *Aeromonas hydrophila*. *Veterinary Immunology and Immunopathology*, **114**, 15–24. doi:10.1016/j.vetimm.2006.06.011

Selvaraj, V., Sampath, K., & Sekar, V. (2009) Administration of lipopolysaccharide increases specific and non-specific immune parameters and survival in carp (*Cyprinus carpio*) infected with *Aeromonas hydrophila*. *Aquaculture*, **286**, 176–183. doi:10.1016/j.aquaculture.2008.09.017

Sepulcre, M. P., Alcaraz-Pérez, F., López-Muñoz, A., *et al.* (2009) Evolution of lipopolysaccharide (LPS) recognition and signaling: fish TLR4 does not recognize LPS and negatively regulates NF-kappaB activation. *Journal of Immunology (Baltimore, Md. : 1950)*, **182**, 1836–1845. doi:10.4049/jimmunol.0801755

Sharma, N., & Tripathi, A. (2008) Effects of *Citrus sinensis* (L.) Osbeck epicarp essential oil on growth and morphogenesis of *Aspergillus niger* (L.) Van Tieghem. *Microbiological Research*, **163**, 337–344. doi:10.1016/j.micres.2006.06.009

Sheikhzadeh, N., Nofouzi, K., Delazar, A., *et al.* (2011) Immunomodulatory effects of decaffeinated green tea (*Camellia sinensis*) on the immune system of rainbow trout (*Oncorhynchus mykiss*). *Fish & Shellfish Immunology*, **31**, 1268–9. doi:10.1016/j.fsi.2011.09.010

Shin, Y. J., Kwon, T. H., Seo, J. Y., *et al.* (2013) Oral immunization of fish against iridovirus infection using recombinant antigen produced from rice callus. *Vaccine*, **31**, 5210–5215. doi:10.1016/j.vaccine.2013.08.085

Silva, M. T., & Correia-Neves, M. (2012) Neutrophils and macrophages: The main partners of phagocyte cell systems. *Frontiers in Immunology*, **3**, 2008–2013. doi:10.3389/fimmu.2012.00174

Siwicki, a K., Anderson, D. P., & Rumsey, G. L. (1994) Dietary intake of immunostimulants by rainbow trout affects non-specific immunity and protection against furunculosis. *Veterinary Immunology and Immunopathology*, **41**, 125–39. Retrieved from http://www.ncbi.nlm.nih.gov/pubmed/8066989

Skalli, A., Castillo, M., Andree, K. B., *et al.* (2013) The LPS derived from the cell walls of the Gram-negative bacteria *Pantoea agglomerans* stimulates growth and immune status of rainbow trout (*Oncorhynchus mykiss*) juveniles. *Aquaculture*, **416–417**, 272–279. doi:10.1016/j.aquaculture.2013.09.037

Skjermo, J., & Bergh, Ø. (2004) High-M alginate immunostimulation of Atlantic halibut (*Hippoglossus hippoglossus* L.) larvae using Artemia for delivery, increases resistance against vibriosis. *Aquaculture*, **238**, 107–113. doi:10.1016/j.aquaculture.2004.05.038

Skjermo, J., Defoort, T., Dehasque, M., *et al.* (1995) Immunostimulation of juvenile turbot (*Scophthalmus maximus* L.) using an alginate with high mannuronic acid content administered via the live food organism Artemia. *Fish & Shellfish Immunology*, **5**, 531–534. doi:10.1016/S1050-4648(95)80053-0

Sommerset, I., Krossøy, B., Biering, E., *et al.* (2005) Vaccines for fish in aquaculture. *Expert Review of Vaccines*, **4**, 89–101. doi:10.1586/14760584.4.1.89

Spitznagel, J. K., Martin, E., & Kinkade, M. (1983) Differential distribution of distinct forms of myoloperoxidase in different azuropholic granule subpopulations from human neutrophils. *Biochemical and Biophysical Research Communications*, **114**, 296–303.

Stroband, H. W. J., & Kroon, A. G. (1981) The development of the stomach in *Clarias lazera* and the intestinal absorption of protein macromolecules. *Cell and Tissue Research*, **215**, 397–415. doi:10.1007/BF00239123

Swain, P., Nayak, S. K., Nanda, P. K., *et al.* (2008) Biological effects of bacterial lipopolysaccharide (endotoxin) in fish: A review. *Fish and Shellfish Immunology*, **25**, 191–201. doi:10.1016/j.fsi.2008.04.009

Tafalla, C., Bøgwald, J., & Dalmo, R. A. (2013) Adjuvants and immunostimulants in fish vaccines: current knowledge and future perspectives. *Fish & Shellfish Immunology*, **35**, 1740–50. doi:10.1016/j.fsi.2013.02.029

Takizawa, F., Araki, K., Ohtani, M., *et al.* (2014) Transcription analysis of two Eomesodermin genes in lymphocyte subsets of two teleost species. *Fish & Shellfish Immunology*, **36**, 215–222. doi:10.1016/j.fsi.2013.11.004

Tanekhy, M. (2016) The role of Toll-like Receptors in innate immunity and infectious diseases of teleost. *Aquaculture Research*, **47**, 1369–1391. doi:10.1111/are.12607

Tang, J., Cai, J., Liu, R., *et al.* (2014) Immunostimulatory effects of artificial feed supplemented with a Chinese herbal mixture on *Oreochromis niloticus* against *Aeromonas hydrophila*. *Fish & Shellfish Immunology*, **39**, 401–6. doi:10.1016/j.fsi.2014.05.028

Thawonsuwan, J., Kiron, V., Satoh, S., *et al.* (2010) Epigallocatechin-3-gallate (EGCG) affects the antioxidant and immune defense of the rainbow trout, *Oncorhynchus mykiss*. *Fish Physiology and Biochemistry*, **36**, 687–697. doi:10.1007/s10695-009-9344-4

Tobar, I., Arancibia S., Torres C., *et al.* (2015) Successive oral immunizations against Piscirickettsia Salmonis and infectious Salmon Anemia Virus are required to maintain a long-term protection in farmed salmonids. *Frontiers in Immunology*, **6**, 1–7.

Torrecillas, S., Makol, A., Caballero, M. J., *et al.* (2007) Immune stimulation and improved infection resistance in European sea bass (*Dicentrarchus labrax*) fed mannan oligosaccharides. *Fish & Shellfish Immunology*, **23**, 969–81. doi:10.1016/j.fsi.2007.03.007

Tort, L. (2011) Stress and immune modulation in fish. *Developmental & Comparative Immunology*, **35**, 1366–75. doi:10.1016/j.dci.2011.07.002

Tu, F. P., Chu, W. H., Zhuang, X. Y., *et al.* (2010) Effect of oral immunization with *Aeromonas hydrophila* ghosts on protection against experimental fish infection. *Letters in Applied Microbiology*, **50**, 13–17. doi:10.1111/j.1472-765X.2009.02746.x

Uncini Manganelli, R. E., Zaccaro, L., & Tomei, P. E. (2005) Antiviral activity *in vitro* of *Urtica dioica* L., *Parietaria diffusa* M. et K. and *Sambucus nigra* L. *Journal of Ethnopharmacology*, **98**, 323–327. doi:10.1016/j.jep.2005.01.021

Vázquez, B., Avila, G., Segura, D., *et al.* (1996) Antiinflammatory activity of extracts from *Aloe vera* gel. *Journal of Ethnopharmacology*, **55**, 69–75.

Vollstad, D., Bøgwald, J., Gåserød, O., *et al.* (2006) Influence of high-M alginate on the growth and survival of Atlantic cod (*Gadus morhua* L.) and spotted wolffish (*Anarhichas minor* Olafsen) fry. *Fish & Shellfish Immunology*, **20**, 548–561. doi:10.1016/j.fsi.2005.07.004

Wang, J.-L., Meng, X., Lu, R., *et al.* (2015) Effects of *Rehmannia glutinosa* on growth performance, immunological parameters and disease resistance to *Aeromonas hydrophila* in common carp (*Cyprinus carpio* L.). *Aquaculture*, **435**, 293–300. doi:10.1016/j.aquaculture.2014.10.004

Wang, T. H., Holland, J. W., Martin, S. A. M., *et al.* (2010) Sequence and expression analysis of two T helper master transcription factors, T-bet and GATA3, in rainbow trout *Oncorhynchus mykiss* and analysis of their expression during bacterial and parasitic infection. *Fish & Shellfish Immunology*, **29**, 705–715. doi:10.1016/j.fsi.2010.06.016

Wang, T., Monte, M. M., Huang, W., *et al.* (2010) Identification of two FoxP3 genes in rainbow trout (*Oncorhynchus mykiss*) with differential induction patterns. *Molecular Immunology*, **47**, 2563–2574. doi:10.1016/j.molimm.2010.06.015

Watanuki, H., Ota, K., Tassakka, A. C. M. a R., *et al.* (2006) Immunostimulant effects of dietary *Spirulina platensis* on carp, *Cyprinus carpio*. *Aquaculture*, **258**, 157–163. doi:10.1016/j.aquaculture.2006.05.003

Weber, J. M., Ruzindana-Umunyana, A., Imbeault, L., *et al.* (2003) Inhibition of adenovirus infection and adenain by green tea catechins. *Antiviral Research*, **58**, 167–173. doi:10.1016/S0166-3542(02)00212-7

Wiart, C., Mogana, S., Khalifah, S., *et al.* (2004) Antimicrobial screening of plants used for traditional medicine in the state of Perak, Peninsular Malaysia. *Fitoterapia*, **75**, 68–73. doi:10.1016/j.fitote.2003.07.013

Xu, Y., Marshall, R. L., & Mukkur, T. K. S. (2006) An investigation on the antimicrobial activity of *Andrographis paniculata* extracts and andrographolide *in vitro*. *Asian Journal of Plant Sciences*. doi:10.3923/ajps.2006.527.530

Xu, Z., Parra, D., Gómez, D., *et al.* (2013) Teleost skin, an ancient mucosal surface that elicits gut-like immune responses. *Proceedings of the National Academy of Sciences*, **110**, 13097–13102. doi:10.1073/pnas.1304319110

Yang, X., Guo, J. L., Ye, J. Y., *et al.* (2015) The effects of *Ficus carica* polysaccharide on immune response and expression of some immune-related genes in grass carp, *Ctenopharyngodon idella*. *Fish & Shellfish Immunology*, **42**, 132–7. doi:10.1016/j.fsi.2014.10.037

Yarahmadi, P., Kolangi Miandare, H., Farahmand, H., *et al.* (2014) Dietary fermentable fiber upregulated immune related genes expression, increased innate immune response and resistance of rainbow trout (*Oncorhynchus mykiss*) against *Aeromonas hydrophila*. *Fish & Shellfish Immunology*, **41**, 326–31. doi:10.1016/j.fsi.2014.09.007

Yeganeh, S., Teimouri, M., & Amirkolaie, A. K. (2015) Dietary effects of *Spirulina platensis* on hematological and serum biochemical parameters of rainbow trout (*Oncorhynchus mykiss*). *Research in Veterinary Science*, **101**, 84–88. doi:10.1016/j.rvsc.2015.06.002

Yin, G., Ardó, L., Thompson, K. D., *et al.* (2009) Chinese herbs (*Astragalus radix* and *Ganoderma lucidum*) enhance immune response of carp, *Cyprinus carpio*, and protection against *Aeromonas hydrophila*. *Fish & Shellfish Immunology*, **26**, 140–145. doi:10.1016/j.fsi.2008.08.015

Yogeshwari, G., Jagruthi, C., Anbazahan, S. M., *et al.* (2015) Herbal supplementation diet on immune response in *Labeo rohita* against *Aphanomyces invadans*. *Aquaculture*, **437**, 351–359. doi:10.1016/j.aquaculture.2014.12.024

Yoon, T. J., Yoo, Y. C., Kang, T. B., *et al.* (1999) Lectins isolated from Korean mistletoe (*Viscum album coloratum*) induce apoptosis in tumor cells. *Cancer Letters*, **136**, 33–40.

Yoon, T. J., Yoo, Y. C., Kang, T. B., *et al.* (2003) Antitumor activity of the korean mistletoe lectin is attributed to activation of macrophages and NK cells. *Archives of Pharmacal Research*, **26**, 861–867.

You, Y.-H., & Lin, Z.-B. (2002) Protective effects of *Ganoderma lucidum* polysaccharides peptide on injury of macrophages induced by reactive oxygen species. *Acta Pharmacologica Sinica*, **23**, 787–791.

Yu, H. H., Han, F., Xue, M., *et al.* (2014) Efficacy and tolerance of yeast cell wall as an immunostimulant in the diet of Japanese seabass (*Lateolabrax japonicus*). *Aquaculture*, **432**, 217–224. doi:10.1016/j.aquaculture.2014.04.043

Yu, H.-H., Seo, S.-J., Kim, Y.-H., *et al.* (2006) Protective effect of *Rehmannia glutinosa* on the cisplatin-induced damage of HEI-OC1 auditory cells through scavenging free radicals. *Journal of Ethnopharmacology*, **107**, 383–388. doi:10.1016/j.jep.2006.03.024

Zanuzzo, F. S., Urbinati, E. C., Rise, M. L., *et al.* (2015) *Aeromonas salmonicida* induced immune gene expression in *Aloe vera* fed steelhead trout,*Oncorhynchus mykiss* (Walbaum). *Aquaculture*, **435**, 1–9. doi:10.1016/j.aquaculture.2014.09.010

Zedlitz, S., Kaufmann, R., & Boehncke, W.-H. (2002) Allergic contact dermatitis from black cumin (*Nigella sativa*) oil-containing ointment. *Contact Dermatitis*, **46**, 188. doi:10.1034/j.1600-0536.2002.460318.x

Zhang, G., Gong, S., Yu, D., *et al.* (2009) Propolis and Herba Epimedii extracts enhance the non-specific immune response and disease resistance of Chinese sucker, *Myxocyprinus asiaticus*. *Fish & Shellfish Immunology*, **26**, 467–472. doi:10.1016/j.fsi.2009.01.011

Zhang, J., Tang, Q., Zimmerman-Kordmann, M., *et al.* (2002) Activation of B lymphocytes by GLIS, a bioactive proteoglycan from *Ganoderma lucidum*. *Life Sciences*, **71**, 623–638. doi:10.1016/S0024-3205(02)01690-9

Zhang, Y.-A., Salinas, I., Li, J., *et al.* (2010) IgT, a primitive immunoglobulin class specialized in mucosal immunity. *Nature Immunology*, **11**, 827–835. doi:10.1038/ni.1913

Zhang, Z., Chi, H., Niu, C., *et al.* (2011) Molecular cloning and characterization of Foxp3 in Atlantic salmon (*Salmo salar*). *Fish & Shellfish Immunology*, **30**, 902–9. doi:10.1016/j.fsi.2011.01.012

Zhong, X., Shi, Y., Chen, J., *et al.* (2014) Polyphenol extracts from *Punica granatum* and *Terminalia chebula* are anti-inflammatory and increase the survival rate of chickens challenged with *Escherichia coli*. *Biological and Pharmaceutical Bulletin*, **37**, 1575–1582. doi:10.1248/bpb.b14-00163

7

Prebiotics and Synbiotics

Seyed Hossein Hoseinifar[1], *Yun-Zhang Sun*[2] *and Zhigzhang Zhou*[3]

[1] *Department of Fisheries, Gorgan University of Agricultural Sciences and Natural Resources, Gorgan, Iran*
[2] *Key Laboratory of Healthy Mariculture for the East China Sea, Ministry of Agriculture, Fisheries College, Jimei University, Xiamen, China*
[3] *Key Laboratory for Feed Biotechnology of the Ministry of Agriculture, Feed Research Institute, Chinese Academy of Agricultural Sciences, Beijing, China*

The Interactions between Feed Additives and Diseases of Fish and Shellfish

Prebiotics and Synbiotics: Definition and History

A variety of useful feed supplements, including probiotics, prebiotics and synbiotics, which have beneficial effects to the host have been used in aquaculture to improve growth and disease resistance, and in some cases, act as an alternative to antimicrobial compounds (Irianto and Austin, 2002), as well as to stimulate immunity response of the host. The successful use of probiotics has laid the foundation for other concepts such as prebiotics. Prebiotics offer an alternative method for manipulating endogenous microbes to improve health. Instead of introducing favourable bacteria with the diet, the aim of prebiotics is to stimulate selected favourable indigenous microbial populations (Dimitroglou *et al.*, 2011).

Classically, prebiotics are defined as non-digestible fibers that benefit the host by selectively stimulating the growth and/or activity of specific health-promoting bacteria that can improve the host health (Pharmaceutiques, 1995). In this regard, prebiotics are used as energy sources for the gut bacteria and can be referred to as functional saccharides (Roberfroid, 1993). According to Gibson *et al.*, only three oligosaccharides, inulin, transgalacto-oligosaccharide (TOS) and lactulose, were originally classified as prebiotics (Gibson *et al.*, 2004). Later, fructo-oligosaccharide (FOS), mannan oligosaccharides (MOS) and beta-glucan have been included in the list (Kocher, 2004). MOS and FOS are perhaps the most well-studied oligosaccharides in fish but some information regarding applications of inulin, galacto-oligosaccharides, xylo-oligosaccharides, arabino-xylo-oligosaccharides and isomalto-oligosaccharides in aquatic animals is also available (Burr *et al.*, 2010; Ibrahem *et al.*, 2010; Merrifield *et al.*, 2010; Ringø *et al.*, 2010).

Diagnosis and Control of Diseases of Fish and Shellfish, First Edition. Edited by Brian Austin and Aweeda Newaj-Fyzul.

Synbiotics are nutritional supplements that combine probiotics and prebiotics in the form of synergism. The concept of synbiotics was proposed to characterize some colonic foods with interesting nutritional properties that make these compounds candidates for classification as health-enhancing functional ingredients (Pharmaceutiques, 1995). Certainly, synbiotics have been widely used in human and veterinary medicine as they could potentially be useful to treat and/or prevent gastrointestinal (GI) disorders (Cheng *et al.*, 2014; Defoirdt *et al.*, 2011). However, there was no research about synbiotics in aquaculture until 2009. Since the first finfish study was published by Rodriguez-Estrada *et al.* (2009), several other studies have emerged (Cerezuela *et al.*, 2011; De *et al.*, 2014; Ringø, *et al.*, 2014).

Mode of Actions on Disease Resistance

Prebiotics modulate composition and/or activity of the gut microbiota through their metabolization by micro-organisms in the gut, thus conferring a beneficial physiological effect on the host. Prebiotics act as a growth factor which can selectively inhibit the adhesion and invasion of pathogenic micro-organisms in the colon epithelium by competing for the same glycoconjugates on the surface of epithelial cells, preferencing the non-specific barrier function and improving the production of mucus, short chain fatty acids and cytokines (Akhter *et al.*, 2015).

Synbiotics, as the combined application of probiotics and prebiotics, are based on the principle of providing a probiont with a competitive advantage over endogenous populations, improving the survival and implantation of the live microbial dietary supplement in the gastrointestinal tract of the host by selectively stimulating the growth and/or by activating the metabolism of one or a limited number of health-promoting bacteria, and thus improving the host 'welfare' (Pharmaceutiques, 1995). The use of synbiotics may give rise to greater benefits than the separate application of individual probionts. Geng *et al.* (2011) demonstrated that diet supplemented with the right level of chitosan and *B. subtilis* significantly enhanced growth, innate immunity and protection against infection for cobia, and established the optimal combination of both ingredients for the assayed conditions and parameters.

Strengthening the Immune Response

The innate immune system, also known as the non-specific immune system, is the first line of defence, comprising cells and mechanisms that defend the host from infection by other organisms. The immunomodulatory activity of prebiotics is mediated through direct interactions with pattern recognition receptors (PRRs), such as beta-glucan receptors and dectin-1 receptors expressed in macrophages (Brown *et al.*, 2002). This type of interaction activates signal transduction molecules, such as NF-kappa-B, which stimulate immune cells (Yadav and Schorey, 2006). Saccharides may also interact with PAMPs, such as teichoic acid, peptidoglycan, glycosylated protein or the capsular polysaccharide of the bacteria, causing an immune response (Bron *et al.*, 2012). On the other hand, prebiotics can selectively increase/decrease specific intestinal bacteria that modulate local cytokine and antibody production, increase intestinal short chain fatty acid production, enhance binding to G-coupled protein receptors on leucocytes, and affect interaction with carbohydrate receptors on intestinal epithelial and immune cells (Seifert and Watzl, 2007).

Conclusion

Prebiotics and synbiotics have important roles in disease control, and they are likely to become more widely used in the future.

References

Akhter, N., Wu, B., Memon, A.M. and Mohsin, M. (2015) Probiotics and prebiotics associated with aquaculture, a review. *Fish and Shellfish Immunology*, **45**, 733–741.

Bron, P.A., van Baarlen, P. and Kleerebezem, M. (2012) Emerging molecular insights into the interaction between probiotics and the host intestinal mucosa. *Nature Reviews Microbiology*, **10**, 66–78.

Brown, G.D., Taylor, P.R., Reid, D.M., *et al.* (2002) Dectin-1 is a major β-glucan receptor on macrophages. *Journal of Experimental Medicine*, **196**, 407–412.

Burr, G., Hume, M., Ricke, S., Nisbet, D. and Gatlin III, D. (2010) In vitro and in vivo evaluation of the prebiotics GroBiotic®-A, inulin, mannanoligosaccharide, and galactooligosaccharide on the digestive microbiota and performance of hybrid striped bass (*Morone chrysops* × *Morone saxatilis*). *Microbial Ecology*, **59**, 187–198.

Cerezuela, R., Meseguer, J. and Esteban, M. (2011) Current knowledge in synbiotic use for fish aquaculture, a review. *Journal of Aquaculture Research and Development*, **1**, 2.

Cheng, G., Hao, H., Xie, S., *et al.* (2014) Antibiotic alternatives, the substitution of antibiotics in animal husbandry? *Frontiers in Microbiology*, **5**, 217.

De, B.C., Meena, D., Behera, B., Das, P., Mohapatra, P.D. and Sharma, A. (2014) Probiotics in fish and shellfish culture, immunomodulatory and ecophysiological responses. *Fish Physiology and Biochemistry*, **40**, 921–971.

Defoirdt, T., Sorgeloos, P. and Bossier, P. (2011) Alternatives to antibiotics for the control of bacterial disease in aquaculture. *Current Opinion in Microbiology*, **14**, 251–258.

Dimitroglou, A., Merrifield, D.L., Carnevali, O., *et al.* (2011) Microbial manipulations to improve fish health and production – a Mediterranean perspective. *Fish and Shellfish Immunology*, **30**, 1–16.

Geng, X., Dong, X.H., Tan, B.P., *et al.* (2011) Effects of dietary chitosan and *Bacillus subtilis* on the growth performance, non-specific immunity and disease resistance of cobia, *Rachycentron canadum*. *Fish and Shellfish Immunology*, **31**, 400–406.

Gibson, G.R., Probert, H.M., van Loo, J., Rastall, R.A. and Roberfroid, M.B. (2004) Dietary modulation of the human colonic microbiota, updating the concept of prebiotics. *Nutrition Research Reviews*, **17**, 259–275.

Ibrahem, M.D., Fathi, M., Mesalhy, S. and El-Aty, A.A. (2010) Effect of dietary supplementation of inulin and vitamin C on the growth, hematology, innate immunity, and resistance of Nile tilapia (*Oreochromis niloticus*). *Fish and Shellfish Immunology*, **29**, 241–246.

Irianto, A. and Austin, B. (2002) Probiotics in aquaculture. *Journal of Fish Diseases*, **25**, 633–642.

Kocher, A. (2004) *The Potential for Immunosaccharides to Maximize Growth Performance. Interfacing Immunity, Gut Health and Performance*. Nottingham University Press, Nottingham.

Merrifield, D.L., Dimitroglou, A., Foey, A., *et al.* (2010) The current status and future focus of probiotic and prebiotic applications for salmonids. *Aquaculture*, **302**, 1–18.

Pharmaceutiques (1995) Dietary modulation of the human colonie microbiota, introducing the concept of prebiotics. *Journal of Nutrition*, **125**, 1401–1412.

Ringø, E., Olsen, R., Gifstad, T., *et al.* (2010) Prebiotics in aquaculture, a review. *Aquaculture Nutrition*, **16**, 117–136.

Ringø, E., Olsen, R.E., Jensen, I., Romero, J. and Lauzon, H.L. (2014) Application of vaccines and dietary supplements in aquaculture, possibilities and challenges. *Reviews in Fish Biology and Fisheries*, **24**, 1005–1032.

Roberfroid, M. (1993) Dietary fiber, inulin, and oligofructose, a review comparing their physiological effects. *Critical Reviews in Food Science and Nutrition*, **33**, 103–148.

Rodriguez-Estrada, U., Satoh, S., Haga, Y., Fushimi, H. and Sweetman, J. (2009) Effects of single and combined supplementation of *Enterococcus faecalis*, mannan oligosaccharide and polyhydroxybutyrate acid on growth performance and immune response of rainbow trout *Oncorhynchus mykiss*. *Suisan zoshoku (Aquaculture Science)*, **57**, 609–617.

Seifert, S. and Watzl, B. (2007) Inulin and oligofructose, review of experimental data on immune modulation. *Journal of Nutrition*, **137**, 2563S–2567S.

Yadav, M. and Schorey, J.S. (2006) The β-glucan receptor dectin-1 functions together with TLR2 to mediate macrophage activation by mycobacteria. *Blood*, **108**, 3168–3175.

8

Probiotics for Disease Control in Aquaculture

S.M. Sharifuzzaman[1] *and Brian Austin*[2]

[1] *Institute of Marine Sciences and Fisheries, University of Chittagong, Chittagong, Bangladesh*
[2] *Institute of Aquaculture, University of Stirling, Stirling, Scotland, UK*

Introduction

Aquaculture is regarded as the fastest growing animal food production system in the world, but outbreaks of infectious diseases remain a key limitation to the expansion of this sector as many microbial pathogens are normal inhabitants of the aquatic environment (Austin and Austin, 2012; Pillay, 2004; Subasinghe, 2005). Taxonomically, the pathogens range from single-stranded RNA viruses, such as infectious salmon anaemia (ISA), to complex parasitic crustaceans, for example sea lice (Murray and Peeler, 2005), and are broadly classified as viruses, bacteria, fungi, parasites, protozoa and metazoans (Austin, 2005; Austin and Austin, 2012; Bondad-Reantaso *et al.*, 2005; Owens, 2003). Both prophylactic and therapeutic measures are available to combat these pathogens (Austin, 2002; Austin and Austin, 2012; Newaj-Fyzul *et al.*, 2014; Vendrell *et al.*, 2006), but the indiscriminate use of antibiotics may lead to the development and spread of antibiotic-resistant bacteria, which may pose a risk to human health (Akinbowale *et al.*, 2006; Alcaide *et al.*, 2005). Thus, the value of preventative measures is recognized and, in consequence, probiotics has garnered attention for disease prevention in aquaculture (Austin *et al.*, 1995; Balcázar *et al.*, 2006; Gatesoupe, 1999; Gobeli *et al.*, 2009; Irianto and Austin, 2002a,b; Newaj-Fyzul and Austin, 2015; Newaj-Fyzul *et al.*, 2014; Sharifuzzaman and Austin, 2009; Spanggaard *et al.*, 2001; Verschuere *et al.*, 2000) (Figure 8.1).

The origin of probiotics use in aquaculture is unclear, but evidence suggests an extensive usage in fish and shellfish culture especially in South America (Ecuador) and Asia (China and India) (Austin and Austin, 2012; Kumar *et al.*, 2006; Nayak *et al.*, 2007; Newaj-Fyzul and Austin, 2015; Preetha *et al.*, 2007; Rengpipat *et al.*, 1998; Vaseeharan and Ramasamy, 2003). However, probiotics led to the control of a range of bacterial pathogens in various fish species. For example, rainbow trout (*Oncorhynchus mykiss*) were protected against *Aeromonas salmonicida* and *Yersinia ruckeri* when administered with dietary *Carnobacterium maltaromaticum* and *C. divergens* at $>10^7$ cells/g for two weeks (Kim and Austin, 2006a). Similarly, reduction of *Lactococcus garvieae*, *Vibrio anguillarum*, *A. hydrophila*, *A. sobria* and *Streptococcus* sp. associated mortalities in rainbow trout, Chinese drum

Diagnosis and Control of Diseases of Fish and Shellfish, First Edition. Edited by Brian Austin and Aweeda Newaj-Fyzul.

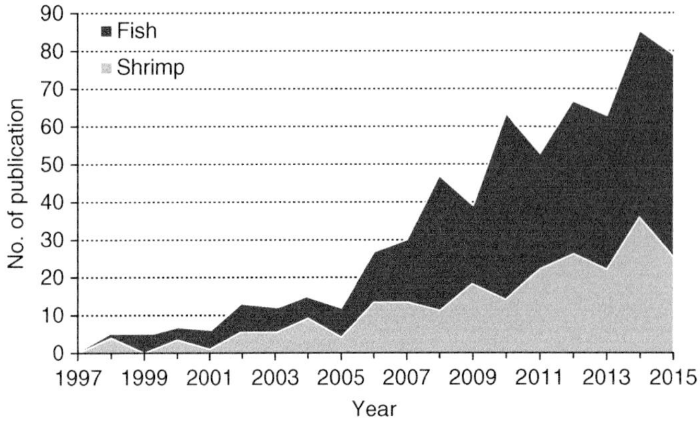

Figure 8.1 Interest in probiotics research for application in aquaculture. Source: search on ISI Web of Knowledge (www.isiknowledge.com) using keywords 'probiotics+fish' and 'probiotics+shrimp'. The search was not exhaustive, but sufficient to illustrate the growing trends in recent years.

(*Miichthys miiuy*), Nile tilapia (*Oreochromis niloticus*), perch (*Perca fluviatilis*) and grouper (*Epinephelus coioides*) was noticeable by the use of probiotics – *A. sobria* (Brunt and Austin, 2005), *Clostridium butyricum* (Pan *et al.*, 2008), *Micrococcus luteus* (El-Rhman *et al.*, 2009), *Pseudomonas chlororaphis* (Gobeli *et al.*, 2009) and *Lactobacillus plantarum* (Son *et al.*, 2009), respectively. In the case of shellfish, probiotics demonstrated effectiveness against *V. alginolyticus*, *V. coralliilyticus*, *V. harveyi*, *V. parahaemolyticus* and *V. splendidus* infections in penaeid shrimp, scallop (*Pecten maximus*) and Pacific oyster (*Crassostrea gigas*) (Kesarcodi-Watson *et al.*, 2012; Li *et al.*, 2008; Preetha *et al.*, 2007; Tseng *et al.*, 2009).

Overall, probiotics have been credited for improved nutrition (Balcázar *et al.*, 2006), some tangible health benefits (Irianto and Austin, 2002b; Nikoskelainen *et al.*, 2003; Panigrahi *et al.*, 2005; Sáenz de Rodrigáñez *et al.*, 2009; Salinas *et al.*, 2005; Silva *et al.*, 2013), reduced disease incidence (Brunt and Austin, 2005; Newaj-Fyzul *et al.*, 2007, Sharifuzzaman and Austin, 2009) as well as food production in an environmentally friendly way (Macey and Coyne, 2005). Thus, the Food and Agriculture Organization of the United Nations (FAO) has now highlighted the use of probiotics in aquaculture as a means of improving the quality of the aquatic environment (Subasinghe *et al.*, 2003).

Definition of Probiotics

The concept of probiotics was introduced by Lilley and Stillwell (1965) to describe 'substances secreted by a micro-organism that stimulate the growth of another organism', and thus 'probiotic', which is derived from the Greek meaning 'for life', is the opposite of antibiotic. Parker (1974) probably first coined the term and definition of probiotics as 'organisms and substances which contribute to intestinal microbial balance'. Since then the description of probiotics has evolved and it is commonly used to indicate bacteria associated with beneficial effects on humans and animals. Fuller (1989) revised probiotics as a 'live microbial feed supplement which beneficially affects the host animal by improving its intestinal microbial balance' – where emphasized the use of live micro-organisms as probiotics. To accommodate the immunostimulatory effect of probiotics, Naidu *et al.* (1999) modified the concept of probiotics as 'a microbial dietary adjuvant that beneficially affects the host physiology by modulating mucosal and systemic immunity, as well as improving nutritional and microbial balance in the intestinal tract'. In the field of aquaculture, Moriarty (1998) widened the definition of probiotics to microbial 'water additives'. Verschuere *et al.* (2000) proposed a broader application of the term as 'a live microbial adjunct which has a beneficial effect on the host by modifying the host-associated or ambient microbial community, by ensuring improved use of the feed or enhancing its nutritional value, by enhancing the host response towards disease, or by improving the quality of its ambient environment'. Salminen *et al.* (1999) proposed probiotics as 'any microbial cell preparation or components of microbial cells that have a beneficial effect on the health and well-being of the host', where dead cells or components of micro-organisms are also included as probiotics.

So, there is a bewildering array of definitions and the 'probiotic concept' remains complex as new findings emerge. The FAO/WHO (2001) has integrated all these definitions and stated that probiotics are 'live micro-organisms which when administered in adequate amounts, confer a health benefit on the host'. However, probiotics in aquaculture can be live or dead preparations, including cellular/extracellular components of micro-organism(s), administered either as feed supplement or to the rearing water, that provide host benefits by improving disease resistance, growth and health status, immunity, feed utilization/conversion, microbial balance and rearing water quality (Hai, 2015; Irianto and Austin, 2002b; Nayak, 2010; Newaj-Fyzul *et al.*, 2014).

Source of Probiotics

The use of host-derived micro-organisms as a source of probiotics has been preferred since the early 1990s (Westerdahl *et al.*, 1991). It is argued that microbiota living in healthy hosts are most likely to be part of the natural defence system and beneficial in multiple ways (Gomez *et al.*, 2013; Lazado *et al.*, 2012; Sharifuzzaman *et al.*, 2014). Most importantly, candidate probionts indigenous to the environment to which they will be exposed are able to survive spontaneously and function physiologically at their optimum level. Thus, comprising a diverse microbial community at high concentration, the gastrointestinal tract of aquatic species has attracted considerable attention in isolating putative strains for probiotics development (Lazado *et al.*, 2015). Micro-organisms occurring in the water and sediment/sand can also be invaluable as probiotics (Irianto and Austin, 2002b; Lauzon *et al.*, 2010).

Because of proven safety and efficacy in human and livestock models, some studies have suggested the use of ubiquitous Lactobacillales (or lactic acid bacteria) found in terrestrial sources for aquaculture (Merrifield *et al.*, 2010a; Nikoskelainen *et al.*, 2003; Picchietti *et al.*, 2007; Ren *et al.*, 2013). An obligately anaerobic bacterium, such as *Cl. butyricum* from the intestine of healthy chickens, has been successfully evaluated as a probiotic for fish species (Pan *et al.*, 2008). Since intrinsic and extrinsic factors influence the functionality of probiotics, the effectiveness of terrestrial probiotics may not always be the same when applied to aquatic hosts due to differences in the biophysicochemical environment. For instance, growth inhibition of bacterial pathogens by a candidate probiotic GP31, isolated from the gut of Atlantic cod (*Gadus morhua*), diminished when the temperature increased from 13 °C to 20 °C (Caipang *et al.*, 2010). This kind of outcome cannot be overlooked if considering the use of terrestrial strains and, in particular, their viability and effectiveness in the marine aquatic environment can be unsatisfactory (Vazquez *et al.*, 2003).

Other sources of probiotics reported in peer-reviewed studies include culture collections (i.e. *L. rhamnosus* GG) and commercial products (i.e. Bactocell®, Calsporin®, Cernivet®LBC, Efinol®L, Sanolife®MIC, Toyocerin®). But the quality control of commercial preparations appears to be poor due to lack of evidence for specific claims, such as identity, composition, number and proper dosage of micro-organisms (Huys *et al.*, 2006; Weese and Martin, 2011). A study by Nimrat and Vuthiphandchai (2011) reported that none of the 12 commercial probiotics marketed for marine shrimp culture in Thailand correctly demonstrate the number/composition of micro-organisms and qualitative extracellular enzymes described on the labels, nor did they inhibit the growth of the shrimp pathogen *V. harveyi*. Evidence of efficacy for commercial probiotic products is thus unclear. Nevertheless, host-derived micro-organisms, particularly microbiota isolated from the gastrointestinal tract of aquatic animals, not only eliminate some of the issues presented above but are also beneficial to the host in several ways, highlighting their great potential to be used as probiotics (Hai, 2015; Irianto and Austin, 2002b; Newaj-Fyzul *et al.*, 2014; Sharifuzzaman and Austin, 2010a).

Application Methods and Options

Probiotics in aquaculture may be applied either directly or indirectly via water or diet, short or long term, in doses containing live or dead preparations either singly or in combination, even as a mixture with prebiotics or immunostimulants. The right choice of route and method of probiotic administration is not clear but they are dependent on many factors surrounding the host, pathogen and culture technique.

Delivery Method

The proposed methods of delivery include:

- bathing the host in a bacterial suspension (Austin *et al.*, 1995; Gram *et al.*, 1999)
- addition of the culture directly to rearing water (Gobeli *et al.*, 2009; Moriarty 1998; Spanggaard *et al.*, 2001)
- supplementation with artificial inert diets (Aly *et al.*, 2008a; Nikoskelainen *et al.*, 2001; Vendrell *et al.*, 2008)
- via bioencapsulation, that is, enrichment of live food artemia/rotifer (Gatesoupe 1994; Planas *et al.*, 2006).

Thus, a feed supplement of *Kocuria* SM1 dosed at $\sim 10^8$ cells/g was effective in controlling infections caused by *V. anguillarum* in rainbow trout (Sharifuzzaman and Austin, 2009). Moreover, turbot (*Scophthalmus maximus*) larvae fed *Roseobacter* 27-4 enriched rotifer were protected against *V. anguillarum* infection (Planas *et al.*, 2006). Similarly, the application of probiotics via rearing water has been successful (Makridis *et al.*, 2008; Ottesen and Olafsen, 2000; Ringø and Vadstein, 1998) and a disease reduction effect was noted by bathing scallop larvae in probiotic suspension (Riquelme *et al.*, 1997). Dietary supplementation of probiotics is more practical than direct application into the rearing medium, although the developmental stage, age and type of host, and culture environment are crucial when choosing an appropriate delivery method.

Dosage, Frequency and Duration of Administration

The dose, which is the cell concentration of probiotics available to the aquatic host, is a principal consideration that determines the efficacy of probiotic products. The FAO/WHO (2001) has emphasized that probiotics should be administered in adequate amounts in order to confer a health benefit on the host. Considering different dose levels (i.e. 10^5–10^9 cells/g feed), Sharifuzzaman (2010) revealed that any dose below or above 10^7 and 10^8 cells/g for probiotics *Kocuria* SM1 and *Rhodococcus* SM2, respectively, did not result in good levels of host protection. Similarly, Newaj-Fyzul *et al.* (2007) demonstrated that doses of *B. subtilis* lower and higher than 10^7 cells/g of feed were less successful at enhancing resistance to *Aeromonas* infection in rainbow trout. Moreover, feeding of rainbow trout with *L. rhamnosus*-supplemented diets at 10^9 cfu/g led to reduced mortality rates, from 52.6% in the control to 18.9% when compared to mortality rates of 46.3% for the dose 10^{12} cfu/g, following challenge with *A. salmonicida* (Nikoskelainen *et al.*, 2001). Probiotic *L. brevis* at 10^9 cells/g was also reported to protect hybrid tilapia against *A. hydrophila* infection (Liu *et al.*, 2013). A dose–effect relationship should be carefully determined to avoid overdosing with resultant lower efficacy and unnecessary costs, or conversely underdosing, which reduces the efficiency of the probiont (Vine *et al.*, 2006).

Frequency of administration is an important factor influencing the proper functioning of probiotics. Daily addition is preferred as probiotic cultures do not show spontaneous primary colonization, but are reported to disappear from the system, either digestive tract or culture medium, on discontinuation of supplementation (Ferguson *et al.*, 2010; Robertson *et al.*, 2000; Sharifuzzaman *et al.*, 2014). As such, continuous or repeated addition of probiotics to the host is recommended (Guo *et al.*, 2009; Skjermo *et al.*, 2015).

Equally, the length of feeding time is fundamentally important when using probiotics. To date, studies with probiotics have involved different feeding durations, for example 1–32-week feeding regimes (Hai, 2015), but the basis for choosing these periods is often unclear. Sharifuzzaman and Austin (2009) demonstrated that rainbow trout fed for two weeks with *Kocuria* SM1 had higher survival against *V. anguillarum* challenge than the control groups and groups with other feeding lengths, such as one-, three- and four-week feeding regimes. Moreover, dietary *L. plantarum* in grouper (Son *et al.*, 2009), *Cl. butyricum* in Chinese drum (Pan *et al.*, 2008) and *Bacillus subtilis*, *L. acidophilus* or a mixture of both in tilapia (Aly *et al.*, 2008a) were beneficial when used for 28, 30 and 60 days, respectively, reducing mortality following challenge with *Streptococcus* sp., *V. anguillarum*, *A. hydrophila*, *Ps. fluorescens* and *S. iniae*. Conversely, one week or less administration time is not suitable because such a short-term supplementation is not capable of improving fish survival nor able to influence microbial community composition appreciably (Qi *et al.*, 2009; Robertson *et al.*, 2000; Sharifuzzaman and Austin, 2009). Nevertheless, probiotics supplementation for two weeks has been comparatively effective in relation to other feeding periods (Balcázar *et al.*, 2007b; Brunt and Austin, 2005; Brunt *et al.*, 2007; Kim and Austin, 2006a; Pieters *et al.*, 2008).

Long-term or extended administration of probiotics can be immunosuppressive (Bricknell and Dalmo, 2005; Sakai, 1999), but a short-term cyclical feeding strategy involving probiotic supplementation for a minimum of two weeks and periodic return to the unsupplemented condition may be beneficial to the host (Bricknell and Dalmo, 2005). In this way, a carry-over effect of probiotics can be realized that maintains a level of protection and immunostimulation for up to four weeks after cessation of supplementation (Sharifuzzaman and Austin, 2010b).

This will help to avoid long-term or continued use of probiotics as well as overstimulation or immunosuppression of the host innate immune response.

Use of Single Strain or Combinations

Many studies have tested single strains of probiotic and documented *in vivo* effectiveness. Robertson *et al.* (2000) confirmed the efficacy of *Carnobacterium* sp. at reducing diseases caused by *A. salmonicida*, *V. ordalii* and *Y. ruckeri* in salmonids. Improved resistance to *V. anguillarum* in cod fry was also reported after addition of *C. divergens* (Gildberg and Mikkelsen, 1998). Formulations of either multistrain or multispecies are suggested to improve the activity of probiotics by triggering synergistic beneficial effects on the health of the host, such as improvement or prolongation of the desirable effects (Timmerman *et al.*, 2004). Aly *et al.* (2008a) noted significantly higher protection in tilapia against several pathogens (*A. hydrophila*, *Ps. fluorescens* and *S. iniae*) when fed mixtures of *B. subtilis* and *L. acidophilus* for one month compared with groups that received either *B. subtilis* or *L. acidophilus* alone. In contrast, tilapia administered a mixture of *M. luteus* and *Pseudomonas* sp. for 90 days did not resist *A. hydrophila* infection, reaching mortality levels of 80% compared with 25% mortality when fed a single culture of *M. luteus* (El-Rhman *et al.*, 2009). Similarly, Irianto and Austin (2002a) did not reveal further benefit by using an equi-mixture of *A. hydrophila*, *V. fluvialis*, *Carnobacterium* sp. and a Gram-positive coccus A1-6, over monospecies preparations of probiotic in controlling *A. salmonicida* in rainbow trout. These data suggest that the level of host protection due to viable probiotics may differ in relation to fish species, the type of probiotic strain and their various combinations.

The concept of a synbiotic, which combines probiotics and prebiotics in a form of synergism with the principal aim of improving the survival of the probiotic supplement in the gastrointestinal tract of the host, is also gaining interest in aquaculture (Gibson and Roberfroid, 1995; Ringø *et al.*, 2014). Feeding with a mixture of *Enterococcus faecalis* and mannan oligosaccharide was reported to enhance growth, immune response and survival of fish which was superior to the use of either probiotic or prebiotic alone (Rodriguez-Estrada *et al.*, 2009). Certainly, dietary inclusion of *B. coagulans* and chitosan oligosaccharides had a synergistic effect that led to improved growth, feed conversion ratio, immunity (peripheral total leucocyte count, respiratory burst, phagocytic, lysozyme and superoxide dismutase activities) and disease resistance against *A. veronii* infection in koi carp, *Cyprinus carpio koi* (Lin *et al.*, 2012). A combination of probiotics with immunostimulants has been studied recently; Guzmán-Villanueva *et al.* (2014) combined beta-1,3/1,6-glucan with probiotic *Shewanella putrefaciens* and the mixture when fed to gilthead seabream (*Sparus aurata*) modulated humoural and cellular innate immunity, expression of immune-related genes and growth of the fish. Also, beta-glucans with bacterial supplements (*B. subtilis*) were reported to induce several immune parameters, including expression of serine protease and prophenoloxidase genes in white shrimp, *Penaeus vannamei* (Wongsasak *et al.*, 2015). The combined use of probiotics and immunostimulants in aquaculture is less well studied and certainly warrants further investigation.

Dead, Inactivated or Cell Component

As an alternative to viable cells, Brunt and Austin (2005) and Pan *et al.* (2008) used formalized, sonicated, heat-killed and cell-free supernatant of probiotics, but these preparations conferred comparatively less protection in rainbow trout and Chinese drum against *S. iniae*, *La. garvieae*, *A. hydrophila* and *V. anguillarum*. Also, Taoka *et al.* (2006b) noted decreased resistance in tilapia to *Edwardsiella tarda* infection after oral administration of dead probiotics. Therefore, the administration of dead/inactivated cells or the supernatant of probiotic cultures does not necessarily reduce bacterial infection, which reinforces the benefit of using live cells.

Abbass *et al.* (2010) observed that subcellular components, such as cell wall proteins (CWPs), whole cell proteins (WCPs), lipopolysaccharides (LPS) and outer membrane proteins (OMPs), of the probiotics *A. sobria* and *B. subtilis*, when administered to rainbow trout, led to 100% survival compared with 10% survival in controls against a new biogroup of *Y. ruckeri* that has been resistant to conventional vaccines. Similarly, the use of CWPs and WCPs of *Kocuria* SM1 and *Rhodococcus* SM2 led to significant resistance to *V. anguillarum* infection in rainbow trout, although extracellular proteins (ECPs) of both probiotics fared less well (Sharifuzzaman *et al.*, 2011). Overall, these results highlight the potential of using cellular components of probiotics in controlling bacterial fish diseases.

Certainly, it is necessary to pick the best possible methods of delivery to the host, including consideration of dose (Brunt and Austin, 2005; Son *et al.*, 2009), feeding duration (Aly *et al.*, 2008a; Sharifuzzaman and Austin, 2009), and composition of the preparation, either single or multiple strains (Aly *et al.*, 2008a; Hai *et al.*, 2009) or in combination with probiotics/immunostimulants (Rodriguez-Estrada *et al.*, 2009; Wongsasak *et al.*, 2015).

Range of Probiotics and their Efficacy

The organisms that offer promise to improve health and/or survival of farmed aquatic species are more diverse and greater in number than those considered for human nutrition (i.e. mostly the lactic acid bacteria) and terrestrial veterinary medicine. Thus, a wide range of Gram-positive and Gram-negative bacteria, bacteriophages, unicellular algae and yeasts as well as beneficial isolates from human [*L. rhamnosus* (Nikoskelainen *et al.* 2003) and *L. plantarum* (Picchietti *et al.*, 2007)] and terrestrial animals [*Cl. butyricum* from the intestine of healthy chickens (Pan *et al.*, 2008)] have been evaluated for use in aquaculture. This is because the mode of action of probiotics is not similar but shows variation in efficacy, suggesting that one probiotic could not be used commonly for all fish species to control single or multiple diseases.

Among the Gram-positive bacteria, *Bacillus* species (such as *B. subtilis*) is the best evaluated genus for use in fish and shellfish farming, followed by various species of *Lactobacillus* (*L. plantarum*, *L. rhamnosus*). Other genera include *Arthrobacter*, *Brevibacillus*, *Brochothrix*, *Clostridium*, *Carnobacterium*, *Enterococcus*, *Kocuria*, *Lactococcus*, *Leuconostoc*, *Microbacterium*, *Micrococcus*, *Pediococcus*, *Rhodococcus*, *Streptococcus*, *Streptomyces*, *Vagococcus* and *Weissella*. Although potential safety concerns due to acquisition of virulence genes by horizontal gene transfer could be an issue in the use of Gram-negative bacteria, yet genera of fish or shellfish pathogens, such as *Aeromonas*, *Pseudomonas* and *Vibrio*, have been evaluated and found beneficial to aquatic hosts. Probiotics of these taxa include *A. hydrophila*, *A. sobria*, *Ps. fluorescens*, *Ps. chlororaphis*, *V. alginolyticus* and *V. proteolyticus*. Amongst other genera, *Agarivorans*, *Alteromonas*, *Bdellovibrio*, *Burkholderia*, *Citrobacter*, *Enterobacter*, *Neptunomonas*, *Phaeobacter*, *Pseudoalteromonas*, *Rhodopseudomonas*, *Roseobacter*, *Shewanella*, *Synechococcus*, *Thalassobacter* and *Zooshikella* have also demonstrated usefulness (Hai 2015; Irianto and Austin, 2002b; Newaj-Fyzul and Austin, 2015; Newaj-Fyzul *et al.*, 2014).

For example, dietary *Bacillus* and *A. sobria* were effective in controlling multiple bacteria, such as *V. anguillarum*, *V. ordalii*, *La. garvieae*, *A. salmonicida*, *S. iniae* and *Y. ruckeri*, in rainbow trout (Brunt *et al.*, 2007). Moreover, Robertson *et al.* (2000) confirmed the efficacy of *Carnobacterium* sp. at reducing diseases caused by *A. salmonicida*, *V. ordalii* and *Y. ruckeri* in salmonids. Improved resistance to *V. anguillarum* in cod fry was also reported after addition of *C. divergens* (Gildberg and Mikkelsen, 1998). The addition of strain JE-34 (*Zooshikella* sp.) in diets enhanced the innate immune response and disease resistance in olive flounder (*Paralichythys olivaceus*) against *S. iniae* (Kim *et al.*, 2010). When applied to water, a mixture of *L. plantarum*, *L. rhamnosus* and *L. salivarius* led to enhanced survival of fish larvae (Talpur *et al.*, 2012). Moreover, *Ps. chlororaphis* induced disease resistance in perch against *A. sobria* (Gobeli *et al.*, 2009). *Bro. thermosphacta* (10^{10} cells/g) fed for 14 days protected rainbow trout from *A. bestiarum* infection (Pieters *et al.*, 2008). In shellfish, *B. subtilis* E20 demonstrated effectiveness in controlling *V. alginolyticus* infection in white shrimp; probiotic supplements at concentrations of 10^6, 10^7 and 10^8 cfu/kg had significantly increased survival rates of 13.3%, 16.7% and 20%, respectively, compared to the control group fed no probiotic (Tseng *et al.*, 2009). Moreover, feeding with probiotic *Synechococcus* increased survival of shrimp (*P. monodon*) postlarvae following challenge with *V. harveyi* (Preetha *et al.*, 2007). Separately, *Pseudoalteromonas* protected scallop larvae against infection with *V. splendidus*, and Pacific oyster against *V. coralliilyticus* (Kesarcodi-Watson *et al.*, 2012). *Arthrobacter* XE-7 significantly enhanced the immune parameters in white shrimp and at the same time significantly reduced host mortality due to *V. parahaemolyticus* (Li et *al.*, 2008). Tables 8.1 and 8.2 provide a list of bacterial probionts used to control fish and shellfish diseases under laboratory conditions.

Other non-bacterial candidates are also being used as probiotics for aquaculture. Bacteriophages from the viral families Myoviridae and Podoviridae, which were isolated from diseased ayu (*Plecoglossus altivelis*), when administered orally have proven to be effective at reducing *Ps. plecoglossicida* infections in medicated fish and numbers of the pathogen in water (Park *et al.*, 2000). Moreover, administration of lytic phage cocktail φSt2 and φGrn1 (obtained from *V. alginolyticus*) directly to live prey artemia (*Artemia salina*) cultures led to a 93% decrease of presumptive *Vibrio* load after four hours of treatment, suggesting that the *Vibrio* population responsible for disease outbreaks in the marine larviculture system can be potentially eliminated by phage therapy (Kalatzis *et al.*, 2016). Microalgae such as *Dunaliella salina*, *D. tertiolecta*, *Isochrysis galbana*, *Phaeodactylum tricornutum* and *Tetraselmis suecica* are also reported to promote growth, survival and health of marine larvae (Cahu *et al.*, 1998; Marques *et al.*, 2006; Nass *et al.*, 1992; Reitan *et al.*, 1997; Supamattaya *et al.*, 2005). For example, *T. suecica*, grown heterotrophically, was used as feed for penaeids and a feed additive for salmonids, and resulted in reduced levels of bacterial diseases (Austin and Day, 1990; Austin *et al.*, 1992). Enhanced protection of gnotobiotic *Artemia* against *V. campbellii* and *V. proteolyticus* was also conferred by the unicellular algal species *D. tertiolecta* (Marques *et al.*, 2006). The freshwater green microalga *Parietochloris incisa*, which is rich in arachidonic acid, was reported to have a health beneficial effect in guppy (*Poecilia reticulata*) when administered as a dietary supplement for a period of 14 days (Dagar *et al.*, 2009).

The use of yeast holds great promise as a probiotic in aquaculture, yet this eukaryotic microbial group has received little attention. Different yeast products, such as cells and beta-glucan of *Saccharomyces cerevisiae*, *Phaffia rhodozyma* and live *S. exiguus* containing xeaxanthin pigment (HPPR1), had a positive effect on juvenile *P. vannamei*, leading to better survival against *V. harveyi* (Scholz *et al.*, 1999). Oral administration of a polyamine

Table 8.1 Range of probiotics effective against fish diseases.

Disease/pathogen	Fish (stage/weight)	Probiotics	Dose/route/duration	Notes/efficacy	Reference
Streptococcosis: *S. iniae*	Rainbow trout (20 g)	*A. sobria*	5×10^7 cells/g; Feed; 14 days	Intraperitoneal challenge; Mortality (↓) 6%	Brunt and Austin (2005)
	Rainbow trout (12 g)	*Bacillus* sp.	2×10^8 cells/g; Feed; 14 days	Intraperitoneal challenge; 100% protection	Brunt *et al.* (2007)
	Nile tilapia (5 g)	*L. acidophilus*	1×10^7 cells/g; Feed; 8 weeks	Intraperitoneal challenge; Relative protection ~47%	Aly *et al.* (2008a)
	Flounder (27.5 g)	*Zooshikella* sp.	~$3.4\times10^{4-8}$ cfu/mL; Feed; 16 weeks	Intramuscular challenge; Mortality (↓) 25–40%	Kim *et al.* (2010)
	Flounder (40 g)	*La. lactis*	$1\times10^{6-8}$ cfu/g; Feed; 14 days	Co-habitation challenge; Survival rate (↑) 66%	Kim *et al.* (2013)
	Rainbow trout (38 g)	*E. casseliflavus*	10^{7-9} cfu/g; Feed; 8 weeks	Intraperitoneal challenge; Mortality reduced to 30–50%	Safari *et al.* (2016)
Lactococcosis: *La. garvieae*	Rainbow trout (20 g)	*A. sobria*	5×10^7 cells/g; Feed; 14 days	Intraperitoneal challenge; 100% protection	Brunt and Austin (2005)
	Rainbow trout (12 g)	*Bacillus* sp.	2×10^8 cells/g; Feed; 14 days	Intraperitoneal challenge; 100% protection	Brunt *et al.* (2007)
	Rainbow trout (27 g)	*Leu. mesenteroides, L. plantarum*	10^6 cfu/g; Feed; 30 days	Co-habitation challenge; Mortality (↓) 46–54%	Vendrell *et al.* (2008)
Furunculosis: *A. salmonicida*	Atlantic salmon (pre smolt)	*Ps. fluorescens*	5×10^5 cfu/mL; via water; 24 hours	Infections (↓) to 0–10%	Smith and Davey (1993)
	Atlantic salmon (21 g)	*V. alginolyticus*	~10^8 cells/mL; via water; 10 min	Immersion challenge; Mortality (↓) to 18%	Austin *et al.* (1995)

(*Continued*)

Table 8.1 (Continued)

Disease/ pathogen	Fish (stage/weight)	Probiotics	Dose/route/duration	Notes/efficacy	Reference
	Atlantic salmon (15 g)	*Carnobacterium* sp.	5×10^7 cells/g; Feed; 14 days	Intraperitoneal challenge; Survival rate (↑) 20%	Robertson *et al.* (2000)
	Rainbow trout (12 g)	*A. hydrophila*, *Carnobacterium* sp., *C. inhibens*, *V. fluvialis*	10^7 cells/g; Feed; 14 days	Intraperitoneal challenge; Mortality (↓) 0–4%	Irianto and Austin (2002a)
	Rainbow trout (25 g)	*C. maltaromaticum*, *C. divergens*	$>10^7$ cells/g; Feed; 14 days	Intraperitoneal challenge; Survival rate (↑) 80%	Kim and Austin (2006a)
	Rainbow trout (40 g)	*La. lactis*, *Leu. mesenteroides*, *L. sakei*	10^6 cfu/g; Feed; 2 weeks	Intraperitoneal challenge; Survival rate (↑) 98–100%	Balcázar *et al.* (2007b)
	Rainbow trout (12 g)	*A. sobria*, *Bacillus* sp.	10^7, 2×10^8 cells/g; Feed; 14 days	Intraperitoneal challenge; 100% protection	Brunt *et al.* (2007)
	Rainbow trout (32 g)	*L. rhamnosus*	10^9 cfu/g; Feed; 51 days	Co-habitation challenge; Mortality (↓) 19%	Nikoskelainen *et al.* (2001)
Vibriosis: *V. anguillarum*	Atlantic salmon (21 g)	*V. alginolyticus*	$\sim10^8$ cells/mL; via water; 10 min	Immersion challenge; Mortality (↓) to 74%	Austin *et al.* (1995)
	Atlantic cod (3 g)	*C. divergens*	2×10^9 cfu/g; Feed; 3 weeks	Mortality (↓) to ~24%	Gildberg *et al.* (1997)
	Rainbow trout (40 g)	*Ps. fluorescens*	10^5 cfu/mL; added to water; 5 days	Immersion challenge; Mortality reduced by 46%	Gram *et al.* (1999)
	Rainbow trout (12 g)	*A. sobria*, *Bacillus* sp.	10^7, 2×10^8 cells/g; Feed; 14 days	Intraperitoneal challenge; Mortality (↓) 6–13%	Brunt *et al.* (2007)
	Chinese drum (200–260 g)	*Cl. butyricum*	10^8 cells/g; Feed; 30 days	Intraperitoneal challenge; Survival rate (↑) 70–78%	Pan *et al.* (2008)
	Rainbow trout (13.2 g)	*E. faecalis*	1% lysed cell; Feed; 12 weeks	Intraperitoneal challenge; Mortality (↓) 23%	Rodriguez-Estrada *et al.* (2009)

	Rainbow trout (10–15 g)	*Kocuria* SM1	10^8 cells/g; Feed; 2 weeks	Intraperitoneal challenge; RPS 81%	Sharifuzzaman and Austin (2010a)
	Rainbow trout (10–15 g)	*Kocuria* SM1, *Rhodococcus* SM2	0.1 mL cell component; i.p. inoculation; 1 week	Intraperitoneal challenge; RPS 80–87%	Sharifuzzaman *et al.* (2011)
	European sea bass (18 g)	*Vagococcus fluvialis*	10^9 cfu/g; Feed; 20 days	Immersion challenge; RPS ~42%	Sorroza *et al.* (2012)
	Grouper (2 g)	*P. pentosaceus*	6×10^8 cfu/g; Feed; 3 weeks	Intraperitoneal challenge; RPS 75–77%	Huang *et al.* (2014)
V. harveyi	Rainbow trout (15 g)	*A. hydrophila* A3-51	10^9 cells/mL; Feed; 6 weeks	Intraperitoneal challenge; RPS 70%	Arijo *et al.* (2008)
V. ordalii	Atlantic salmon (21 g)	*V. alginolyticus*	~10^8 cells/mL; via water; 10 min	Immersion challenge; Mortality (↓) to 74%	Austin *et al.* (1995)
	Atlantic salmon (15 g)	*Carnobacterium* sp.	5×10^7 cells/g; Feed; 14 days	Intraperitoneal challenge; Survival rate (↑) 74%	Robertson *et al.* (2000)
	Rainbow trout (12 g)	*A. sobria*, *Bacillus* sp.	10^7, 2×10^8 cells/g; Feed; 14 days	Intraperitoneal challenge; 100% protection	Brunt *et al.* (2007)
	Rainbow trout (10–15 g)	*Kocuria* SM1	10^8 cells/g; Feed; 2 weeks	Intraperitoneal challenge; RPS 73%	Sharifuzzaman and Austin (2010a)
ERM: *Y. ruckeri*	Atlantic salmon (15 g)	*Carnobacterium* sp.	5×10^7 cells/g; Feed; 14 days	Intraperitoneal challenge; Survival rate (↑) 71%	Robertson *et al.* (2000)
	Rainbow trout (1.5 g)	*B. licheniformis*, *B. subtilis*	4×10^4 spores/g; Feed; 42 days	Intraperitoneal challenge; RPS ~35%	Raida *et al.* (2003)
	Rainbow trout (25 g)	*C. maltaromaticum*, *C. divergens*	>10^7 cells/g; Feed; 14 days	Intraperitoneal challenge; Survival rate (↑) 73–80%	Kim and Austin (2006a)
	Rainbow trout (12 g)	*A. sobria*, *Bacillus* sp.	10^7, 2×10^8 cells/g; Feed; 14 days	Intraperitoneal challenge; Mortality (↓) to 0–6%	Brunt *et al.* (2007)
	Rainbow trout (110 g)	*Ent. cloacae*, *B. mojavensis*	1×10^8 cells/g; Feed; 60 days	Immersion challenge; Survival rate (↑) to 99%	Capkin and Altinok (2009)

(*Continued*)

Table 8.1 (Continued)

Disease/ pathogen	Fish (stage/weight)	Probiotics	Dose/route/duration	Notes/efficacy	Reference
Haemorrhagic septicaemia: *Aeromonas* sp.	Rainbow trout (30 g)	*B. subtilis*	10^7 cells/g; Feed; 14 days	Intraperitoneal challenge; 100% protection	Newaj-Fyzul *et al.* (2007)
	Nile tilapia (5 g)	*B. subtilis*	1×10^7 cells/g; Feed; 8 weeks	Intraperitoneal challenge; Relative protection ~48%	Aly *et al.* (2008a)
A. hydrophila	Indian major carp (15 g)	*B. subtilis*	1.5×10^7 cfu/g; Feed; 2 weeks	Intraperitoneal challenge; Survival rate (↑) to 87.5%	Kumar *et al.* (2006)
	Chinese drum (200–260 g)	*Cl. butyricum*	10^8 cells/g; Feed; 30 days	Intraperitoneal challenge; Survival rate (↑) 83–84%	Pan *et al.* (2008)
	Nile tilapia (2.35 g)	*M. luteus*	10^7 cells/g; Feed; 90 days	Intraperitoneal challenge; Mortality (↓) to 25%	El-Rhman *et al.* (2009)
	Catla (~6.5 g)	*B. circulans*	2×10^5 cells 100/g; Feed; 60 days	Immersion challenge; Survival rate (↑) to ~97%	Bandyopadhyay and Mohapatra (2009)
	Common carp (25 g)	*E. faecium*	10^8 cfu/g; Feed; 30 or 60 days	Intramuscular injection; RPS 50–78%	Gopalakannan and Arul (2011)
A. sobria	Perch (10–15 g)	*Ps. chlororaphis*	1×10^7 cfu/mL; via rearing water; 22 hours	Bath challenge; Mortality (↓) to 16%	Gobeli et al. (2009)
A. veronii	Snakehead (120 g)	*Bacteriovorax* sp.	1×10^4 PFU/mL; via tank water; immediately	Bath challenge; RPS 75%	Cao *et al.* (2014)
Fin rot: *A. bestiarum*	Rainbow trout (25 g)	*A. sobria*, *Bro. thermosphacta*	10^8, 10^{10} cells/g; Feed; 14 days	Intramuscular injection; Survival rate (↑) to 76–88%	Pieters *et al.* (2008)
White spot or Ich: *Ichthyophthirius multifiliis*	Rainbow trout (25 g)	*A. sobria*	10^8 cells/g; Feed; 14 days	Immersion challenge; 100% survival	Pieters *et al.* (2008)

Pseudomonas: *Ps. fluorescens*	Nile tilapia (5 g)	*B. subtilis*	1×10^{7} cells/g; Feed; 8 weeks	Intraperitoneal challenge; Relative protection ~43%	Aly *et al.* (2008a)
Edwardsiellosis: *Ed. tarda*	European eel (30 g)	*E. faecium* (from Cernivet®LBC)	1 g Cernivet® in 100 mL sprayed over 1000 g; Feed; 2 weeks	Challenged anally; Survival rate (↑) to 73%	Chang and Liu (2002)
	Nile tilapia (60–70 g)	*L. rhamnosus*	$10^{8,10}$ cfu/g; Feed; 2 weeks	Intraperitoneal challenge; Mortality (↓) to 3.3–16.7%	Pirarat *et al.* (2006)
Ed. ictaluri	Channel catfish (13 g)	*B. subtilis* AP143 or AB01	8×10^{7} cfu/g; Feed; 2 weeks	Immersion challenge; Mortality (↓) to ~83–85%	Ran *et al.* (2012)
	Striped catfish (~14 g)	*B. subtilis* AP79	$\sim10^{7}$ cfu/g; Feed; 2 weeks	Immersion challenge; Mortality (↓) to 9.7%	Ran *et al.* (2012)
CWD or RTFS: *Flavobacterium psychrophilum*	Rainbow trout (5 g)	*Enterobacter* sp., *Ent. amnigenus*	10^{6-8} cells/g; Feed; 10 days	Subcutaneous challenge; Mortality (↓) to ~27–49%	Burbank *et al.* (2011)
	Rainbow trout (~2–3 g)	*Pseudomonas* M174 or M162	$\sim2\times10^{5-9}$ cfu/g; Feed; 2 weeks	Intramuscular injection; RPS ~28–49%	Korkea-Aho *et al.* (2011, 2012)
Photobacteriosis: *Photobacterium damselae* subsp. *piscicida*	Senegalese sole (~23–26 g)	*Sh. putrefaciens* Pdp11	10^{9} cells/g; Feed; 8 weeks	Intraperitoneal challenge; RPS ~25–44%	De la Banda *et al.* (2012)
	Cobia (4.6 g)	*P. pentosaceus*	10^{9} cfu/g; Feed; 2 weeks	Immersion challenge; RPS ~74%	Xing *et al.* (2013)
VCCS	Rainbow trout (fry stage)	*P. acidilactici*	1.5×10^{6} cfu/g; Feed; 5 months	Reduced the occurrence of VCCS to 4%	Aubin *et al.* (2005)

Bacterial genus: *A., Aeromonas, B., Bacillus, Bro., Brochothrix, C., Carnobacterium, Cl., Clostridium, E., Enterococcus, Ed., Edwardsiella, Ent., Enterobacter, L., Lactobacillus, La., Lactococcus, Leu., Leuconostoc, P., Pediococcus, Ps., Pseudomonas, S., Streptococcus, Sh., Shewanella, V., Vibrio.*

Fish species: Atlantic salmon (*Salmo salar*), Channel catfish (*Ictalurus punctatus*), Cobia (*Rachycentron canadum*), European eel (*Anguilla anguilla*), Indian major carp (*Labeo rohita*), Snakehead (*Ophiocephalus argus*), Senegalese sole (*Solea senegalensis*), Striped catfish (*Pangasianodon hypophthalmus*).

CWD or RTFS, coldwater disease or rainbow trout fry syndrome; ERM, enteric redmouth; i..p., intraperitoneal; RPS, relative percent survival; VCCS, vertebral column compression syndrome.

Table 8.2 Range of probiotics effective against shellfish diseases.

Disease/pathogen	Shellfish (stage/weight)	Probiotics	Dose/route/duration	Notes/efficacy	Reference
Vibriosis: *V. anguillarum*	Chilean scallop (veliger larvae)	*Vibrio* sp. *Alt. haloplanktis*	10^3 cells/mL; Water; 1 hour	Immersion challenge; Mortality (↓) to ~2–6%	Riquelme *et al.* (1997)
	Shrimp (5–6 g)	*B. subtilis*	10^6 cfu/mL; Water; 5 days	Bath challenge; Mortality (↓) to 32%	Vaseeharan and Ramasamy (2003)
V. coralliilyticus	Scallop (larvae)	*Alt. macleodii*, *Neptunomonas* sp., *Ph. gallaeciensis*, *Pseudoalteromonas* sp.	$10^{3,4,5}$ cfu/mL; Water; 20 hours	Immersion challenge; Survival rate (↑) to ~85–97%	Kesarcodi-Watson *et al.* (2012)
	Flat oyster (larvae)	*Ph. gallaeciensis*	10^5 cfu/mL; Water; 20 hours	Immersion challenge; Survival rate (↑) to ~92%	Kesarcodi-Watson *et al.* (2012)
	Pacific oyster (larvae)	*Ph. gallaeciensis*, *Pseudoalteromonas* sp.	$10^{3,4}$ cfu/mL; Water; 20 hours	Immersion challenge; Survival rate (↑) to ~87–97%	Kesarcodi-Watson *et al.* (2012)
V. harveyi	Shrimp (PL-30; 0.7–0.8 g)	*Bacillus*	~10^{10} cfu/g; Feed; 100 days	Immersion challenge; 100% survival	Rengpipat *et al.* (1998)
	White shrimp (1.2 g)	*B. subtilis*	10^5 cfu/g; Feed; 28 days	Immersion challenge; Mortality (↓) to ~18%	Balcázar and Rojas-Luna (2007)
	Shrimp (PL-20; 0.1–0.15 g)	*Synechocystis* MCCB 114 or 115	1:1 ratio; Feed; 20 days	Oral challenge; RPS ~59–74%	Preetha *et al.* (2007)
	Shrimp (PL-10)	*S. phocae*, *E. faecium*	10^7 cfu/mL; Water	Immersion challenge; Mortality (↓) to 8–16%	Swain *et al.* (2009)
	Shrimp (PL-33)	*Streptomyces* CLS-28	1% (v/w) cell mass; Feed; 15 days	Bath challenge; Mortality (↓) to ~31%	Das *et al.* (2010)
	Shrimp (protozoea I)	*Bacillus*, *Pseudomonas*, *Arthrobacter*	10^6 cfu/mL; Rearing water; 38 days	Bath challenge; Mortality (↓) to <10%	Pai *et al.* (2010)
	White shrimp (juvenile)	*B. subtilis*	10^8 cfu/g; Feed; 8 weeks	Intramuscular injection; Mortality (↓) to 20%	Zokaeifar *et al.* (2012)

V. parahaemolyticus	White shrimp (2.2 g)	*B. subtilis, V. alginolyticus, R. gallaeciensis, Ps. aestumarina*	10^5 cfu/g; Feed; 28 days	Immersion challenge; Mortality (↓) to 17–22%	Balcázar *et al.* (2007c)
	White shrimp (1.75 g)	*Arthrobacter*	$10^{8,10}$ cfu/g; Feed; 49 days	Bath challenge; Mortality (↓) to ~52%	Li *et al.* (2008)
	Shrimp (PL-7)	*E. faecium*	10^7 cfu/g; Feed	Immersion challenge; Survival rate (↑) to 40%	Swain *et al.* (2009)
V. pectenicida	Flat oyster (larvae)	*Alt. macleodii, Neptunomonas* sp., *Ph. gallaeciensis*	$10^{5,6}$ cfu/mL; Water; 20 hours	Immersion challenge; Survival rate (↑) to ~77–98%	Kesarcodi-Watson *et al.* (2012)
V. splendidus	Greenshell mussel (D-veliger larvae)	*Alt. macleodii, Neptunomonas* sp. *Ph. gallaeciensis,*	10^8 cfu/mL; Water; 7 days	Immersion challenge; Survival rate (↑) to ~65%	Kesarcodi-Watson *et al.* (2010)
	Scallop (larvae)	*Pseudoaltermonas* sp.	$10^{3,5}$ cfu/mL; Water; 20 hours	Immersion challenge; Survival rate (↑) to ~76–95%	Kesarcodi-Watson *et al.* (2012)
V. tubiashii	Pacific oyster (larvae)	*Aeromonas media* A199	10^4 cfu/mL; Water	Immersion challenge; Survival rate (↑) to ~72–98%	Gibson (1999)
WSSV	White shrimp (1.75 g)	*Bacillus*	10^{10} cfu/g; Feed; 28 days	Oral challenge; Survival rate (↑) to >80%	Li *et al.* (2009)
	White shrimp (~7 g)	*P. pentosaceus, Staphylococcus haemolyticus*	1–2×10^6 cfu/g; Feed; 10 days	Natural infection; Lower WSSV prevalence (~8–17%)	Leyva-Madrigal *et al.* (2011)

Shellfish species: Greenshell mussel (*Perna canaliculus*), Chilean scallop (*Argopecten purpurutus*), Flat oyster (*Ostrea edulis*).
Bacterial genus: *Alt., Alteromonas, Ph., Phaeobacter, R., Roseobacter.*
PL, postlarvae; WSSV, white spot syndrome virus.

(spermine and spermidine)-producing yeast, *Debaryomyces hansenii*, improved survival but reduced the growth of European sea bass (*Dicentrarchus labrax*) larvae (Tovar *et al.*, 2002). A mixture of yeasts (isolates SS1, AY1) and bacteria (isolate SY9), which was added to dry feed at 10^7 cfu/g and fed to abalone (*Haliotis midae*) for 14 days, led to 62% survival after challenge with *V. anguillarum* compared to 25% survival of the controls (Macey and Coyne, 2005). Also, marine yeast (*Yarrowia lipolytica*) supplementation (with microalgae) was effective in improving survival and growth of juvenile pearl oyster, *Pinctada mazatlanica* (Aguilar-Macias *et al.*, 2010). Indeed, *S. cerevisiae* was documented as a probiotic for catla (*Catla catla*) (Mohanty *et al.*, 1996), hybrid striped bass (*Morone chrysops* × *M. saxatilis*) (Li and Gatlin, 2004), flounder (Taoka *et al.*, 2006a), Nile tilapia (Lara-Flores *et al.*, 2003; Taoka *et al.*, 2006b) and common carp (*Cyprinus carpio*) (Faramarzi *et al.*, 2011).

Modes of Action

The relationship between probiotic bacteria and their hosts is complex, and thus mechanisms of action of probiotics are not completely understood. However, their effect on disease reduction may be linked to a combination of factors, as illustrated in Figure 8.2. One of the earliest notions was that probiotics are involved in competitive exclusion of potential pathogens – upon entering the host digestive tract, the beneficial micro-organism(s) produce inhibitory molecules and/or compete for adhesion site, nutrient, chemical or energy sources that can interfere with pathogen growth and/or activities (Balcázar *et al.*, 2006; Brunt *et al.*, 2007; Chabrillón *et al.*, 2005b; Decamp *et al.*, 2008; Irianto and Austin, 2002b; Verschuere *et al.*, 2000; Vine *et al.*, 2004b).

Incidentally, beneficial isolates from the intestine of both marine and freshwater species have demonstrated antagonistic activity against several fish and shellfish pathogens. For example, extracellular products of five candidate probionts recovered from the stomach and intestine of common clownfish (*Amphiprion percula*) were inhibitory against *A. hydrophila*, *A. salmonicida*, *V. harveyi*, *V. anguillarum*, *V. damsela* [= *Photobacterium damselae*], *V. alginolyticus* and *C. piscicola* (Vine *et al.*, 2004a). *Aeromonas media* (strain A199), which was isolated from the rearing water of eel culture, was also strongly inhibitory to *Saprolegnia* sp. (Lategan *et al.*, 2004). *B. amyloliquefaciens* was found to produce diffusible inhibitors to *A. hydrophila*, *Ed. tarda*, *V. harveyi* and *V. parahaemolyticus* (Das *et al.*, 2013). Substances that are known to induce bactericidal or bacteriostatic effects include bacteriocins, lysozymes, hydrogen peroxide, proteases, carbon dioxide and siderophores, among many others. In addition, the production of organic acids and volatile fatty acids (e.g. lactic, acetic, butyric and propionic acids) can alter gut pH (Gram and Melchiorsen, 1996; Ringø and Gatesoupe, 1998; Sugita *et al.*, 1998; Tinh *et al.*, 2008; Verschuere *et al.*, 2000; Vine *et al.*, 2006). In this way, probiotics may outcompete the proliferation of opportunistic pathogenic micro-organisms *in vivo*.

Some probiotic micro-organisms are also capable of preventing pathogen growth on the gut surface by competing for attachment sites (Chabrillón *et al.*, 2005a; Gueimonde *et al.*, 2006; Mukai *et al.*, 2002). In agreement with this statement, Balcázar *et al.* (2008) demonstrated that adhesion of the fish pathogens *A. hydrophila*, *A. salmonicida*, *V. anguillarum* and *Y. ruckeri* to intestinal mucus of rainbow trout was reduced by lactic acid bacteria *La. lactis*, *L. plantarum* and *L. fermentum*, respectively, under *in vitro* conditions. This antiadhesion activity may be explained by the secretion of antimicrobial substances, such as antibiotics or siderophores (Balcázar *et al.*, 2008; Mukai *et al.*, 2002). Indeed, by competing for free iron, the

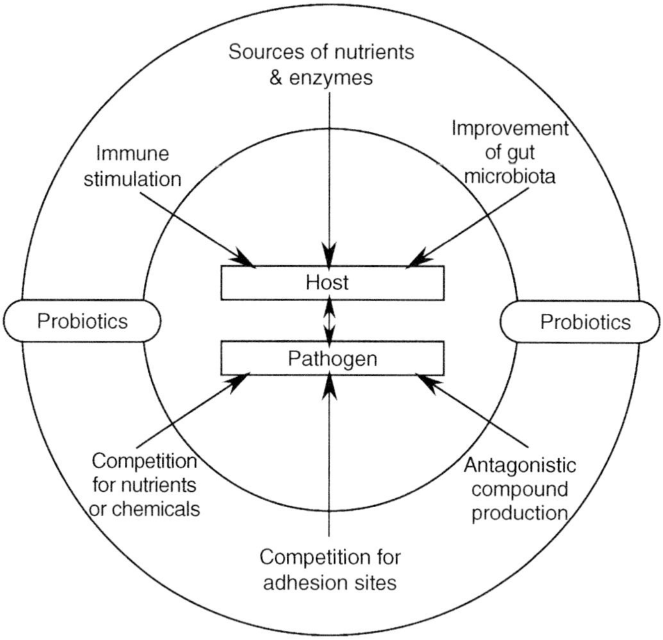

Figure 8.2 Possible modes of action of probiotics. Source: adapted from de Schryver *et al.* (2012).

siderophore-producing probiont *Ps. fluorescens* was able to inhibit the growth of *V. anguillarum* (Gram *et al.*, 1999). In addition, probiotics are reported to colonize the intestine of an aquatic host when administered orally. Sharifuzzaman *et al.* (2014) noted colonization of *Kocuria* SM1 and *Rhodococcus* SM2 in the gut of rainbow trout after two weeks of feeding when the two organisms accounted for ~90–100% of the total culturable bacterial population. Probiotic cultures do not show spontaneous primary colonization in the digestive tract, instead sustaining a transient state as long as the bacteria are introduced via the feed and then disappearing upon switching to regular feed (Newaj-Fyzul *et al.*, 2007; Robertson *et al.*, 2000; Sharifuzzaman *et al.*, 2014). However, the ability of probiotics to adhere to and grow in mucus and epithelial cells as well as colonize the gastrointestinal tract is considered to be a first line of defence against invasion by pathogens (de Schryver *et al.*, 2012).

Another promising aspect of using probiotics is the potential improvement in feed efficiency, which may be reflected through improved feed utilization and better growth rate of the animal. Sáenz de Rodrigáñez *et al.* (2009) reported significantly higher growth and nutrient utilization in juvenile sole (10–15 g) after dietary supplementation with probiotics (i.e. Alteromonadaceae family) for 60 days. Likewise, weight gain and specific growth rate (SGR) improved significantly when prawn (*Macrobrachium rosenbergii*) juveniles were reared either in water supplemented with *Bacillus* NL110 (1.15×10^6 cfu/mL) or with feed (4.34×10^9 cfu/g) and water (1.25×10^6 cfu/mL) supplemented with *Vibrio* NE17 compared to controls (Rahiman *et al.*, 2010). Moreover, a significant improvement of feed conversion ratio (FCR), SGR and protein efficiency ratio was observed in rainbow trout (~45 g), previously treated with antibiotic, after 70 days feeding on mixed *B. subtilis* and *B. licheniformis* supplemented diets (Merrifield *et al.*, 2010b). Surprisingly, in a similar experiment keeping most of the parameters identical, Merrifield *et al.* (2010a) observed no statistical improvements of SGR in rainbow trout (~70 g) fed with probiotics, although an enhanced SGR was noted compared to the controls. However, some probiotic strains may be a source of essential nutrients, such as fatty acids (Vine *et al.*, 2006), biotin and vitamin B_{12} (Sugita *et al.*, 1991, 1992), and their activity in the digestive tract may also stimulate the specific and/or total activities of digestive enzymes, such as amylase, chitinase, lipase and protease (Balcázar *et al.*, 2006; Newaj-Fyzul and Austin, 2015; Newaj-Fyzul *et al.*, 2014; Sáenz de Rodrigáñez *et al.*, 2009), thereby improving the whole digestive process and enhancing the digestibility of feed and the effective utilization of nutritive supplies, leading to improvement of FCR.

Certainly, immunostimulation has been identified as the dominant mode of action for a range of probiotics, including representatives of both Gram-positive and Gram-negative bacterial taxa (Austin and Austin, 2012), and many studies have provided evidence of this (Irianto and Austin, 2002b; Newaj-Fyzul and Austin, 2015; Newaj-Fyzul *et al.*, 2014). For example, in finfish, there is often stimulation of innate and cellular immunity, including enhancement of:

- number of vital immune competent cells in the blood: erythrocyte (Brunt and Austin, 2005; El-Rhman *et al.*, 2009; Sharifuzzaman and Austin, 2010a), granulocyte (Irianto and Austin, 2002a; Kumar *et al.*, 2008), leucocyte (Brunt and Austin, 2005; Huang *et al.*, 2014; Korkea-Aho *et al.*, 2012; Merrifield *et al.*, 2010a,b; Newaj-Fyzul *et al.*, 2007; Sharifuzzaman and Austin, 2010a; Standen *et al.*, 2013), lymphocyte (Aly *et al.*, 2008b; Irianto and Austin 2002a; Kumar *et al.*, 2008; Newaj-Fyzul *et al.*, 2007), macrophage (Irianto and Austin, 2002a; Kumar *et al.*, 2008) and monocyte (Aly *et al.*, 2008b; Standen *et al.*, 2013)
- macrophage phagocytosis (Brunt and Austin, 2005; Newaj-Fyzul *et al.*, 2007; Pan *et al.*, 2008; Panigrahi *et al.*, 2005; Pieters *et al.*, 2008; Reyes-Becerril *et al.*, 2008; Salinas *et al.*, 2008; Sharifuzzaman and Austin, 2009,2010a; Son *et al.*, 2009)
- respiratory burst (Aly *et al.*, 2008a; Brunt and Austin, 2005; Brunt *et al.*, 2007; Giri *et al.*, 2013; Heo *et al.*, 2013; Kim and Austin, 2006a; Korkea-Aho *et al.*, 2011; Kumar *et al.*, 2008; Newaj-Fyzul *et al.*, 2007; Nikoskelainen *et al.*, 2003; Pieters *et al.*, 2008; Sharifuzzaman and Austin, 2010a,b; Zhou *et al.*, 2010; Xing *et al.*, 2013)
- peroxidase content (Heo *et al.*, 2013; Newaj-Fyzul *et al.*, 2007; Reyes-Becerril *et al.*, 2008, 2013; Rodríguez *et al.*, 2003; Salinas *et al.*, 2008; Sharifuzzaman and Austin, 2009, 2010b; Wang *et al.*, 2008)
- myeloperoxidase (Das *et al.*, 2013; Lee *et al.*, 2013)
- superoxide dismutase (Cha *et al.*, 2013; Giri *et al.*, 2013; Ridha and Azad, 2012; Sun *et al.*, 2010; Zhou *et al.*, 2010)
- complement activity (Balcázar *et al.*, 2007a; Choi and Yoon, 2008; Giri *et al.*, 2013; Neissi *et al.*, 2013;Nikoskelainen *et al.*, 2003; Panigrahi *et al.*, 2004; Reyes-Becerril *et al.*, 2013; Sharifuzzaman and Austin, 2010a; Sun *et al.*, 2010),
- lysozyme activity (Aly *et al.*, 2008a; Kim and Austin, 2006a; Pan *et al.*, 2008; Panigrahi *et al.*, 2005; Rodríguez *et al.*, 2003; Sharifuzzaman and Austin, 2009, 2010a,2010b; Son *et al.*, 2009)
- serum/plasma bactericidal activity (Aly *et al.*, 2008a; Kumar *et al.*, 2008; Sharifuzzaman and Austin, 2010b; Taoka *et al.*, 2006b)
- antiprotease (Brunt *et al.*, 2007; Heo *et al.*, 2013; Newaj-Fyzul *et al.*, 2007; Sharifuzzaman and Austin, 2009)
- immunoglobulin (Al-Dohail *et al.*, 2009; Balcázar *et al.*, 2007a; Mandiki *et al.*, 2011; Nayak *et al.*, 2007; Neissi *et al.*, 2013; Nikoskelainen *et al.*, 2003; Panigrahi *et al.*, 2004, 2005; Ridha and Azad, 2012; Sharifuzzaman *et al.*, 2011; Sun *et al.*, 2010; Xing *et al.*, 2013)

- total protein (Das *et al.*, 2013; Nayak *et al.*, 2007; Newaj-Fyzul *et al.*, 2007; Sharifuzzaman and Austin, 2009, 2010a,2010b) and albumin (Sharifuzzaman and Austin 2010a; Wang *et al.*, 2008).

Application of '-omics' tools has also been employed to further the understanding of probiotic functionality. Brunt *et al.* (2008) carried out proteome analysis of serum from fish fed a diet containing *Bacillus* JB-1 and noted an increased expression of transferrin that is known to have a function in immunity. Using real-time PCR, Pérez-Sánchez *et al.* (2011) identified upregulated expression of interleukin (IL)-1-beta, IL-10 and tumour necrosis factor (TNF)-gene in the head kidney of rainbow trout when administered *L. plantarum* orally. Other studies noted the induction of a variety of cytokines (= cellular immunity) such as IL-1-beta, IL-8, TNF-alpha, beta-defensin and transforming growth factor (TGF)-beta (Kim and Austin, 2006b; Panigrahi *et al.*, 2007; Reyes-Becerril *et al.*, 2013; Standen *et al.*, 2013), IL-12 and interferon (IFN)-gamma (Kim *et al.*, 2013), and generation of an increased memory T-cell population (Picchietti *et al.*, 2009) in naïve fish or fish previously exposed to probiotic-supplemented diets.

At the gut level, probiotics are capable of modulating immune responses via the gut-associated lymphoid tissue (Newaj-Fyzul and Austin, 2015), and an enhanced number of goblet cells (Standen *et al.*, 2013), immunoglobulin positive (Ig^+) cells, T-cells, acidophilic granulocytes, and lysozyme and phagocytic activities have also been described (Nayak, 2010; Picchietti *et al.*, 2007, 2008; Salinas *et al.*, 2008). With shrimp or prawn, improvements in total haemocyte count, phagocytosis, phenoloxidase, plasma protein concentration, respiratory burst or superoxide dismutase, lysozyme and antibacterial activities have been reported (Hai and Fotedar, 2009; Li *et al.*, 2009; NavinChandran *et al.*, 2014; Pattukumar *et al.*, 2014; Rahiman *et al.*, 2010; Rengpipat *et al.*, 2000; Wang and Gu, 2010).

In contrast, some studies failed to detect any specific change in serum lysozyme level after supplementation of *L. sakei*, *La. lactis* subsp. *lactis*, *Leu. mesenteroides*, *L. rhamnosus* and *A. sobria* in fish (Balcázar *et al.*, 2007a,b; Brunt *et al.*, 2007; Panigrahi *et al.*, 2005). The phagocytic activity of head kidney macrophages and bactericidal activity of serum were also not modified by the use of *La. lactis* in turbot (Villamil *et al.*, 2002), suggesting that different probiotics may produce differing immunostimulatory effects. Nevertheless, probiotics, even in some cases the inactivated or cellular preparations (Irianto and Austin, 2003; Sharifuzzaman *et al.*, 2011), have been shown to stimulate host immunity. Evidently the non-specific defence of vertebrates has evolved towards recognition of preserved microbial components such as yeast/fungal cell wall beta-glucan, bacterial polysaccharide and peptidoglycan, bacterial DNA and viral double-stranded RNA (Abbass *et al.*, 2010). Thus, LPS, OMPs, CWPs and WCPs of probiotics were immunostimulatory to fish (Arijo *et al.*, 2008; Sakai, 1999; Sharifuzzaman *et al.*, 2011).

Example of Commercial-Scale Application

Many companies are manufacturing different types of probiotics, either as single or multiple species in a concentrated or encapsulated form, that are often claimed to provide multiple benefits such as improvement of water quality, enhancement of growth rate and prevention of disease (Qi *et al.*, 2009), although data on their use and efficacy in commercial-scale aquaculture operation are insufficient. In a field trial at Thailand, Rengpipat *et al.* (2003) used *Bacillus* S11 (~10^{10} cfu/g) as a feed supplement for 100 days to rear black tiger shrimp (0.6–0.9 g) in cages, and noted significantly (p <0.05) higher growth and survival of stocks compared to a group receiving non-supplemented feed. Moreover, when challenged with luminescent bacterium *V. harveyi*, probiotic S11 delayed the onset of mortality. The authors concluded that annual shrimp production (i.e. two 100-day crops) may be increased to 49% by using probiotics.

In China, Wang *et al.* (2005) tested commercial probiotics (mixture of *Bacillus* sp., photosynthetic bacteria, *S. cerevisiae*, *Nitrosomonas* sp. and *Nitrobacter* sp.) directly in pond water for culturing white shrimp, at a density of 0.75 million juveniles/ha. At the end of the 109-day culture period, the results indicated a noticeable positive effect on shrimp survival (from 48.67% ± 3.51% to 81.00% ± 6.25%) and yields (from 4985 ± 503 kg/ha to 8215 ± 265 kg/ha), including improvement of water quality as reflected by higher population density of beneficial bacterial flora, lower presumptive *Vibrio* counts and reduced total inorganic nitrogen levels.

Decamp *et al.* (2008) reported the outcome of the commercial probiotic Sanolife®MIC (mixture of *Bacillus* strains; 1–5 × 10^4 cfu/mL) used in Asian and Latin American hatcheries. When applied to 175 L tank water, Sanolife®MIC resulted in an increased biomass (from 18.6 ± 15.6 g/tank to 58.3 ± 28.7 g/tank) and survival of *P. monodon* postlarvae in a Thai hatchery. Similarly, daily application of Sanolife®MIC to a 20 MT tank with a stocking density of 5 million white shrimp nauplii led to the improvement of larvae survival (from ~30% to ~90%) in a Brazilian hatchery.

Safety and Regulatory Issues

Uncertainty over the fate of probiotics after application remains an important issue. Specifically, concerns have been voiced about possible acquisition of antibiotic resistance and virulence genes via horizontal gene transfer (HGT) by the Gram-negative probiont (Newaj-Fyzul *et al.*, 2014). Although there are no documented studies of this notion, antibiotic-resistant bacteria have often been reported from aquaculture sites (di Cesare *et al.*, 2012; Tamminen *et al.*, 2011) and this situation could potentially lead to safety problems if using live probiotics in an open aquatic environment. Inactivated or encapsulated preparations of probiotics may be an alternative to overcome the problem of HGT. In addition, probiotics can affect host tissues such as the gills, skin, surface mucus and intestinal tract (Harris, 1993), and thus Salma *et al.* (2011) reported severe cell damage when the distal intestine of beluga (*Huso huso*) was exposed to *L. plantarum* isolated from cheese made from sheep milk. This signifies that probiotic strains must also be recognized as safe for the cellular integrity of host. Moreover, probiotic products predominantly marketed in developing countries lack labelling information on species or strain, concentrations of different species in case of mixed products, and accurate cell numbers, thus highlighting serious product quality issues (Nimrat and Vuthiphandchai, 2011). Therefore, regulatory scrutiny may be the best way to improve the quality and efficacy of commercial aquaculture probiotics.

Conclusion

A large number of beneficial micro-organisms have been isolated from the environment, terrestrial or aquatic hosts, the latter being the preferred source, many of which have led to enhanced disease resistance in fish and shellfish species (Newaj-Fyzul *et al.*, 2014; Sharifuzzaman and Austin, 2009; Vendrell *et al.*, 2008), even against multiple pathogens

(Brunt *et al.*, 2007). Probiotics can be composed of single strains or mixtures with probiotics/immunostimulants and administered via water or as a dietary supplement for a minimum of two weeks. In contrast to typical viable cells, the inactivated/dead preparations (Brunt and Austin, 2005; Irianto and Austin, 2003; Pan *et al.*, 2008; Taoka *et al.*, 2006b) or cellular components such as LPS, OMPs, CWPs and WCPs of probiotics have also been reported to protect the host from diseases (Abbass *et al.*, 2010; Arijo *et al.*, 2008; Sharifuzzaman *et al.*, 2011).

The possible modes of action of probiotics are multifactorial and largely depend on probiont–pathogen–host interactions, but predominantly reflect stimulation of host cellular and humoral innate immunity. However, there are often uncertainties about the longevity of protection conferred by probiotics and their ultimate fate in the aquatic environment when used as viable formulations (Newaj-Fyzul and Austin, 2015; Newaj-Fyzul *et al.*, 2014). The manufacturing and marketing of probiotics also need to be standardized and regulated to maintain product quality as well as determining efficacy in large-scale aquaculture operations in order to produce organic aquatic food and higher economic returns. Overall, further in-depth investigations of these issues alongside an environmental impact assessment of probiotics are key requirements to realize desirable outcomes in aquaculture.

Clearly, there is a role for probiotics in fish and shellfish disease control strategies, and their use can not only help to replace some of the inhibitory chemicals currently used in aquaculture but also promote food and health safety.

References

Abbass, A., Sharifuzzaman, S.M. and Austin, B. (2010) Cellular components of probiotics control *Yersinia ruckeri* infection in rainbow trout, *Oncorhynchus mykiss* (Walbaum). *Journal of Fish Diseases*, **33**, 31–37.

Aguilar-Macias, O.L., Ojeda-Ramirez, J.J., Campa-Cordova, A.I. and Saucedo, P.E. (2010) Evaluation of natural and commercial probiotics for improving growth and survival of the pearl oyster, *Pinctada mazatlanica*, during late hatchery and early field culturing. *Journal of the World Aquaculture Society*, **41**, 447–454.

Akinbowale, O.L., Peng, H. and Barton, M.D. (2006) Antimicrobial resistance in bacteria isolated from aquaculture sources in Australia. *Journal of Applied Microbiology*, **100**, 1103–1113.

Alcaide, E., Blasco, M.D. and Esteve, C. (2005) Occurrence of drug-resistant bacteria in two European eel farms. *Applied and Environmental Microbiology*, **71**, 3348–3350.

Al-Dohail, M.A., Hashim, R. and Aliyu-Paiko, M. (2009) Effects of the probiotic, *Lactobacillus acidophilus*, on the growth performance, haematology parameters and immunoglobulin concentration in African Catfish (*Clarias gariepinus*, Burchell 1822) fingerling. *Aquaculture Research*, **40**, 1642–1652.

Aly, S.M., Ahmed, Y.A.G., Ghareeb, A.A.A.and Mohamed, M.F. (2008a) Studies on *Bacillus subtilis* and *Lactobacillus acidophilus*, as potential probiotics, on the immune response and resistance of *Tilapia nilotica* (*Oreochromis niloticus*) to challenge infections. *Fish and Shellfish Immunology*, **25**, 128–136.

Aly, S.M., Mohamed, M.F. and John, G. (2008b) Effect of probiotics on the survival, growth and challenge infection in Tilapia nilotica (*Oreochromis niloticus*). *Aquaculture Research*, **39**, 647–656.

Arijo, S., Brunt, J., Chabrillón, M., Diaz-Rosales, P. and Austin, B. (2008) Subcellular components of *Vibrio harveyi* and probiotics induce immune responses in rainbow trout, *Oncorhynchus mykiss* (Walbaum), against *V. harveyi*. *Journal of Fish Diseases*, **31**, 579–590.

Aubin, J., Gatesoupe, F.J., Labbé, L. and Lebrun, L. (2005) Trial of probiotics to prevent the vertebral column compression syndrome in rainbow trout (*Oncorhynchus mykiss*, Walbaum). *Aquaculture Research*, **36**, 758–767.

Austin, B. (2002) Fish need doctoring too! *Microbiology Today*, **29**, 171–173.

Austin, B. (2005) Bacterial pathogens of marine fish, in *Oceans and Health, Pathogens in the Marine Environment* (eds S. Belkin and R.R. Colwell), Springer, New York.

Austin, B. and Austin, D.A. (2012) *Bacterial Fish Pathogens: Disease of Farmed and Wild Animals*, 5th edn, Springer, Dordrecht.

Austin, B. and Day, J.G. (1990) Inhibition of prawn pathogenic *Vibrio* spp. by a commercial spray-dried preparation of *Tetraselmis suecica*. *Aquaculture*, **90**, 389–392.

Austin, B., Baudet, E. and Stobie, M.B.C. (1992) Inhibition of bacterial fish pathogens by *Tetraselmis suecica*. *Journal of Fish Diseases*, **15**, 55–61.

Austin, B., Stuckey, L.F., Robertson, P.A.W., Effendi, I. and Griffith, D.R.W. (1995) A probiotic strain of *Vibrio alginolyticus* effective in reducing diseases caused by *Aeromonas salmonicida*, *Vibrio anguillarum* and *Vibrio ordalii*. *Journal of Fish Diseases*, **18**, 93–96.

Balcázar, J.L. and Rojas-Luna, T. (2007) Inhibitory activity of probiotic *Bacillus subtilis* UTM 126 against *Vibrio* species confers protection against Vibriosis in juvenile shrimp (*Litopenaeus vannamei*). *Current Microbiology* **55**, 409–412.

Balcázar, J.L., de Blas, I., Ruiz-Zarzuela, I., Cunningham, D., Vendrell, D. and Múzquiz, J.L. (2006) The role of probiotics in aquaculture. *Veterinary Microbiology*, **114**, 173–186.

Balcázar, J.L., de Blas, I., Ruiz-Zarzuela, I., *et al.* (2007a) Changes in intestinal microbiota and humoral immune response following probiotic administration in brown trout (*Salmo trutta*). *British Journal of Nutrition*, **97**, 522–527.

Balcázar, J.L., de Blas, I., Ruiz-Zazuela, I., Vandrell, D., Gironés, O. and Muzquiz, J.L. (2007b) Enhancement of the immune response and protection induced by probiotic lactic acid bacteria against furunculosis in rainbow trout (*Oncorhynchus mykiss*). *FEMS Immunology and Medical Microbiology*, **51**, 185–193.

Balcázar, J.L., Rojas-Luna, T. and Cunningham, D.P. (2007c) Effect of the addition of four potential probiotic strains on the survival of pacific white shrimp (*Litopenaeus vannamei*) following immersion challenge with *Vibrio parahaemolyticus*. *Journal of Invertebrate Pathology*, **96**, 147–150.

Balcázar, J.L., Vendrell, D., de Blas, I., Ruiz-Zarzuela, I., Muzquiz, J.L. and Girones, O. (2008) Characterization of probiotic properties of lactic acid bacteria isolated from intestinal microbiota of fish. *Aquaculture*, **278**, 188–191.

Bandyopadhyay, P. and Mohapatra, P.K.D. (2009) Effect of a probiotic bacterium *Bacillus circulans* PB7 in the formulated diets: on growth, nutritional quality and immunity of *Catla catla* (Ham.). *Fish Physiology and Biochemistry*,**35**, 467–478.

Bondad-Reantaso, M.G., Subasinghe, R.P., Arthur, J.R., *et al.* (2005) Disease and health management in Asian aquaculture. *Veterinary Parasitology*, **132**, 249–272.

Bricknell, I. and Dalmo, R.A. (2005) The use of immunostimulants in fish larval aquaculture. *Fish and Shellfish Immunology*, **19**, 457–472.

Brunt, J. and Austin, B. (2005) Use of a probiotic to control lactococcosis and streptococcosis in rainbow trout, *Oncorhynchus mykiss* (Walbaum). *Journal of Fish Diseases*, **28**, 693–701.

Brunt, J., Newaj-Fyzul, A. and Austin, B. (2007) The development of probiotics for the control of multiple bacterial diseases of rainbow trout, *Oncorhynchus mykiss* (Walbaum). *Journal of Fish Diseases*, **30**, 573–579.

Brunt, J., Hansen, R., Jamieson, D.J. and Austin, B. (2008) Proteomic analysis of rainbow trout (*Oncorhynchus mykiss*, Walbaum) serum after administration of probiotics in diets. *Veterinary Immunology and Immunopathology*, **121**, 199–205.

Burbank, D.R., Shah, D.H., LaPatra, S.E., Fornshell, G. and Cain, K.D. (2011) Enhanced resistance to coldwater disease following feeding of probiotic bacterial strains to rainbow trout (*Oncorhynchus mykiss*). *Aquaculture*, **321**, 185–190.

Cahu, C.L., Zambonino Infante, J.L., Pıres, A., Quazuguel, P. and Le Gall, M.M. (1998) Algal addition in sea bass (*Dicentrarchus labrax*) larvae rearing: effect on digestive enzymes. *Aquaculture*, **161**, 479–489.

Caipang, C.M.A., Brinchmann, M.F. and Kiron, V. (2010) Antagonistic activity of bacterial isolates from intestinal microbiota of Atlantic cod, *Gadus morhua*, and an investigation of their immunomodulatory capabilities. *Aquaculture Research*, **41**, 249–256.

Cao, H., Hou, S., He, S., Lu, L. and Yang, X. (2014) Identification of a *Bacteriovorax* sp. isolate as a potential biocontrol bacterium against snakehead fish-pathogenic *Aeromonas veronii*. *Journal of Fish Diseases*, **37**, 283–289.

Capkin, E. and Altinok, I. (2009) Effects of dietary probiotic supplementations on prevention/treatment of yersiniosis disease. *Journal of Applied Microbiology*, **106**, 1147–1153.

Cha, J.H., Rahimnejad, S., Yang, S.Y., Kim, K.W. and Lee, K.J. (2013) Evaluations of *Bacillus* spp. as dietary additives on growth performance, innate immunity and disease resistance of olive flounder (*Paralichthys olivaceus*) against *Streptococcus iniae* and as water additives. *Aquaculture*, **402**, 50–57.

Chabrillón, M., Rico, R.M., Balebona, M.C. and Moriñigo, M.A. (2005a) Adhesion to sole, *Solea senegalensis* Kaup, mucus of microorganisms isolated from farmed fish, and their interaction with *Photobacterium damselae* subsp. *piscicida*. *Journal of Fish Diseases*, **28**, 229–237.

Chabrillón, M., Rico, R.M., Arijo, S., Díaz-Rosales, P., Balebona, M.C. and Moriñigo, M.A. (2005b) Interactions of microorganisms isolated from gilthead sea bream, *Sparus aurata* L., on *Vibrio harveyi*, a pathogen of farmed Senegalese sole, *Solea senegalensis* (Kaup). *Journal of Fish Diseases*, **28**, 531–537.

Chang, C.I. and Liu,W.Y. (2002) An evaluation of two probiotic bacterial strains, *Enterococcus faecium* SF68 and *Bacillus toyoi*, for reducing edwardsiellosis in cultured European eel, *Anguilla anguilla*, L. *Journal of Fish Diseases*, **25**, 311–315.

Choi, S.H. and Yoon, T.J. (2008) Non-specific immune response of rainbow trout (*Oncorhynchus Mykiss*) by dietary heat-inactivated potential probiotics. *Immune Network*, **8**, 67–74.

Dagar, A., Zilberg, D., Cohen, Z., Boussiba, S. and Khozin-Goldberg, I. (2009) Short-term dietary supplementation with the microalga *Parietochloris incisa* enhances stress resistance in guppies *Poecilia reticulata*. *Aquaculture Research*, **41**, 267–277.

Das, A., Nakro, K., Chowdhury, S. and Kamilya, D. (2013) Effects of potential probiotic *Bacillus amyloliquefaciens* FPTB16 on systemic and cutaneous mucosal immune responses and disease resistance of catla (*Catla catla*). *Fish and Shellfish Immunology*, **35**, 1547–1553.

Das, S.,Ward, L.R. and Burke, C. (2010) Screening of marine *Streptomyces* spp. for potential use as probiotics in aquaculture. *Aquaculture*, **305**, 32–41.

Decamp, O., Moriarty, D.J.W. and Lavens, P. (2008) Probiotics for shrimp larviculture: review of field data from Asia and Latin America. *Aquaculture Research*, **39**, 334–338.

De la Banda, I.G., Lobo, C., Chabrillón, M., *et al.* (2012) Influence of dietary administration of a probiotic strain *Shewanella putrefaciens* on Senegalese sole (*Solea senegalensis*, Kaup 1858) growth, body composition and resistance *to Photobacterium damselae* subsp *piscicida*. *Aquaculture Research*, **43**, 662–669.

De Schryver, P., Defoirdt, T., Boon, N., Verstraete, W. and Bossier, P. (2012) Managing the microbiota in aquaculture systems for disease prevention and control, in *Infectious Disease in Aquaculture: Prevention and Control* (ed. B. Austin), Woodhead, pp.393–418.

Di Cesare, A., Vignaroli, C., Luna, G.M., Pasquaroli, S. and Biavasco, F. (2012) Antibiotic-resistant enterococci in seawater and sediments from a coastal fish farm. *Microbial Drug Resistance*, **18**, 502–509.

El-Rhman, A.M.A., Khattab, Y.A.E. and Shalaby, A.M.E. (2009) *Micrococcus luteus* and *Pseudomonas* species as probiotics for promoting the growth performance and health of Nile tilapia, *Oreochromis niloticus*. *Fish and Shellfish Immunology*, **27**, 175–180.

FAO/WHO (2001) *Health and Nutritional Properties of Probiotics in Food Including Powder Milk With Live Lactic Acid Bacteria*, Food and Agriculture Organization of the United Nations/World Health Organization Joint Report, Córdoba, Argentina.

Faramarzi, M., Kiaalvandi, S. and Iranshahi, F. (2011) The effect of probiotics on growth performance and body composition of common carp (*Cyprinus carpio*). *Journal of Animal and Veterinary Advances*, **10**, 2408–2413.

Ferguson, R.M.W., Merrifield, D.L., Harper, G.M., Rawling, M.D. and Mustafa, S. (2010) The effect of *Pediococcus acidilactici* on the gut microbiota and immune status of on-growing red tilapia (*Oreochromis niloticus*). *Journal of Applied Microbiology*, **109**, 851–862.

Fuller, R. (1989) Probiotic in man and animals. *Journal of Applied Bacteriology*, **66**, 365–378.

Gatesoupe, F.J. (1994) Lactic acid bacteria increase the resistance of turbot larvae, *Scophthalmus maximus*, against pathogenic *Vibrio*. *Aquatic Living Resources*, **7**, 277–282.

Gatesoupe, F.J. (1999) The use of probiotics in aquaculture. *Aquaculture*, **180**, 147–165.

Gibson, G.R. and Roberfroid, M.B. (1995) Dietary modulation of the human clonic microbiota: introducing the concept of prebiotics. *Journal of Nutrition*, **125**, 1401–1405.

Gibson, L.F. (1999) Bacteriocin activity and probiotic activity of *Aeromonas media*. *Journal of Applied Microbiology*, **85**, S243–S248.

Gildberg, A. and Mikkelsen, H. (1998) Effect of supplementing the feed of Atlantic cod (*Gadus morhua*) fry with lactic acid bacteria and immunostimulating peptides during a challenge trial with *Vibrio anguillarum*. *Aquaculture*, **167**, 103–113.

Gildberg, A., Mikkelsen, H., Sandaker, E. and Ringø, E. (1997) Probiotic effect of lactic acid bacteria in the feed on growth and survival of fry of Atlantic cod (*Gadus morhua*). *Hydrobiologia*, **352**, 279–285.

Giri, S.S., Sukumaran, V. and Oviya, M. (2013) Potential probiotic *Lactobacillus plantarum* VSG3 improves the growth, immunity, and disease resistance of tropical freshwater fish, *Labeo rohita*. *Fish and Shellfish Immunology*, **34**, 660–666.

Gobeli, S., Goldschmidt-Clermont, E., Frey, J. and Burr, S.E. (2009) *Pseudomonas chlororaphis* strain JF3835 reduces mortality of juvenile perch, *Perca fluviatilis* L., caused by *Aeromonas sobria*. *Journal of Fish Diseases*, **32**, 597–602.

Gomez, D., Sunyer, J.O. and Salinas, I. (2013) The mucosal immune system of fish: the evolution of tolerating commensals while fighting pathogens. *Fish and Shellfish Immunology*, **35**, 1729–1739.

Gopalakannan, A. and Arul, V. (2011) Inhibitory activity of probiotic *Enterococcus faecium* MC13 against *Aeromonas hydrophila* confers protection against hemorrhagic septicemia in common carp *Cyprinus carpio*. *Aquaculture International*, **19**, 973–985.

Gram, L. and Melchiorsen, J. (1996) Interaction between fish spoilage bacteria *Pseudomonas* sp. and *Shewanella putrefaciens* in fish extracts and on fish tissue. *Journal of Applied Bacteriology*, **80**, 589–595.

Gram, L., Melchiorsen, J., Spanggaard, B., Huber, I. and Nielsen, T.F. (1999) Inhibition of *Vibrio anguillarum* by *Pseudomonas fluorescens* AH2, a possible probiotic treatment of fish. *Applied and Environmental Microbiology*, **65**, 969–973.

Gueimonde, M., Jalonen, L., He, F., Hiramatsu, M. and Salminen, S. (2006) Adhesion and competitive inhibition and displacement of human enteropathogens by selected lactobacilli. *Food Research International*, **39**, 467–471.

Guo, J.J., Liu, K.F., Cheng, S.H., *et al.* (2009) Selection of probiotic bacteria for use in shrimp larviculture. *Aquaculture Research*, **40**, 609–618.

Guzman-Villanueva, T., Tovar-Ramirez, D., Gisbert, E., *et al.* (2014) Dietary administration of β-1,3/1,6-glucan and probiotic strain *Shewanella putrefaciens*, single or combined, on gilthead seabream growth, immune responses and gene expression. *Fish and Shellfish Immunology*, **39**, 34–41.

Hai, N.V. (2015) The use of probiotics in aquaculture. *Journal of Applied Microbiology*, **119**, 917–935.

Hai V.N. and Fotedar, R. (2009) Comparison of the effects of the prebiotics (Bio-Mos® and b-1,3-D-glucan) and the customised probiotics (*Pseudomonas synxantha* and *P. aeruginosa*) on the culture of juvenile western king prawns (*Penaeus latisulcatus* Kishinouye, 1896). *Aquaculture*, **289**, 310–316.

Hai, N.V., Buller, N. and Fotedar, R. (2009) The use of customised probiotics in the cultivation of western king prawns (*Penaeus latisulcatus* Kishinouye, 1896). *Fish and Shellfish Immunology*, **27**, 100–104.

Harris, J.M. (1993) The presence, nature, and role of gut microflora in aquatic invertebrates: a synthesis. *Microbial Ecology*, **25**, 195–231.

Heo, W.S., Kim, Y.R., Kim, E.Y., Bai, S.C. and Kong, I.S. (2013) Effect of dietary probiotic, *Lactococcus lactis* subsp. *lactis* I2, supplementation on the growth and immune response of olive flounder (*Paralichthys olivaceus*). *Aquaculture*, **376**, 20–24.

Huang, J.B., Wu, Y.C. and Chi, S.C. (2014) Dietary supplementation of *Pediococcus pentosaceus* enhances innate immunity, physiological health and resistance to *Vibrio anguillarum* in orange-spotted grouper (*Epinephelus coioides*). *Fish and Shellfish Immunology*, **39**, 196–205.

Huys, G., Vancanneyt, M., D'Haene, K., Vankerckhoven, V., Goossens, H. and Swings, J. (2006) Accuracy of species identity of commercial bacterial cultures intended for probiotic or nutritional use. *Research in Microbiology*, **157**, 803–810.

Irianto, A. and Austin, B. (2002a) Use of probiotics to control furunculosis in rainbow trout, *Oncorhynchus mykiss* (Walbaum). *Journal of Fish Diseases*, **25**, 333–342.

Irianto, A. and Austin, B. (2002b) Probiotics in aquaculture. *Journal of Fish Diseases*, **25**, 633–642.

Irianto, A. and Austin, B. (2003) Use of dead probiotic cells to control furunculosis in rainbow trout, *Oncorhynchus mykiss* (Walbaum). *Journal of Fish Diseases*, **26**, 59–62.

Kalatzis, P.G., Bastías, R., Kokkari, C. and Katharios, P. (2016) Isolation and characterization of two lytic bacteriophages, φSt2 and φGrn1; phage therapy application for biological control of *Vibrio alginolyticus* in aquaculture live feeds. *PLoS One*, **11**(3), e0151101.

Kesarcodi-Watson, A., Kaspar, H., Lategan, M.J. and Gibson, L. (2010) *Alteromonas macleodii* 0444 and *Neptunomonas* sp. 0536, two novel probiotics for hatchery-reared Greenshell (TM) mussel larvae, *Perna canaliculus*. *Aquaculture*, **309**, 49–55.

Kesarcodi-Watson, A., Miner, P., Nicolas, J.L. and Robert, R. (2012) Protective effect of four potential probiotics against pathogen-challenge of the larvae of three bivalves: Pacific oyster

(*Crassostrea gigas*), flat oyster (*Ostrea edulis*) and scallop (*Pecten maximus*). *Aquaculture*, **344**, 29–34.

Kim, D., Beck, B.R., Heo, S.B., *et al.* (2013) *Lactococcus lactis* BFE920 activates the innate immune system of olive flounder (*Paralichthys olivaceus*), resulting in protection against *Streptococcus iniae* infection and enhancing feed efficiency and weight gain in large-scale field studies. *Fish and Shellfish Immunology*, **35**, 1585–1590.

Kim, D.H. and Austin, B. (2006a) Innate immune responses in rainbow trout (*Oncorhynchus mykiss*, Walbaum) induced by probiotics. *Fish and Shellfish Immunology*, **21**, 513–524.

Kim, D.H. and Austin, B. (2006b) Cytokine expression in leucocytes and gut cells of rainbow trout, *Oncorhynchus mykiss* Walbaum, induced by probiotics. *Veterinary Immunology and Immunopathology*, **114**, 297–304.

Kim, J.S., Harikrishnan, R., Kim, M.C., Balasundaram, C. and Heo, M.S. (2010) Dietary administration of *Zooshikella* sp. to enhance the innate immune response and disease resistance of *Paralichthys olivaceus* against *Streptococcus iniae*. *Fish and Shellfish Immunology*, **29**, 104–110.

Korkea-Aho, T.L., Heikkinen, J., Thompson, K.D., von Wright, A. and Austin, B. (2011) *Pseudomonas* sp. M174 inhibits the fish pathogen *Flavobacterium psychrophilum*. *Journal of Applied Microbiology*, **111**, 266–277.

Korkea-Aho, T.L., Papadopoulou, A., Heikkinen, J., *et al.* (2012) *Pseudomonas* M162 confers protection against rainbow trout fry syndrome by stimulating immunity. *Journal of Applied Microbiology*, **113**, 24–35.

Kumar, R., Mukherjee, S.C., Prasad, K.P. and Pal, A.K. (2006) Evaluation of *Bacillus subtilis* as a probiotic to Indian major carp *Labeo rohita* (Ham.). *Aquaculture Research*, **37**, 1215–1221.

Kumar, R., Mukherjee, S.C., Ranjan, R. and Nayak, S.K. (2008) Enhanced innate immune parameters in *Labeo rohita* (Ham.) following oral administration of *Bacillus subtilis*. *Fish and Shellfish Immunology*, **24**, 168–172.

Lara-Flores, M., Olvera-Novoa, M.A., Guzmán-Méndez, B.E. and López-Madrid, W. (2003) Use of the bacteria *Streptococcus faecium* and *Lactobacillus acidophilus*, and the yeast *Saccharomyces cerevisiae* as growth promoters in Nile tilapia (*Oreochromis niloticus*). *Aquaculture*, **216**, 193–201.

Lategan, M.J., Torpy, F.R. and Gibson, L.F. (2004) Control of saprolegniosis in the eel *Anguilla australis* Richardson, by *Aeromonas* media strain A199. *Aquaculture*, **240**, 19–27.

Lauzon, H.L., Gudmundsdottir, S., Steinarsson, A., *et al.* (2010) Effects of bacterial treatment at early stages of Atlantic cod (*Gadus morhua* L.) on larval survival and development. *Journal of Applied Microbiology*, **108**, 624–632.

Lazado, C.C., Caipang, C.M.A. and Kiron, V. (2012) Enzymes from the gut bacteria of Atlantic cod, *Gadus morhua* and their influence on intestinal enzyme activity. *Aquaculture Nutrition*, **18**, 423–431.

Lazado, C.C., Caipang, C.M.A.and Estante, E.G. (2015) Prospects of host-associated microorganisms in fish and penaeids as probiotics with immunomodulatory functions. *Fish and Shellfish Immunology*, **45**, 2–12.

Lee, B.J., Kim, S.S., Song, J.W., *et al.* (2013) Effects of dietary supplementation of citrus by0products fermented with a probiotic microbes on growth performance, innate immunity and disease resistance *against Edwardsiella tarda* in juvenile olive flounder, *Paralichthys olivaceus* (Temminck and Schlegel). *Journal of Fish Diseases*, **36**, 617–628.

Leyva-Madrigal, K.Y., Luna-González, A., Escobedo-Bonilla, C.M., Fierro-Coronado, J.A. and Maldonado-Mendoza, I.E. (2011) Screening for potential probiotic bacteria to reduce prevalence of WSSV and IHHNV in whiteleg shrimp (*Litopenaeus vannamei*) under experimental conditions. *Aquaculture*, **322–323**, 16–22.

Li, J., Tan, B. and Mai, K. (2009) Dietary probiotic *Bacillus* OJ and isomaltooligosaccharides influence the intestine microbial populations, immune responses and resistance to white spot syndrome virus in shrimp (*Litopenaeus vannamei*). *Aquaculture*, **291**, 35–40.

Li, J.Q., Tan, B.P., Mai, K.S., *et al.* (2008) Immune responses and resistance against *Vibrio parahaemolyticus* induced by probiotic bacterium *Arthrobacter* XE-7 in Pacific white shrimp, *Litopenaeus vannamei*. *Journal of the World Aquaculture Society*, **39**, 477–489.

Li, P. and Gatlin, D.M.I.I.I. (2004) Dietary brewers yeast and the prebiotic Grobiotic™ AE influence growth performance, immune responses and resistance of hybrid striped bass (*Morone chrysops* × *M. saxatilis*) to *Streptococcus iniae* infection. *Aquaculture*, **231**, 445–456.

Lilley, D.M. and Stillwell, R.H. (1965) Probiotics: growth promoting factors produced by microorganisms. *Science*, **147**, 747–748.

Lin, S., Mao, S., Guan, Y., Luo, L., Luo, L. and Pan, Y. (2012) Effects of dietary chitosan oligosaccharides and *Bacillus coagulans* on the growth, innate immunity and resistance of kopi (*Cyprinus carpio koi*). *Aquaculture*, **342–343**, 36–41.

Liu, W.S., Ren, P.F., He, S.X., *et al.* (2013) Comparison of adhesive gut bacteria composition, immunity, and disease resistance in juvenile hybrid tilapia fed two different *Lactobacillus* strains. *Fish and Shellfish Immunology*, **35**, 54–62.

Macey, B.M. and Coyne, V.E. (2005) Improved growth rate and disease resistance in farmed *Haliotis midae* through probiotic treatment. *Aquaculture*, **245**, 249–261.

Makridis, P., Martins, S., Reis, J. and Dinis, M.T. (2008) Use of probiotic bacteria in the rearing of Senegalese sole (*Solea senegalensis*) larvae. *Aquaculture Research*, **39**, 627–634.

Mandiki, S.N.M., Milla, S.,Wang, N., *et al.* (2011) Effects of probiotic bacteria on growth parameters and immune defence in Eurasian perch *Perca fluviatilis* L. larvae under intensive culture conditions. *Aquaculture Research*, **42**, 693–703.

Marques, A., Thanh, T.H., Sorgeloos, P. and Bossier, P. (2006) Use of microalgae and bacteria to enhance protection of gnotobiotic *Artemia* against different pathogens. *Aquaculture*, **258**, 116–126.

Merrifield, D.L., Dimitroglou, A., Foey, A., *et al.* (2010a) The current status and future focus of probiotic and prebiotic applications for salmonids. *Aquaculture*, **302**, 1–18.

Merrifield, D.L., Bradley, G., Baker, R.T.M. and Davies, S.J. (2010b) Probiotic applications for rainbow trout (*Oncorhynchus mykiss* Walbaum). II. Effects on growth performance, feed utilization, intestinal microbiota and related health criteria postantibiotic treatment. *Aquaculture Nutrition*, **16**, 496–503.

Mohanty, S.N., Swain, S.K. and Tripathi, S.D. (1996) Rearing of catla (*Catla catla* Ham.) spawn on formulated diets. *Journal of Aquaculture in the Tropics*, **11**, 253–258.

Moriarty, D.J.W. (1998) Control of luminous *Vibrio* species in penaeid aquaculture ponds. *Aquaculture*, **164**, 351–358.

Mukai, T., Asasaka, T., Sato, E., Mori, K., Matsumoto, M. and Ohori, H. (2002) Inhibition of binding of *Helicobacter pylori* to the glycolipid receptors by probiotic *Lactobacillus reuteri*. *FEMS Immunology and Medical Microbiology*, **35**, 105–110.

Murray, A.G. and Peeler, E.J. (2005) A framework for understanding the potential for emerging diseases in aquaculture. *Preventive Veterinary Medicine*, **67**, 223–235.

Naidu, A.S., Bidlack, W.R. and Clemens, R.A. (1999) Probiotic spectra of lactic acid bacteria (LAB). *Critical Reviews of Food Science and Nutrition*, **39**, 13–126.

Nass, K., Naess, T. and Harboe, T. (1992) Enhanced first feeding of halibut larvae *Hippoglossus hippoglossus* L. in green water. *Aquaculture,* **105**, 143–156.

NavinChandran, M., Iyapparaj, P., Moovendhan, S., *et al.* (2014) Influence of probiotic bacterium *Bacillus cereus* isolated from the gut of wild shrimp *Penaeus monodon* in turn as a potent growth promoter and immune enhancer in *P. monodon*. *Fish and Shellfish Immunology,* **36**, 38–45.

Nayak, S.K. (2010) Probiotics and immunity: a fish perspective. *Fish and Shellfish Immunology,* **29**, 2–14.

Nayak, S.K., Swain, P. and Mukherjee, S.C. (2007) Effect of dietary supplementation of probiotic and vitamin C on the immune response of Indian major carp, *Labeo rohita* (Ham). *Fish and Shellfish Immunology,* **23**, 892–896.

Neissi, A., Rafiee, G., Nematollahi, M. and Safari, O. (2013) The effect of *Pediococcus acidilactici* bacteria used as probiotic supplement on the growth and non-specific immune responses of green terror, *Aequidens rivulatus*. *Fish and Shellfish Immunology,* **35**, 1976–1980.

Newaj-Fyzul, A. and Austin, B. (2015) Probiotics, immunostimulants, plant products and oral vaccines, and their role as feed supplements in the control of bacterial fish diseases. *Journal of Fish Diseases,* **38**, 937–955.

Newaj-Fyzul, A., Adesiyun, A.A., Mutani, A., Ramsubhag, A., Brunt, J. and Austin, B. (2007) *Bacillus subtilis* AB1 controls *Aeromonas* infection in rainbow trout (*Oncorhynchus mykiss*, Walbaum). *Journal of Applied Microbiology,* **103**, 1699–1706.

Newaj-Fyzul, A., Al-Harbi, A.H. and Austin, B. (2014) Review: Developments in the use of probiotics for disease control in aquaculture. *Aquaculture,* **431**, 1–11.

Nikoskelainen, S., Ouwehand, A., Salminen, S. and Bylund, G. (2001) Protection of rainbow trout (*Oncorhynchus mykiss*) from furunculosis by *Lactobacillus rhamnosus*. *Aquaculture,* **198**, 229–236.

Nikoskelainen, S., Ouwehand, A.C., Bylund, G., Salminen, S. and Lilius, E.M. (2003) Immune enhancement in rainbow trout (*Oncorhynchus mykiss*) by potential probiotic bacteria (*Lactobacillus rhamnosus*). *Fish and Shellfish Immunology,* **15**, 443–452.

Nimrat, S. and Vuthiphandchai, V. (2011) *In vitro* evaluation of commercial probiotic products used for marine shrimp cultivation in Thailand. *African Journal of Biotechnology,* **10**, 4643–4650.

Ottesen, O.H. and Olafsen, J.A. (2000) Effects on survival and mucous cell proliferation of Atlantic halibut, *Hippoglossus hippoglossus* L., larvae following microflora manipulation. *Aquaculture,* **187**, 225–238.

Owens, L. (2003) Diseases, in *Aquaculture: Farming Aquatic Animals and Plants* (eds J.S. Lucas and P.C. Southgate), Fishing News Books, Oxford, pp. 199–214.

Pai, S.S., Anas, A., Jayaprakash, N.S., *et al.* (2010) *Penaeus monodon* larvae can be protected from *Vibrio harveyi* infection by pre-emptive treatment of a rearing system with antagonistic or non-antagonistic bacterial probiotics. *Aquaculture Research,* **41**, 847–860.

Pan, X., Wu, T., Song, Z., Tang, H. and Zhao, Z. (2008) Immune responses and enhanced disease resistance in Chinese drum, *Miichthys miiuy* (Basilewsky), after oral administration of live or dead cells of *Clostridium butyricum* CB2. *Journal of Fish Diseases,* **31**, 679–686.

Panigrahi, A., Kiron, V., Kobayashi, T., Puangkaew, J., Satoh, S. and Sugita, H. (2004) Immune responses in rainbow trout *Oncorhynchus mykiss* induced by a potential probiotic bacteria *Lactobacillus rhamnosus* JCM 1136. *Veterinary Immunology and Immunopathology,* **102**, 379–388.

Panigrahi, A., Kiron, V., Puangkaew, J., Kobayashi, T., Satoh, S. and Sugita, H. (2005) The viability of probiotic bacteria as a factor influencing the immune response in rainbow trout *Oncorhynchus mykiss*. *Aquaculture*, **243**, 241–254.

Panigrahi, A., Kiron, V., Satoh, S., Hirono, I., Kobayashi, T. and Sugita, H. (2007) Immune modulation and expression of cytokine genes in rainbow trout *Oncorhynchus mykiss* upon probiotic feeding. *Developmental and Comparative Immunology*, **31**, 372–382.

Park, S.C., Shimamura, I., Fukunaga, M., Mori, K. and Nakai, T. (2000) Isolation of bacteriophages specific to a fish pathogen, *Pseudomonas plecoglossicida*, as a candidate for disease control. *Applied and Environmental Microbiology*, **66**, 1416–1422.

Parker, R.B. (1974) Probiotics, the other half of the antibiotics story. *Animal Nutrition and Health*, **29**, 4–8.

Pattukumar, V., Kanmani, P., Kumar R.S., Yuvaraj, N., Paari, A. and Arul, V. (2014) Enhancement of innate immune system, survival and yield in *Penaeus monodon* reared in ponds using *Streptococcus phocae* PI80. *Aquaculture Nutrition*, **20**, 505–513.

Pérez-Sánchez, T., Balcazar, J.L.,Merrifield, D.L., *et al.* (2011) Expression of immune-related genes in rainbow trout (*Oncorhynchus mykiss*) induced by probiotic bacteria during *Lactococcus garvieae* infection. *Fish and Shellfish Immunology*, **31**, 196–201.

Picchietti, S., Mazzini, M., Taddei, A.R., *et al.*. (2007) Effects of administration of probiotic strains on GALT of larval gilthead seabream: immunohistochemical and ultrastructural studies. *Fish and Shellfish Immunology*, **22**, 57–67.

Picchietti, S., Guerra, L., Selleri, L., *et al.* (2008) Compartmentalisation of T cells expressing CD8α and TCR β in developing thymus of sea bass *Dicentrarchus labrax* (L.). *Developmental and Comparative Immunology*, **32**, 92–99.

Picchietti, S., Fausto, A.M., Randelli, E., *et al.* (2009) Early treatment with *Lactobacillus delbrueckii* strain induces an increase in intestinal T-cells and granulocytes and modulates immune-related genes of larval *Dicentrarchus labrax* (L.). *Fish and Shellfish Immunology*, **26**, 368–376.

Pieters, N., Brunt, J., Austin, B. and Lyndon, A.R. (2008) Efficacy of in-feed probiotics against *Aeromonas bestiarum* and *Ichthyophthirius multifiliis* skin infections in rainbow trout (*Oncorhynchus mykiss*, Walbaum). *Journal of Applied Microbiology*, **105**, 723–732.

Pillay, T.V.R. (2004) Pathogens in the aquatic environment, in *Aquaculture and the Environment*, 2nd edn (ed. T.V.R. Pillay), Blackwell, Oxford, pp. 92–96.

Pirarat, N., Kobayashi, T., Katagiri, T., Maita, M. and Endo, M. (2006) Protective effects and mechanisms of a probiotic bacterium *Lactobacillus rhamnosus* against experimental *Edwardsiella tarda* infection in tilapia (*Oreochromis niloticus*). *Veterinary Immunology and Immunopathology*, **113**, 339–347.

Planas, M., Pérez-Lorenzo, M., Hjelm, M., *et al.* (2006) Probiotic effect *in vivo* of *Roseobacter* strain 27-4 against *Vibrio (Listonella) anguillarum* infections in turbot (*Scophthalmus maximus* L.) larvae. *Aquaculture*, **255**, 323–333.

Preetha, R., Jayaprakash, N.S. and Singh, I.S.B. (2007) *Synechocystis* MCCB 114 and 115 as putative probionts for *Penaeus monodon* post-larvae. *Diseases of Aquatic Organisms*, **74**, 243–247.

Qi, Z., Zhang, X.H, Boon, N. and Bossier, P. (2009) Probiotics in aquaculture of China – current state, problems and prospect. *Aquaculture*, **290**, 15–21.

Rahiman, K.M.M., Jesmi, Y., Thomas, A.P. and Hatha, A.A.M. (2010) Probiotic effect of *Bacillus* NL110 and *Vibrio* NE17 on the survival, growth performance and immune response of *Macrobrachium rosenbergii* (de Man). *Aquaculture Research*, **41**, e120–e134.

Raida, M.K., Larsen, J.L., Nielsen, M.E. and Buchmann, K. (2003) Enhanced resistance of rainbow trout, *Oncorhynchus mykiss* (Walbaum), against *Yersinia ruckeri* challenge following oral administration of *Bacillus subtilis* and *B. licheniformis* (BioPlus2B). *Journal of Fish Diseases*, **26**, 495–498.

Ran, C., Carrias, A., Williams, M.A., *et al.* (2012) Identification of *Bacillus* strains for biological control of catfish pathogens. *PLoS One*, **7**(9), e45793.

Reitan, K., Rainuzzo, J., Oie, G. and Olsen, Y. (1997) A review of the nutritional effects of algae in marine fish larvae. *Aquaculture*, **155**, 207–221.

Ren, P., Xu, L., Yang, Y., *et al.* (2013) *Lactobacillus planarum* subsp. *plantarum* JCM 1149 *vs. Aeromonas hydrophila* NJ-1 in the anterior intestine and posterior intestine of hybrid tilapia *Oreochromis niloticus* ♀ × *Oreochromis aureus* ♂: an *ex vivo* study. *Fish and Shellfish Immunology*, **35**, 146–153.

Rengpipat, S., Phianphak, W., Piyatiratitivorakul, S. and Menasveta, P. (1998) Effects of a probiotic bacterium in black tiger shrimp *Penaeus monodon* survival and growth. *Aquaculture*, **167**, 301–313.

Rengpipat, S., Rukpratanporn, S., Piyatiratitivorakul, S. and Menasaveta, P. (2000) Immunity enhancement in black tiger shrimp (*Penaeus monodon*) by a probiont bacterium (*Bacillus* S11). *Aquaculture*, **191**, 271–288.

Rengpipat, S., Tunyanun, A., Fast, A.W., Piyatiratitivorakul, S. and Menasveta, P. (2003) Enhanced growth and resistance to *Vibrio* challenge in pond-reared black tiger shrimp *Penaeus monodon* fed a *Bacillus* probiotic. *Diseases of Aquatic Organisms*, **55**, 169–173.

Reyes-Becerril, M., Salinas, I., Cuesta, A., *et al.* (2008) Oral delivery of live yeast *Debaryomyces hansenii* modulates the main innate immune parameters and the expression of immune–relevant genes in the gilthead sea bream (*Sparus aurata* L.). *Fish and Shellfish Immunology*, **25**, 731–739.

Reyes-Becerril, M., Guardiola, F., Rojas, M., Ascencio-Valle, F. and Esteban, M.A. (2013) Dietary administration of microalgae *Navicula* sp. affects immune status and gene expression of gilthead seabream (*Sparus aurata*). *Fish and Shellfish Immunology*, **35**, 883–889.

Ridha, M.T. and Azad, I.S. (2012) Preliminary evaluation of growth performance and immune response of Nile tilapia *Oreochromis niloticus* supplemented with two putative probiotic bacteria. *Aquaculture Research*, **43**, 843–852.

Ringø, E. and Gatesoupe, F.J. (1998) Lactic acid bacteria in fish: a review. *Aquaculture*, **160**, 177–203.

Ringø, E. and Vadstein, O. (1998) Colonization of *Vibrio pelagius* and *Aeromonas caviae* in early developing turbot (*Scopthalmus maximus* L.) larvae. *Journal of Applied Microbiology*, **84**, 227–233.

Ringø, E., Olsen, R.E., Jensen, I., Romero, J. and Lauzon, H.L. (2014) Application of vaccines and dietary supplements in aquaculture: possibilities and challenges. *Reviews in Fish Biology and Fisheries*, **24**, 1005–1032.

Riquelme, C., Araya, R., Vergara, N., Rojas, A., Guaita, M. and Candia M. (1997) Potential probiotic strains in the culture of the Chilean scallop *Argopecten purpuratus* (Lamarck, 1819). *Aquaculture*, **154**, 17–26.

Robertson, P.A.W., O'Dowd, C., Burrells, C., Williams, P. and Austin, B. (2000) Use of *Carnobacterium* sp. as a probiotic for Atlantic salmon (*Salmo salar* L.) and rainbow trout (*Oncorhynchus mykiss* Walbaum). *Aquaculture*, **185**, 235–243.

Rodríguez, A., Cuesta, A., Ortuño, J., Esteban, M.A. and Meseguer, J. (2003) Immunostimulant properties of a cell wall-modified whole *Saccharomyces cerevisiae* strain administered by diet to seabream (*Sparus aurata* L.). *Veterinary Immunology and Immunopathology*, **96**, 183–192.

Rodriguez-Estrada, U., Satoh, S., Haga, Y., Fushimi, H. and Sweetman, J. (2009) Effects of single and combined supplementation of *Enterococcus faecalis*, mannan oligosaccharide and polyhydrobutyric acid on growth performance and immune response of rainbow trout *Oncorhynchus mykiss*. *Aquaculture Science*, **57**, 609–617.

Sáenz de Rodrigáñez, M.A., Díaz-Rosales, P., Chabrillón, M., *et al.* (2009) Effect of dietary administration of probiotics on growth and intestine functionally of juvenile Senegalese sole (*Solea senegalensis*, Kaup 1858). *Aquaculture Nutrition*, **15**, 177–185.

Safari, R., Adel, M., Lazado, C.C., Caipang, C.M.A. and Dadar, M. (2016) Host-derived probiotics *Enterococcus casseliflavus* improves resistance against *Streptococcus iniae* infection in rainbow trout (*Oncorhynchus mykiss*) via immunomodulation. *Fish and Shellfish Immunology*, **52**, 198–205.

Sakai, M. (1999) Current research status of fish immunostimulants. *Aquaculture*, **172**, 63–92.

Salinas, I., Cuesta, A., Esteban, M.Á. and Meseguer, J. (2005) Dietary administration of *Lactobacillus delbrueckii* and *Bacillus subtilis*, single or combined, on gilthead seabream cellular innate immune responses. *Fish and Shellfish Immunology*, **19**, 67–77.

Salinas, I., Abelli, L., Bertoni, F., *et al.* (2008) Monospecies and multispecies probiotic formulations produce different systemic and local immunostimulatory effects in the gilthead seabream (*Sparus aurata* L.). *Fish and Shellfish Immunology*, **25**, 114–123.

Salma, W., Zhou, Z., Wang, W., *et al.* (2011) Histological and bacteriological changes in intestine of beluga (*Huso huso*) following *ex vivo* exposure to bacterial strains. *Aquaculture*, **314**, 24–33.

Salminen, S., Ouwehand, A., Benno, Y. and Lee, Y.K. (1999) Probiotics: how should they be defined? *Trends in Food Science and Technology*, **10**, 107–110.

Scholz, U., Garcia Diaz, G., Ricque, D., Cruz Suarez, L.E., Vargas Albores, F. and Latchford, J. (1999) Enhancement of vibriosis resistance in juvenile *Penaeus vannamei* by supplementation of diets with different yeast products. *Aquaculture*, **176**, 271–283.

Sharifuzzaman, S.M. (2010) Studies on probiotics for the control of vibriosis in rainbow trout (*Oncorhynchus mykiss*, Walbaum). PhD thesis, Heriot-Watt University, Edinburgh.

Sharifuzzaman, S.M. and Austin, B. (2009) Influence of probiotic feeding duration on disease resistance and immune parameters in rainbow trout. *Fish and Shellfish Immunology*, **27**, 440–445.

Sharifuzzaman, S.M. and Austin, B. (2010a) *Kocuria* SM1 controls vibriosis in rainbow trout (*Oncorhynchus mykiss*, Walbaum). *Journal of Applied Microbiology*, **108**, 2162–2170.

Sharifuzzaman, S.M. and Austin, B. (2010b) Development of protection in rainbow trout (*Oncorhynchus mykiss*, Walbaum) to *Vibrio anguillarum* following use of the probiotic *Kocuria* SM1. *Fish and Shellfish Immunology*, **29**, 212–216.

Sharifuzzaman, S.M., Abbass, A., Tinsley, J.W. and Austin, B. (2011) Subcellular components of probiotics *Kocuria* SM1 and *Rhodococcus* SM2 induce protective immunity in rainbow trout (*Oncorhynchus mykiss*, Walbaum) against *Vibrio anguillarum*. *Fish and Shellfish Immunology*, **30**, 347–353.

Sharifuzzaman, S.M., Al-Harbi, A.H. and Austin, B. (2014) Characteristics of growth, digestive system functionality, and stress factors of rainbow trout fed probiotics *Kocuria* SM1 and *Rhodococcus* SM2. *Aquaculture*, **418**/419, 55–61.

Silva, E.F., Soares, M.A., Calazans, N.F., *et al.* (2013) Effect of probiotic (*Bacillus* spp.) addition during larvae and postlarvae culture of the white shrimp *Litopenaeus vannamei*. *Aquaculture Research*, **44**, 13–21.

Skjermo, J., Bakke, I., Dahle, S.W. and Vadstein, O. (2015) Probiotic strains introduced through live feed and rearing water have low colonizing success in developing Atlantic cod larvae. *Aquaculture*, **438**, 17–23.

Smith, P. and Davey, S. (1993) Evidence for the competitive exclusion of *Aeromonas salmonicida* from fish with stress-inducible furunculosis by a fluorescent pseudomonad. *Journal of Fish Diseases*, **16**, 521–524.

Son, V.M., Changa, C.C., Wu, M.C., Guu, Y.K., Chiu, C.H. and Cheng, W. (2009) Dietary administration of the probiotic, *Lactobacillus plantarum*, enhanced the growth, innate immune responses, and disease resistance of the grouper *Epinephelus coioides*. *Fish and Shellfish Immunology*, **26**, 691–698.

Sorroza, L., Padilla, D., Acosta, F., *et al.* (2012) Characterization of the probiotic strain *Vagococcus fluvialis* in the protection of European sea bass (*Dicentrarchus labrax*) against vibriosis by *Vibrio anguillarum*. *Veterinary Microbiology*, **155**, 369–373.

Spanggaard, B., Huber, I., Nielsen, J., *et al.* (2001) The probiotic potential against vibriosis of the indigenous microflora of rainbow trout. *Environmental Microbiology*, **3**, 755–765.

Standen, B.T., Rawling, M.D., Davies, S.J., *et al.* (2013) Probiotic *Pediococcus acidilactici* moderates both localized intestinal- and peripheral-immunity in tilapia (*Oreochromis niloticus*). *Fish and Shellfish Immunology*, **35**, 1097–1104.

Subasinghe, R.P. (2005) Epidemiological approach to aquatic animal health management: opportunities and challenges for developing countries to increase aquatic production through aquaculture. *Preventive Veterinary Medicine*, **67**, 117–124.

Subasinghe, R.P., Curry, D., McGladdery, S.E. and Bartley, D. (2003) *Recent Technological Innovations in Aquaculture, Review of the State of World Aquaculture*, FAO Fisheries Circular, p. 59–74.

Sugita, H., Miyajima, C. and Deguchi, H. (1991) The vitamin B12-producing ability of the intestinal microflora of freshwater fish. *Aquaculture*, **92**, 267–276.

Sugita,H., Takahashi, J. and Deguchi, H. (1992) Production and consumption of biotin by the intestinal microflora of cultured freshwater fishes. *Bioscience, Biotechnology, and Biochemistry*, **56**, 1678–1679.

Sugita, H., Hirose, Y., Matsuo, N. and Deguchi, Y. (1998) Production of the antibacterial substance by *Bacillus* sp. strain NM12, an intestinal bacterium of Japanese coastal fish. *Aquaculture*, **165**, 269–280.

Sun, Y.Z., Yang, H.L., Ma, R.L. and Lin, W.Y. (2010) Probiotic applications of two dominant gut *Bacillus* strains with antagonistic activity improved the growth performance and immune responses of grouper *Epinephelus coioides*. *Fish and Shellfish Immunology*, **29**, 803–809.

Supamattaya, K., Kiriratnikom, S., Boonyaratpalin, M. and Borowitzka, L. (2005) Effect of a *Dunaliella* extract on growth performance, health condition, immune response and disease resistance in black tiger shrimp (*Penaeus monodon*). *Aquaculture*, **248**, 207–216.

Swain, S.M., Singh, C. and Arul, V. (2009) Inhibitory activity of probiotics *Streptococcus phocae* PI80 and *Enterococcus faecium* MC13 against vibriosis in shrimp *Penaeus monodon*. *World Journal of Microbiology and Biotechnology*, **25**, 697–703.

Talpur, A.D., Memon, A.J., Khan, M.I., Ikhwanuddin, M., Daniel, M.M.D. and Abol-Munafi, A.B. (2012) Inhibition of pathogens by lactic acid bacteria and application as water additive multi isolates in early stages larviculture of *P. pelagicus* (Linnaeus, 1758). *Journal of Animal and Plant Sciences*, **22**, 54–64.

Tamminen, M., Karkman, A., Lõhmus, A., *et al.* (2011) Tetracycline resistance genes persist at aquaculture farms in the absence of selection pressure. *Environmental Science and Technology*, **45**, 386–391.

Taoka, Y., Maeda, H., Jo, J., *et al.* (2006a) Growth, stress tolerance and non-specific immune response of Japanese flounder *Paralichthys olivaceus* to probiotics in a closed recirculating system. *Fisheries Science*, **72**, 310–321.

Taoka, Y., Maeda, H., Jo, J.Y., *et al.* (2006b) Use of live and dead probiotic cells in tilapia *Oreochromis niloticus*. *Fisheries Science*, **72**, 755–766.

Timmerman, H.M., Koning, C.J.M., Mulder, L., Rombout, F.M. and Beynen, A.C. (2004) Monospecies, multistrain and multispecies probiotics: a comparison of functionality and efficacy. *International Journal of Food Microbiology*, **96**, 219–233.

Tinh, N.T.N., Dierckens, K., Sorgeloos, P. and Bossier, P. (2008) A review of the functionality of probiotics in the larviculture food chain. *Marine Biotechnology*, **10**, 1–12.

Tovar, D., Zambonino, J., Cahu, C., Gatesoupe, F.J., Vazquez-Juarez, R. and Lesel, R. (2002) Effect of yeast incorporation in compound diet on digestive enzyme activity in sea bass (*Dicentrarchus labrax*) larvae. *Aquaculture*, **204**, 113–123.

Tseng, D.Y., Ho, P.L., Huang, S.Y., *et al.* (2009) Enhancement of immunity and disease resistance in the white shrimp, *Litopenaeus vannamei*, by the probiotic, *Bacillus subtilis* E20. *Fish and Shellfish Immunology*, **26**, 339–344.

Vaseeharan, B. and Ramasamy, P. (2003) Control of pathogenic *Vibrio* spp. by *Bacillus subtilis* BT23, a possible probiotic treatment for black tiger shrimp *Penaeus monodon*. *Letters in Applied Microbiology*, **36**, 83–87.

Vazquez, J.A., Cabo, M.L., Gonzalez, M.P. and Murado, M.A. (2003) Survival of lactic acid bacteria in seawater: a factorial study. *Current Microbiology*, **47**, 508–513.

Vendrell, D., Balcázar, J.L., Ruiz-Zarzuela, I., de Blas, I., Gironés, O. and Múzquiz, J.L. (2006) *Lactococcus garvieae* in fish: a review. *Comparative Immunology, Microbiology and Infectious Diseases*, **29**, 177–198.

Vendrell, D., Balcazar, J.L., de Blas, I., Ruiz-Zarzuela, I., Girones, O. and Muzquiz, J.L. (2008) Protection of rainbow trout (*Oncorhynchus mykiss*) from lactococcosis by probiotic bacteria. *Comparative Immunology, Microbiology and Infectious Diseases*, **31**, 337–345.

Verschuere, L., Rombaut, G., Sorgeloos, P. and Verstraete, W. (2000) Probiotic bacteria as biological control agents in aquaculture. *Microbiology and Molecular Biology Reviews*, **64**, 655–671.

Villamil, L., Tafalla, C., Figueras, A. and Novoa, B. (2002) Evaluation of immunomodulatory effects of lactic acid bacteria in turbot (*Scophthalmus maximus*). *Clinical and Diagnostic Laboratory Immunology*, **9**, 1318–1323.

Vine, N.G., Leukes, W.D. and Kaiser, H. (2004a) *In vitro* growth characteristics of five candidate aquaculture probiotics and two fish pathogens grown in fish intestinal mucus. *FEMS Microbiology Letters*, **231**, 145–152.

Vine, N.G., Leukes, W.D., Kaiser, H., Daya, S., Baxter, J. and Hecht, T. (2004b) Competition for attachment of aquaculture candidate probiotic and pathogenic bacteria on fish intestinal mucus. *Journal of Fish Diseases*, **27**, 319–326.

Vine, N.G., Leukes, W.D. and Kaiser, H. (2006) Probiotics in marine larviculture. *FEMS Microbiology Reviews*, **30**, 404–427.

Wang, Y.B. and Gu, Q. (2010) Effect of probiotics on white shrimp (*Penaeus vannamei*) growth performance, and immune response. *Marine Biology Research*, **6**, 327–332.

Wang, Y.B., Xu, Z.R. and Xia, M.S. (2005) The effectiveness of commercial probiotics in northern white shrimp *Penaeus vannamei* ponds. *Fisheries Science*, **71**, 1036–1041.

Wang, Y.B., Tian, Z.Q., Yao, J.T. and Li, W.F. (2008) Effect of probiotics, *Enteroccus faecium*, on tilapia (*Oreochromis niloticus*) growth performance and immune response. *Aquaculture*, **277**, 203–207.

Weese, J.S. and Martin, H. (2011) Assessment of commercial probiotic bacterial contents and label accuracy. *Canadian Veterinary Journal*, **52**, 43–46.

Westerdahl, A., Olsson, J.C., Kjelleberg, S. and Conway, P.L. (1991) Isolation and characterization of turbot (*scophthamus maximus*)-associated bacteria with inhibitory effects against *Vibrio anguillarum*. *Applied and Environmental Microbiology*, **57**, 2223–2228.

Wongsasak, U., Chaijamrus, S., Kumkhong, S. and Boonanuntanasarn, S. (2015) Effects of dietary supplementation with β-glucan and synbiotics on immune gene expression and immune parameters under ammonia stress in Pacific white shrimp. *Aquaculture*, **436**, 179–187.

Xing, C.F., Hu, H.H., Huang, J.B., *et al.* (2013) Diet supplementation of *Pediococcus pentosaceus* in cobia (*Rachycentron canadum*) enhances growth rate, respiratory burst and resistance against photobacteriosis. *Fish and Shellfish Immunology*, **35**, 1122–1128.

Zhou, X.X., Tian, Z.Q., Wang, Y.B. and Li, W.F. (2010) Effect of treatment with probiotics as water additives on tilapia (*Oreochromis niloticus*) growth performance and immune response. *Fish Physiology and Biochemistry*, **36**, 501–509.

Zokaeifar, H., Balcazar, J.L., Saad, C.R., *et al.* (2012) Effects of *Bacillus subtilis* on the growth performance, digestive enzymes, immune gene expression and disease resistance of white shrimp, *Litopenaeus vannamei*. *Fish and Shellfish Immunology*, **33**, 683–689.

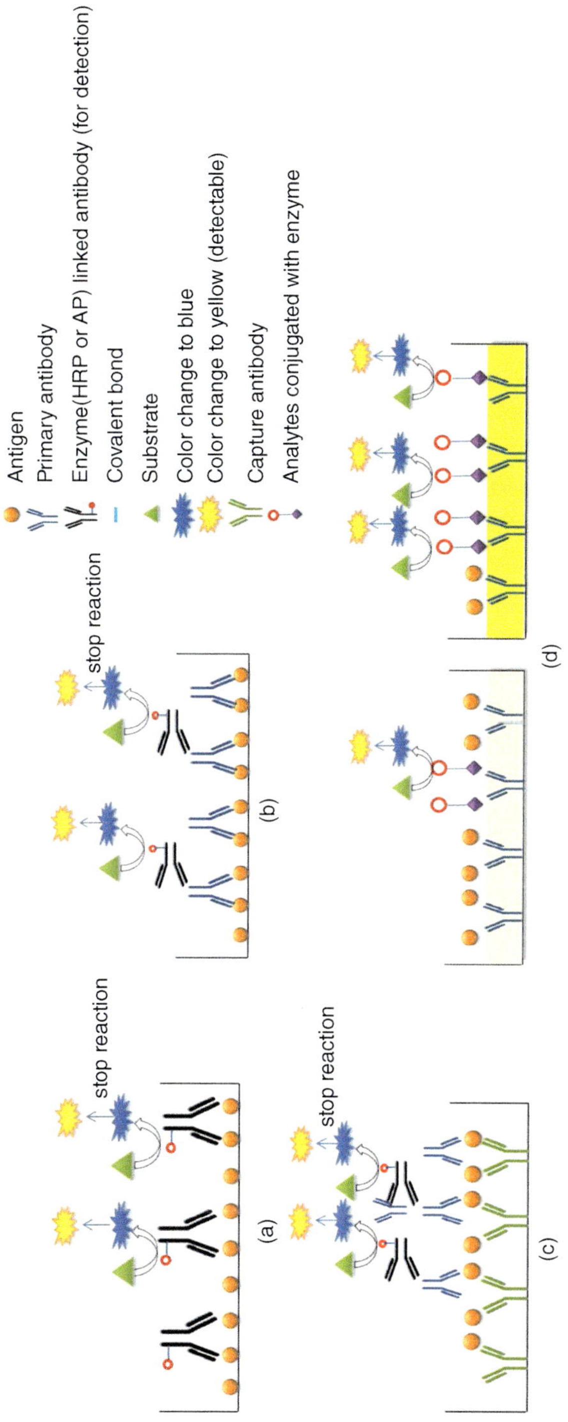

Figure 5.2 ELISAs according to detection method. (a) Direct ELISA; (b) indirect ELISA; (c) sandwich ELISA; (d) competitive ELISA.

Diagnosis and Control of Diseases of Fish and Shellfish, First Edition. Edited by Brian Austin and Aweeda Newaj-Fyzul.

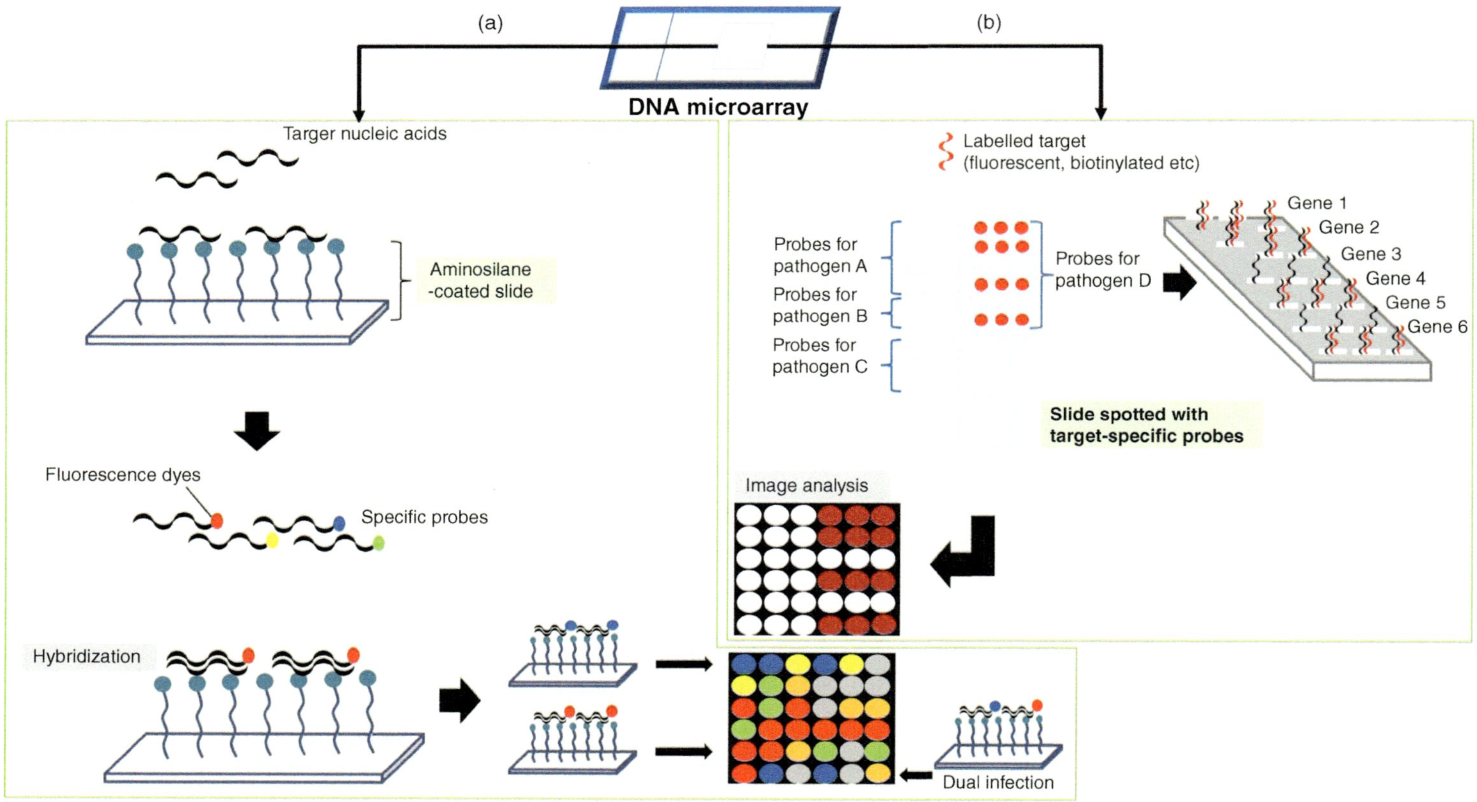

Figure 5.6 Schematic diagram of DNA microarray. (a) Nucleic acids (including cDNA through RT-PCR) extracted from the sample are printed on an aminosilane-coated slide. After UV cross-linking, specific fluorescent probes for targets are hybridized to the DNA microarray. (b) Labelled targets prepared by PCR amplification are hybridized to the microarray consisting of pathogen-specific probes (species or strain specific) immobilized onto a solid surface. This test can also detect the presence of specific virulence genes for a target (e.g. pathogen D).

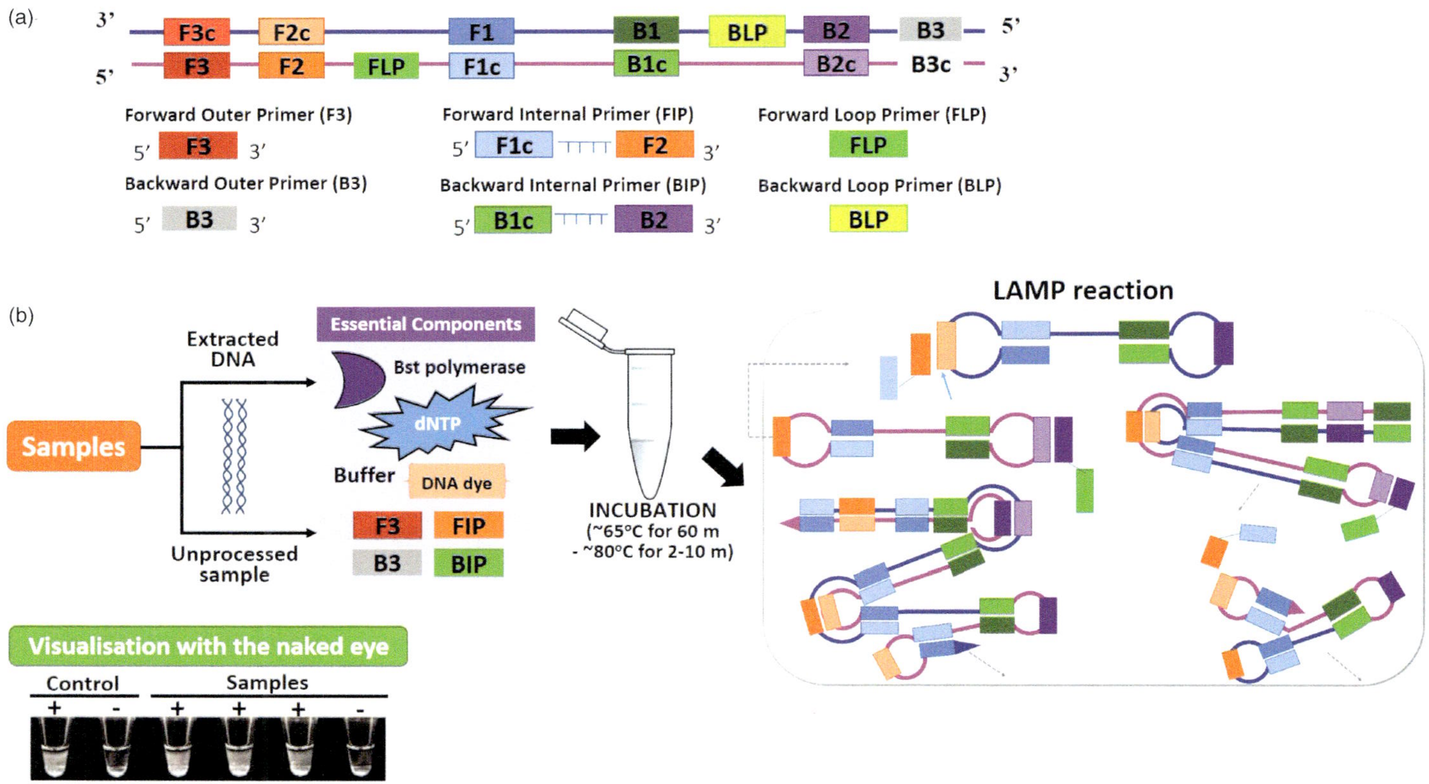

Figure 5.7 Schematic diagram of loop-mediated isothermal amplification (LAMP) diagnostics. (a) Primers used in the LAMP method, showing six primers (two optional: FLP and BLP) hybridizing to eight regions of a target gene. (b) LAMP assay protocol.

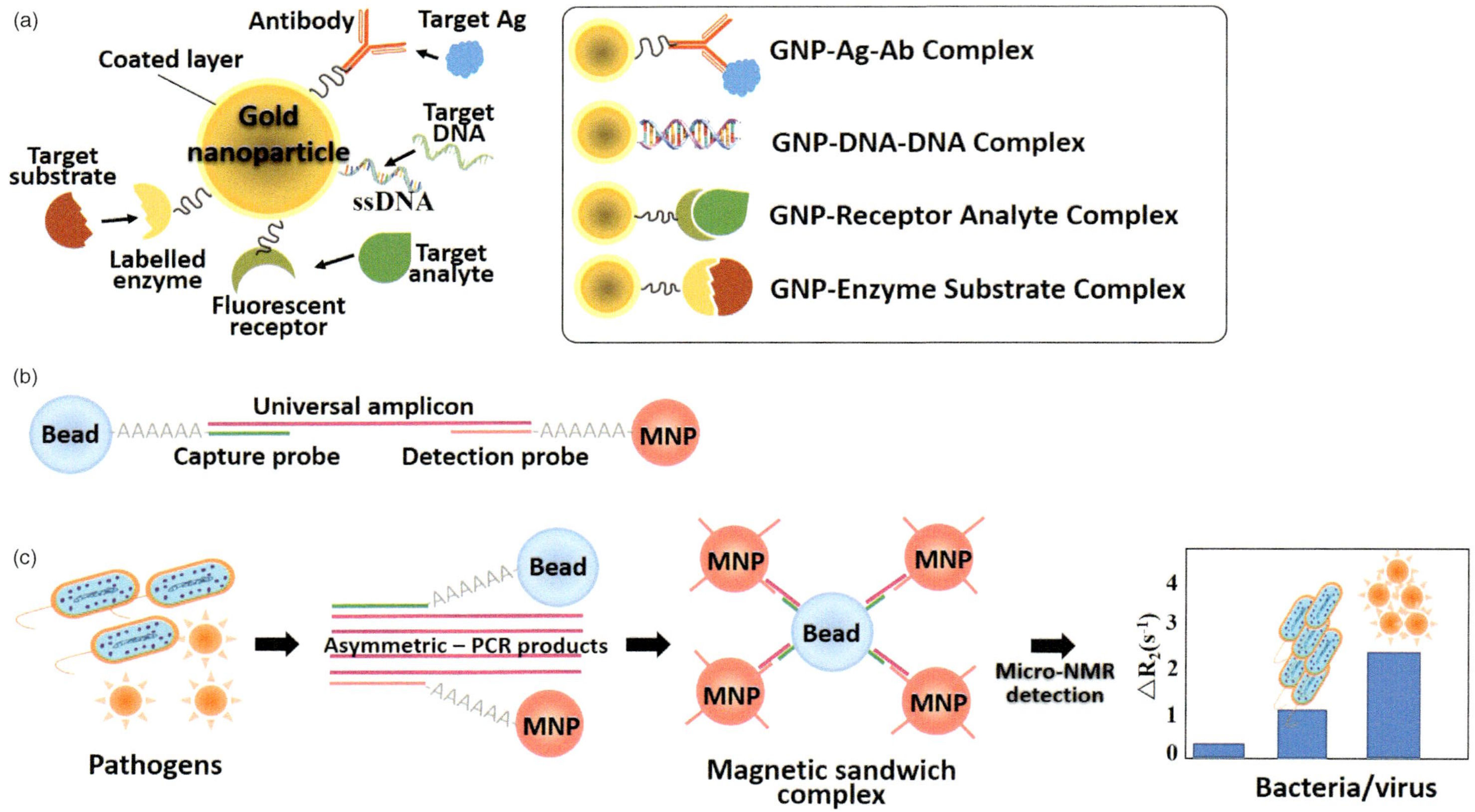

Figure 5.8 Potential detection of pathogens using nanoparticles. (a) Functionalization of gold nanoparticles in biomedical applications. (b) Schematic universal probes targeting a conserved region of bacterial 16S rRNA and conjugated to bead and magnetic nanoparticles (MNPs) at the end of each probe in the magneto-DNA assay. (c) Main steps of the assay procedure including amplification of target 16S rRNA; the binding of target DNA to capture probes conjugated to beads; hybridization of target DNA-capture probe with magnetic nanoparticles (MNPs) to form a magnetic sandwich complex. The results are then analysed by using a micronuclear magnetic resonance (μNMR) system.

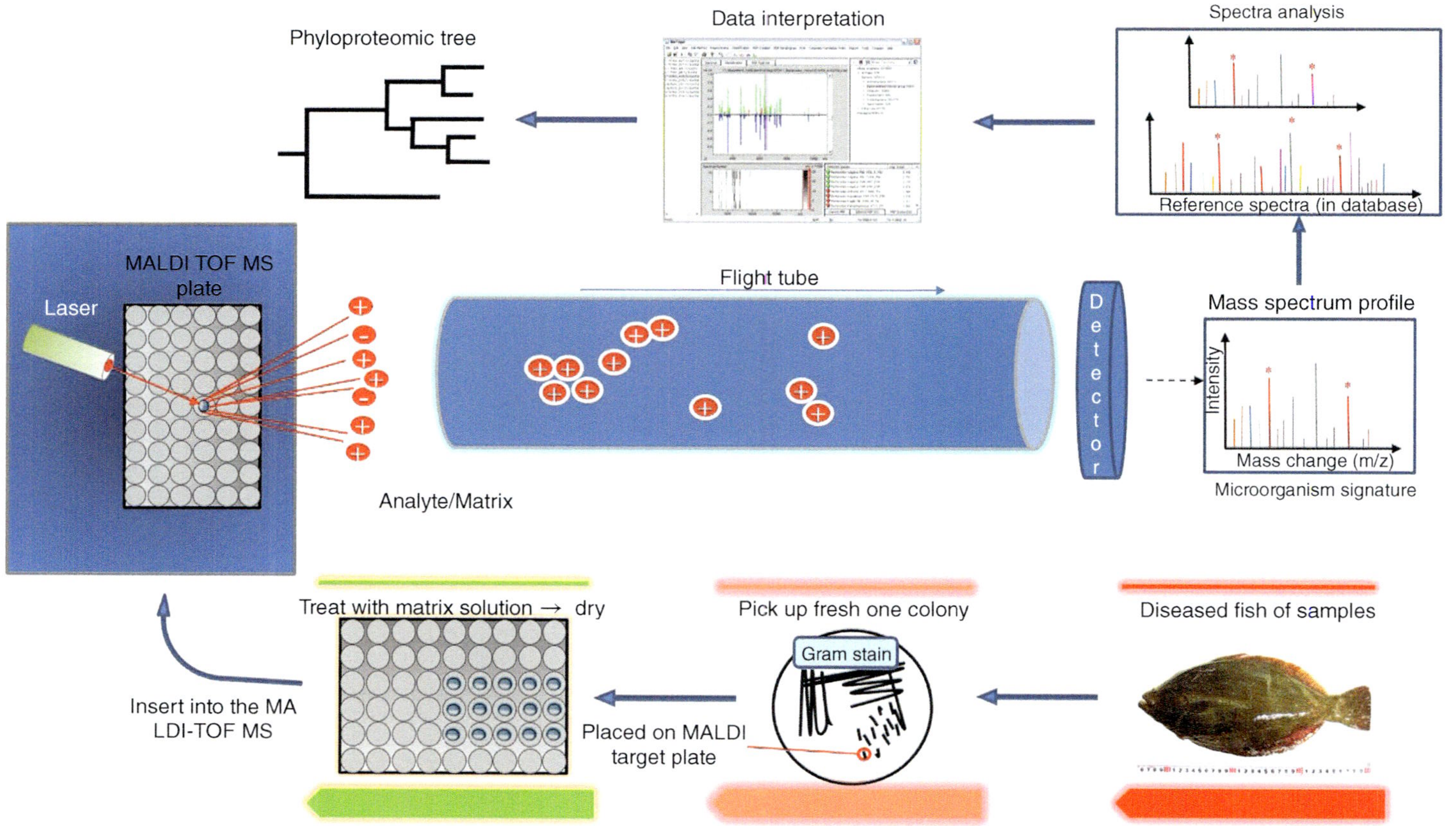

Figure 5.9 Principle of MALDI-TOF MS for bacterial identification. Microbial samples are deposited on a conductive metallic target plate and overlaid with a matrix solution composed of an organic acid. Once placed in the instrument, the samples are ionized by short laser followed by acceleration of variably charged particles through an electric field.

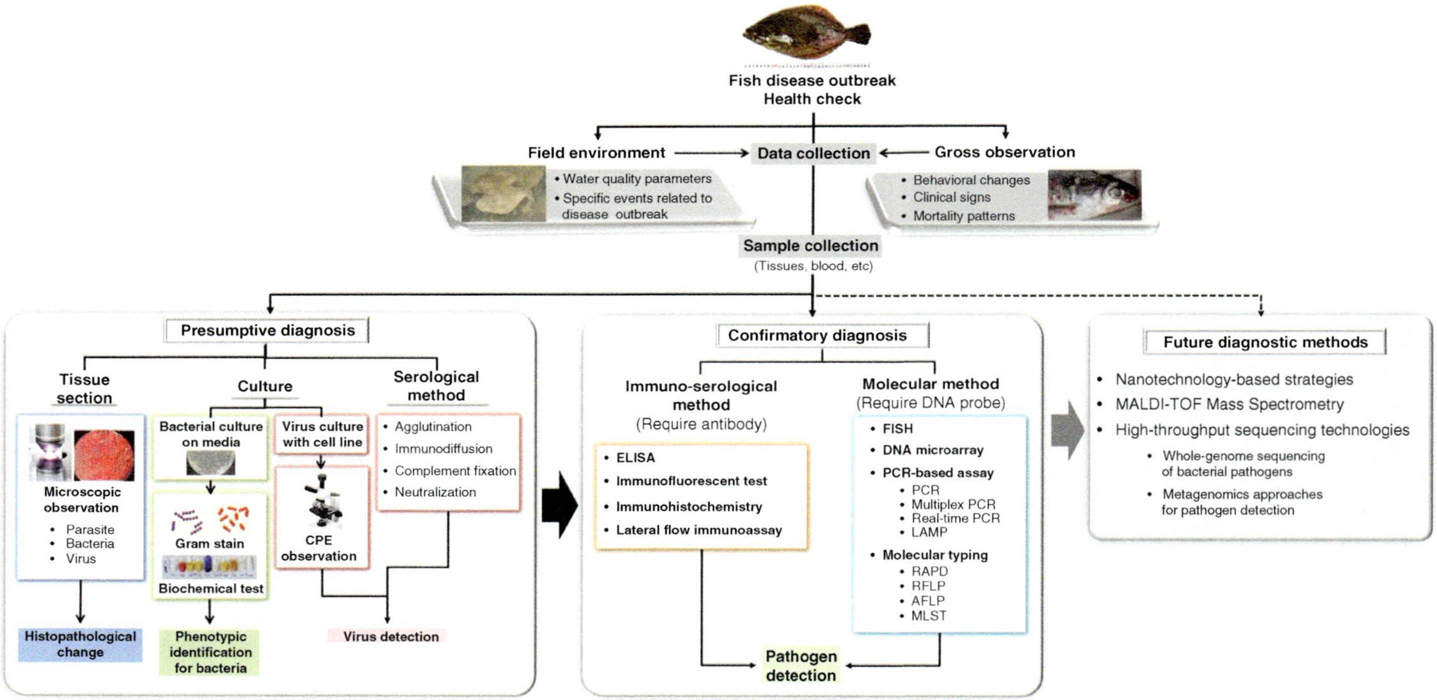

Figure 5.10 Conventional and modern diagnostic methods that can be used in aquatic animal health laboratories.

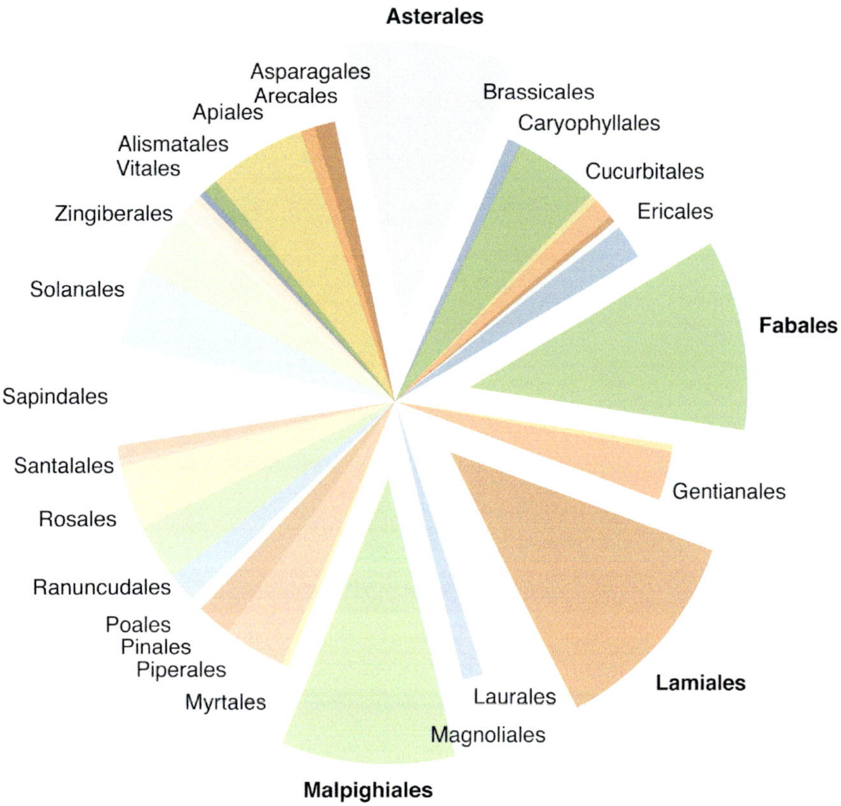

Figure 9.2 Orders of plants used in aquaculture.

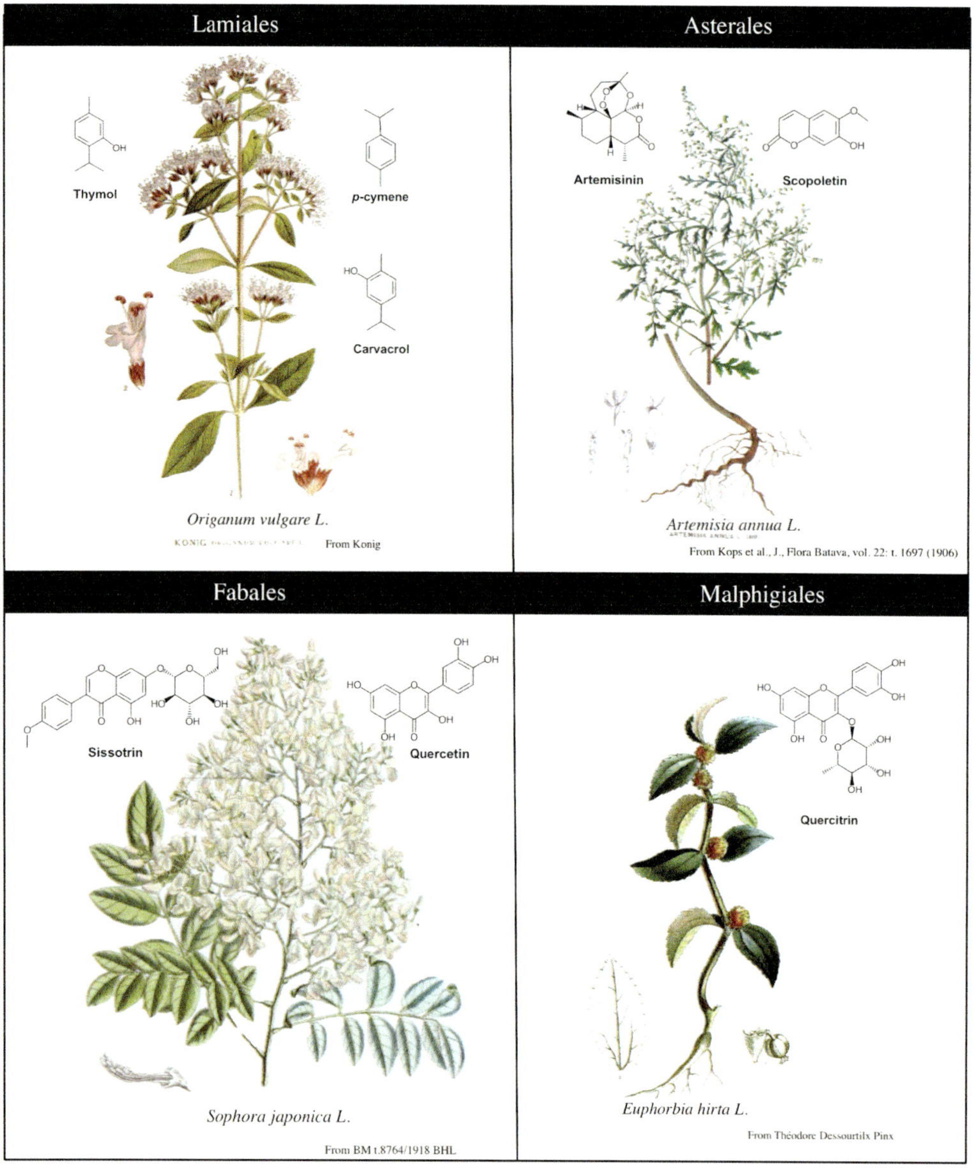

Figure 9.3 Plant examples and isolated molecules from the plant orders most used in aquaculture.

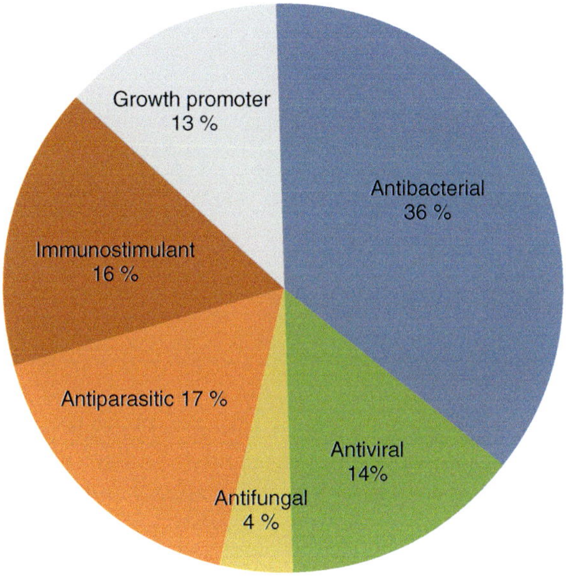

Figure 9.4 Plant bioactivities in aquaculture.

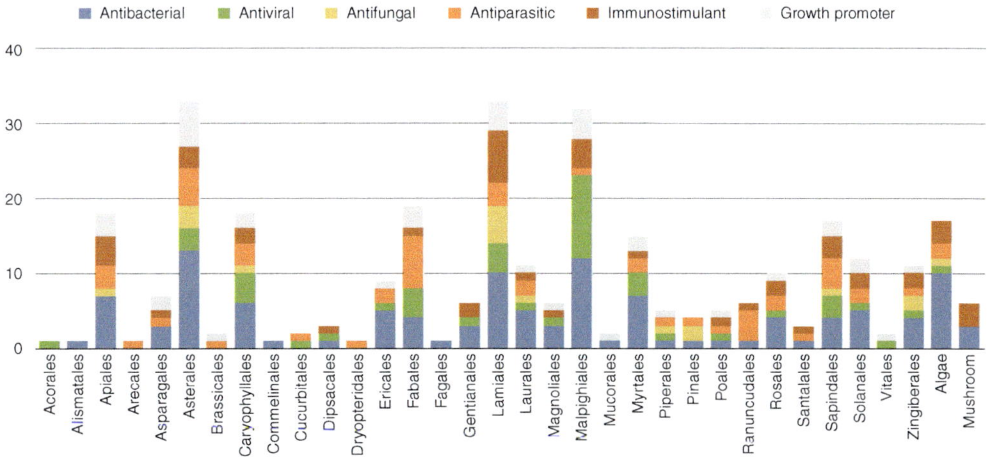

Figure 9.5 Bioactivities of plant orders in aquaculture.

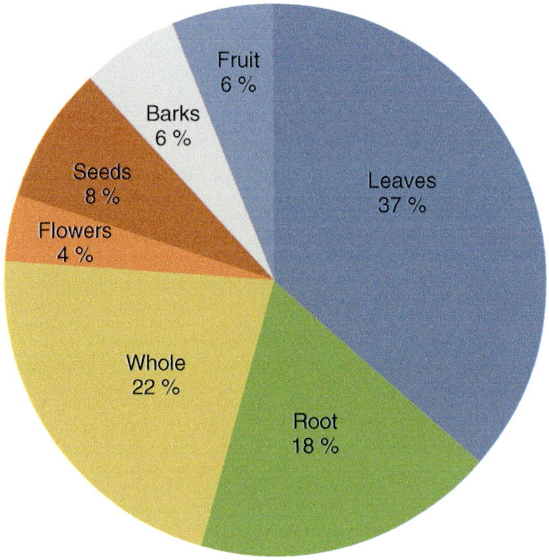

Figure 9.6 Parts of plants used in aquaculture.

9

Use of Medicinal Plants in Aquaculture

Miriam Reverter[1,2], *Nathalie Tapissier-Bontemps*[1,2], *Pierre Sasal*[1,2] *and Denis Saulnier*[2,3]

[1] *CRIOBE, Paris Sciences et Lettres (PSL), University of Perpignan Via Domitia, Perpignan, France*
[2] *Laboratoire d'Excellence "CORAIL", Moorea, French Polynesia*
[3] *Ifremer, Taravao, Tahiti, French Polynesia*

Introduction

For thousands of years, civilizations throughout the world have used medicinal plants to treat a variety of diseases. The oldest written evidence of medicinal plant usage was found on a Sumerian clay slab, approximately 5000 years old (Petrovska, 2012). Nowadays, traditional medicinal plants continue to be the primary source of healthcare in many developing countries and rural regions (Calixto, 2005). Ethnobotanical studies have proved to be very useful in identifying bioactive plants, and numerous research studies have been conducted on the biological activities and chemical composition of ethnomedicinal plants (Ayyanar *et al.*, 2011; Banskota *et al.*, 2003). Interest in medicinal plants for human and veterinary health has been fuelled by the countless side effects and rising costs of prescription drugs (Hoareau and Da-Silva, 1999). Plants also possess a complex chemical composition which displays varied biological activities, making plants suitable for the treatment of multifactorial diseases, and makes plants a suitable alternative to antibiotics with little risk for development of resistance (Gostner *et al.*, 2012; Srivastava *et al.*, 2014).

Aquaculture is the fastest growing animal food-producing sector, with an average annual increase of 6.2% per year in the period 2000–2012 (FAO, 2014). However, aquaculture growth is often linked to culture intensification, leading to overcrowding and poor water quality, facilitating the spread of pathogens and increasing disease outbreaks and mortality (Bondad-Reantaso *et al.*, 2005). In order to avoid economic losses related to sanitary shortcomings, veterinary drugs are commonly used in aquaculture to prevent and treat disease outbreaks (Rico *et al.*, 2013).

The intensive use of synthetic drugs presents numerous disadvantages, for both the environment and health. Intensive use of antibiotics has resulted in accumulation in muscle of commercialized animals (Cabello *et al.*, 2006; Romero-Ormazabal *et al.*, 2012) and the development of resistant bacteria strains (Miranda and Zemelman, 2002; Seyfried *et al.*, 2010). Also, the use of antiparasitic drugs like trichlorfon or praziquantel in bath treatments is hazardous for animals and the environment and can also result in the development of resistance (Forwood *et al.*, 2013; Umeda *et al.*, 2006). Vaccines, considered to be the most effective method to prevent disease outbreaks in aquaculture, are too expensive for widespread use

Diagnosis and Control of Diseases of Fish and Shellfish, First Edition. Edited by Brian Austin and Aweeda Newaj-Fyzul.

by fish producers and since it is extremely difficult to develop multiple strain vaccines, most vaccines are only effective against one type of pathogen (Pasnik *et al.*, 2005; Sakai, 1999).

Considering the numerous disadvantages of synthetic drugs, there is an increasing need for the development of alternative strategies in aquaculture disease management. Moreover, disease outbreaks in aquaculture are often associated with animal fitness and health, most pathogens being opportunistic and taking advantage of immunocompromised or stressed fish. Thus, alternative solutions should maximize fish immunity and fitness as a strategy to face pathogen infections (Ashley *et al.*, 2007; Davis *et al.*, 2002; Iguchi *et al.*, 2003). Medicinal plants can therefore provide a cheaper and more sustainable alternative to chemotherapy in aquaculture, since they have been reported to display numerous bioactivity such as antistress, immunostimulant and antiparasitic (bacterial, fungus, virus and ectoparasites) effects (Reverter *et al.*, 2014).

Medicinal Plants in Aquaculture

Although interest in the use of medicinal plants and plant extracts in aquaculture has exploded recently, medicinal plants have long been used by rural fish farmers. Caruso *et al.* (2013) found that 46% of the fish farmers surveyed in West Java (Indonesia) used plants in their farms, most of which were also traditionally used in the human pharmacopoeia. In most cases, fresh plants were directly introduced into the rearing water and used to improve water quality, reduce fish stress, increase fish resistance to pathogens and treat fish diseases. This study showed that fish farmers used plants and doses depending on their personal experience and ethnic origin.

Numerous scientific studies endorse the use of medicinal plants in aquaculture (Bhuvansewari and Balasundaram, 2006; Harikrishnan *et al.*, 2011a). Plants have been reported to produce various effects such as antistress, growth promotion, appetite stimulation, immunostimulation, aphrodisiac and to have antipathogen properties in fish and shrimp aquaculture due to their varied active principles such as alkaloids, terpenoids, tannins, saponins and flavonoids (Chakraborty and Hancz, 2011; Citarasu, 2010).

Biological Activity of Medicinal Plants in Aquaculture

Several plant extracts are reported to stimulate appetite and promote weight gain when administered to cultured fish (Pavaraj *et al.*, 2011; Takaoka *et al.*, 2011). For example, grouper (*Epinephelus tauvina*) fed with a supplemented diet of a mixture of methanolic herb extracts (*Cynodon dactylon, Piper longum, Phyllanthus niruri, Tridax procumbens* and *Zingiber officinalis*) displayed 41% higher weight than control fish (Punitha *et al.*, 2008). Other studies have reported that administration of plant extracts improves digestibility and availability of nutrients, resulting in an increase in feed conversion and leading to higher protein synthesis (Putra *et al.*, 2013; Talpur *et al.*, 2013).

Numerous studies have shown that fish treated with medicinal plants presented enhanced immune parameters (Dügenci *et al.*, 2003; Yuan *et al.*, 2007). For example, Nile tilapia (*Oreochromis niloticus*) fed with a diet containing mistletoe (*Viscum album coloratum*) for a period of 80 days displayed higher lysozyme, respiratory burst, alternative complement and phagocytic activity, which resulted in 42% increased survivability when they were challenged with the bacterial pathogen *Aeromonas hydrophila* (Park and Choi, 2012). Studies on fish haematological parameters have shown that fish treated with plants displayed higher levels of erythrocytes, lymphocytes, monocytes and haemoglobin than control fish, indicating better fish fitness (Haghighi and Rohani, 2013; Harikrishnan *et al.*, 2012a).

In vitro and *in vivo* studies have shown the potential of medicinal plants against a wide range of marine pathogens (bacteria, virus, fungus and ectoparasites) (Chitmanat *et al.*, 2005; Direkbusarakom *et al.*, 1996; Ji *et al.*, 2012). Antibacterial properties of medicinal plants are by far the best studied biological activities, with abundant *in vitro* studies reporting antibacterial activity in numerous plants against both Gram-positive and Gram-negative marine bacteria (Castro *et al.*, 2008; Roomiani *et al.*, 2013). *In vivo* studies in Indian major carp (*Labeo rohita*) fed with diets enriched with prickly chaff flower (*Achyrantes aspera*, 0,2%) and Indian ginseng (*Withania somnifera*, 0,5%) showed a reduction in mortality of 41% and 49% respectively when fish were challenged with *A. hydrophila* (Sharma *et al.*, 2010; Vasudeva-Rao *et al.*, 2006).

Antiviral and antifungal activities of medicinal plants are also able to prevent high mortality rates in aquaculture. Balasubramanian *et al.* (2008a,2008b) showed that black tiger shrimp (*Penaeus monodon*) challenged with white spot syndrome virus (WSSV) while being treated with Bermuda grass (*Cynodon dactylon*) displayed no mortality and no signs of disease compared to 100% mortality observed in control groups. Several studies have shown *in vitro* antifungal activities of several plants like conidinium fruit (*Cnidium monnieri*), magnolia bark (*Magnolia officinalis*), aucklandia root (*Aucklandia lappa*) and common rue (*Ruta graveolens*) (Hashemi *et al.*, 2012; Xue-Gang *et al.*, 2013).

Medicinal plants also seem to be an effective alternative for treating ectoparasites. Several studies have shown antiparasitic activities of medicinal plants when added to water or administered orally (Fu *et al.*, 2014; Huang *et al.*, 2013; Yi *et al.*, 2012). Methanol extract of bupleurum root (*Radix bupleuri chinensis*), aqueous and methanol extracts of cinnamon (*Cinnamomum cassia*), methanol extract of Chinese spice bush (*Lindera aggregata*) and methanol and ethyl acetate extracts of golden larch (*Pseudolarix kaempferi*) had 100% *in vivo* efficacy against monogenean *Dactylogyrus intermedium* in infected goldfish (*Carassius auratus*) (Ji *et al.*, 2012; Wu *et al.*, 2011). Harikrishnan *et al.* (2012c) showed 40% mortality decrease and enhanced immunity in olive flounder (*Paralichthys olivaceus*) infected by the protozoan ciliate *Miamiensis avidus* when fish were fed with a diet supplemented with *Suaeda maxima*.

Application of Medicinal Plants in Aquaculture

Plants can be administered as a whole plant or parts (leaf, root, seed, fruit) and can either be used fresh or as prepared herbal extracts with different solvents (water, methanol, chloroform, ethyl acetate) (van Hai, 2015). Biological activity and chemical composition of plants and extracts can vary greatly depending on the part used and type of extract, and thus knowledge of the plant's bioactive compounds is required. In addition, seasonal variations in production of bioactive metabolites has also been observed in different plants and algae, so study of the plant's production of bioactive molecules is desirable (Chaves *et al.*, 2013; Manilal *et al.*, 2009).

To date, most scientific studies on the use of medicinal plants in aquaculture have focused on identification of biological activity rather than natural product determination (Balasubramanian *et al.*, 2007; Cox *et al.*, 2010; Ji *et al.*, 2012). Exploratory studies on the potential of medicinal plants in aquaculture can therefore be misleading if the wrong part or wrong solvent is used. Also, suitable dosing is crucial to obtain the desired effects, since inappropriate doses can display toxic effects in fish (Ekanem *et al.*, 2007; Kavitha *et al.*, 2012; Sambasivam *et al.*, 2003). For example, grouper (*Epinephelus coioides*) fed with a diet supplemented with 1% ethanol katuk extract (*Sauropus androgynous*) showed enhanced growth and improved food utilization, whereas at 2.5% and 5% of katuk extract they presented lower growth levels (Putra *et al.*, 2013). Treatment length is another important parameter in medicinal plant application in aquaculture, since it directly influences treatment effectiveness. For example, Militz *et al.* (2013) showed that farmed barramundii (*Lates calcarifer*) fed with an enriched diet of garlic (*Allium sativum*) for 30 days displayed 70% decreased *Neobenedenia* sp. infection success compared to control and short-term treatment (10 days).

Medicinal plants can be administered to fish and shellfish by injection (intramuscular and intraperitoneal), oral administration and through immersion or baths (Ji *et al.*, 2012; Putra *et al.*, 2013; Wu *et al.*, 2010). Although intraperitoneal injection has proved to be the most rapid and efficient method of administration, it is expensive, laborious and stressful for fish, especially for very young specimens (Anderson, 1992; Yoshida *et al.*, 1995). Baths are extensively used for the treatment of ectoparasites (Forwood *et al.*, 2013; Whittington, 2012) but this method is also expensive and laborious and involves the release of exogenous molecules in the marine environment, and thus can present some undesired environmental side effects (Umeda *et al.*, 2006). Hence, oral administration seems to be the most suitable for aquaculture, since medicinal plants can induce physiological changes in fish to improve their fitness and reinforce their resistance to pathogens.

Finally, determining natural plant products helps to better understand their mode of action. For example, chelerythrine and chelidonine are two benzo[c]phenanthridines with antimicrobial, antifungal and anti-inflammatory activities isolated from greater celandine (*Chelidonium majus* L.) (Malikova *et al.*, 2006; Waltérova *et al.*, 1995). Several studies have shown that chelerythrine exhibits high cytotoxic potency against a large number of cells, through multiple apoptosis-inducing pathways, indicating that a direct action on mitochondria may be involved in the eradication of parasites (Kaminskyy *et al.*, 2008; Kemény-Beke *et al.*, 2006; Slaninová *et al.*, 2001). Other studies have shown that the mechanism of action of chelidonine against the monogenean ectoparasite *Dactylogyrus intermedium* may be through the mitochondrial cell death pathway activated via caspase-9 (Philchenkov *et al.*, 2008). Therefore, it is of high importance to identify the bioactive molecules for the observed bioactivities and standardize extraction procedures depending on the molecules identified, application procedures and doses, duration of treatments and type of pathogen (Reverter *et al.*, 2014).

It is important to state that modes of action and toxicity of many plants are still poorly understood, so more research is needed before they can be safely used in aquaculture. Many of the plant bioactive molecules can also be toxic or antinutritional in fish, decreasing efficient utilization of feed nutrients or causing intestinal dysfunction, so their effect on fish physiology and adequate dosing needs to be studied (Krogdahl *et al.*, 2010). In order to fill in the gaps in current knowledge, a structured research plan should be followed, focused on, first, bioactivity, compounds and modes of actions of the plants, and second on the plant effect on the organism's physiology and its appropriate use. In Figure 9.1, we propose some directions for research on medicinal plant utilization in aquaculture. *In vitro* tests should be performed in order to determine plant bioactivity, together with bioassay-guided fractionation to identify and characterize the bioactive natural products. *In vitro* tests should also be carried out to test the cytotoxicity of plant extracts on fish cells. Then *in vivo* tests on model species should be performed, first to understand the plant effects on animal physiology and determine the best conditions for plant application (mode of application, plant part and preparation, dose and length of treatment), and second, to estimate plant efficiency in organism survival against different pathogenic infections. Haematology indicators such as haematocrit, haemoglobin,

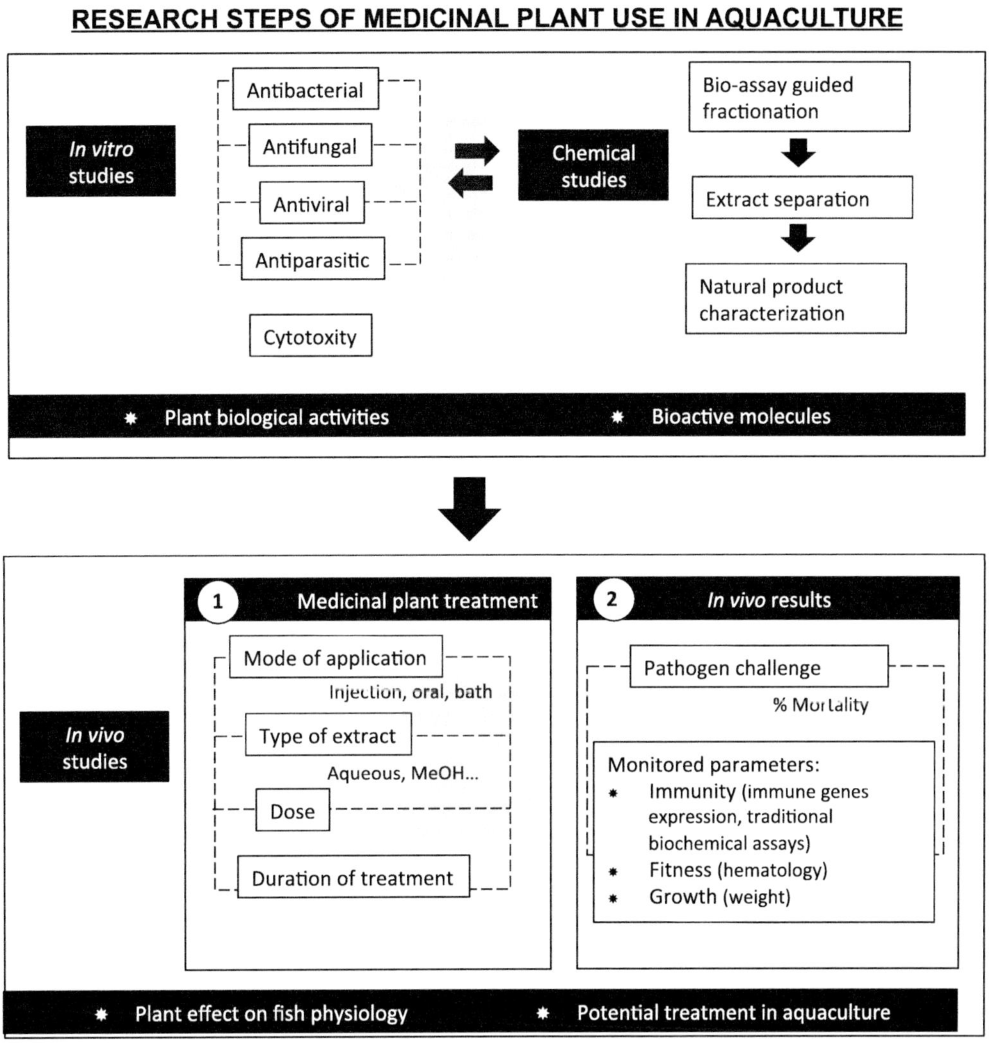

Figure 9.1 Research steps for medicinal plant utilization in aquaculture.

erythrocyte and lymphocyte levels can be used to determine fish fitness (Haghighi and Rohani, 2013; Kanani *et al.*, 2014).

Fish immunity is often analysed to determine the immunomodulatory power of plants and this can be studied via classic biochemical approaches (lysozyme, phagocytic or respiratory burst activity) or by the study of immune gene expression (e.g. Lys, TNF-alpha, IL-1, IL-10 genes) (Chakrabarti *et al.*, 2014; Harikrishnan *et al.*, 2011a; Kumar *et al.*, 2013).

Analysis of Plants Used in Aquaculture

An extensive literature review was performed on the published studies on plant use in aquaculture in order to identify the most common studied plants and their activities (Table 9.1).

Table 9.1 Plants, algae and mushrooms used or studied for potential application in aquaculture.

Order	Family	Species	Activities	Part used	Reference
Acorales	Acoraceae	*Acorus calamus*	AV	R	Sivasankar *et al.*, 2015
Alismatales	Araceae	*Alocasia macrorrhizos*	NA	L	Caruso *et al.*, 2013
Alismatales	Araceae	*Colocasia esculenta*	AB	R	Wei *et al.*, 2010
Apiales	Apiaceae	*Angelica membranaceus*	IM	R	Jian and Wu, 2004
Apiales	Apiaceae	*Angelica sinensis*	IM	R	Wang *et al.*, 2011
Apiales	Apiaceae	*Angelica pubsecens*	AF	R	Xue-Gang *et al.*, 2013
Apiales	Apiaceae	*Bupleurum chinense*	AP	W	Wu *et al.*, 2011
Apiales	Apiaceae	*Centella asiatica*	AB	R	Rattanachaikunsopon and Phumkhachorn, 2010
Apiales	Apiaceae	*Cnidium officinale*	AB,GP	L, Fr	Takaoka *et al.*, 2007b
Apiales	Apiaceae	*Corandrium sativum*	AB	NA	Innocent *et al.*, 2011
Apiales	Apiaceae	*Heracleum lasiopetalum*	AB	R	Pirbalouti *et al.*, 2011
Apiales	Apiaceae	*Radix peucedani*	AP	W	Wu *et al.*, 2011
Apiales	Araliaceae	*Kalopanax pictus*	AP, IM	S	Harikrishnan *et al.*, 2011e
Apiales	Araliaceae	*Panax ginseng*	IM	R	Gooda, 2008
Apiales	Araliaceae	*Eleutherococcus senticosus*	AB, IM	R	Won *et al.*, 2008
Apiales	Araliaceae	*Panax quinquefolium*	GP	W	Abdel-Tawwab, 2012
Apiales	Umberlliferae	*Carum carvi*	GP	L	Abdel-Tawwab, 2011
Arecales	Arecaceae	*Area catechu*	AP	L	Caruso *et al.*, 2013
Arecales	Arecaceae	*Phoenix dactylifera*	NA	L	Hoseinfar, 2015
Asparagales	Amaryllidaceae	*Allium sativum*	AB, AP, IM, GP	W	Aly *et al.*, 2008; Nya and Austin, 2009; Militz *et al.*, 2013; Sahu *et al.*, 2007
Asparagales	Amaryllidaceae	*Allium tuberosum*	AB, GP	L	Rattanachaikunsopon and Phumkhachorn, 2009a
Asparagales	Xanthorrhoeacea	*Aloe vera*	AB	W	Alishani *et al.*, 2010 ; Kim *et al.*, 1999
Asterales	Asteraceae	*Ageratum conzyoides*	NA	L	Caruso *et al.*, 2013
Asterales	Asteraceae	*Artemisia annua*	AP	L	Martins *et al.*, 2002
Asterales	Asteraceae	*Artemisia argyi*	AB, AF, AP	NA	Ekanem and Brisibe (2010)
Asterales	Asteraceae	*Artemisia capillaries*	AB, GP	W	Ji *et al.*, 2007b

Table 9.1 (Continued)

Order	Family	Species	Activities	Part used	Reference
Asterales	Asteraceae	*Artemisia cina*	AB, GP	W	Abdelhadi *et al.*, 2010
Asterales	Asteraceae	*Artemisia vulgaris*	AB, AV, AP	NA	El-Deen and Mohamed, 2009
Asterales	Asteraceae	*Aucklandia lappa*	AV	NA	Xue-Gang *et al.*, 2013
Asterales	Asteraceae	*Austroeupatorium inulifolium*	NA	NA	Caruso *et al.*, 2013
Asterales	Asteraceae	*Chamaemelum nobile*	AB	NA	Syahidah *et al.*, 2015
Asterales	Asteraceae	*Chrysanthemum cinerariaefolium*	AP, IM, GP	NA	Harikrishnan *et al.*, 2010d
Asterales	Asteraceae	*Cosmos caudatus*	AB	NA	Caruso *et al.*, 2013, Syahidah *et al.*, 2015
Asterales	Asteraceae	*Echinacea purpura*	AB, AP	L, F	Aly and Mohamed, 2010; Caruana *et al.*, 2012
Asterales	Asteraceae	*Eclipta alba*	AB, GP	L,S	Christybapita *et al.*, 2007
Asterales	Asteraceae	*Erechtites valerianifolia*	NA	NA	Caruso *et al.*, 2013
Asterales	Asteraceae	*Eupatorium fortunei*	AP	S	Huang *et al.*, 2013
Asterales	Asteraceae	*Gynura procumbens*	NA	NA	Caruso *et al.*, 2013
Asterales	Asteraceae	*Lactuca indica*	AB, IM	NA	Harikrishnan *et al.*, 2011c
Asterales	Asteraceae	*Matricaria chamomilla*	AB, GP	NA	Abdelhadi *et al.*, 2010
Asterales	Asteraceae	*Mikania scandens*	NA	NA	Caruso *et al.*, 2013
Asterales	Asteraceae	*Siegesbeckia glabrescens*	AB, IM	W	Harikrishnan *et al.*, 2012b
Asterales	Asteraceae	*Spagneticola calendulacea*	AB	NA	Direkbysarakom *et al.*, 2004
Asterales	Asteraceae	*Tagetes erecta*	AB, AV	L	Caruso *et al.*, 2013
Asterales	Asteraceae	*Tithonia diversifolia*	NA	NA	Caruso *et al.*, 2013
Asterales	Asteraceae	*Tridax procumbens*	AV, GP	W	Sivasankar *et al.*, 2015
Asterales	Asteraceae	*Vernonia amygdaluna*	AF	NA	Syahidah *et al.*, 2015
Brassicales	Caricaceae	*Carica papaya*	AP, GP	NA	Ekanem *et al.*, 2004
Brassicales	Moringaceae	*Moringa oleifera*	NA	W	Caruso *et al.*, 2013

(*Continued*)

Table 9.1 (Continued)

Order	Family	Species	Activities	Part used	Reference
Caryophyllales	Amaranthaceae	*Acyranthes aspera*	AB, IM	NA	Vasudeva-Rao *et al.*, 2006
Caryophyllales	Amaranthaceae	*Alteranthera sessilis*	GP	L, S, Fr	Radhakrishnan *et al.*, 2014
Caryophyllales	Amaranthaceae	*Kochia scoparia*	AP	NA	Lu *et al.*, 2012
Caryophyllales	Amaranthaceae	*Suaeda maritima*	AP, IM	NA	Harikrishnan *et al.*, 2011c
Caryophyllales	Cactaceae	*Opuntia stricta*	NA	L, F	Khem, 2015
Caryophyllales	Caryophyllaceae	*Stellaria aquatica*	AB, AV	NA	Shangliang *et al.*, 1990 (siva)
Caryophyllales	Molluginaceae	*Glinus oppositifolius*	AV	Fr	Sivasankar *et al.*, 2015
Caryophyllales	Plumbaginaceae	*Aegialitis rotundifolia*	AB	L, W	Choudhury *et al.*, 2005
Caryophyllales	Polygonaceae	*Polyonum hydropipper*	AB, AV, AF	B	Direkbysarakom *et al.*, 2004
Caryophyllales	Polygonaceae	*Rheum officinale*	AB, AV, GP	NA	Xie *et al.*, 2008
Caryophyllales	Polygonaceae	*Rumex obtusifolius*	AP	L	Caruana *et al.*, 2012
Caryophyllales	Portulacaceae	*Portulaca oleracea*	AB	F	Direkbysarakom *et al.*, 2004
Commelinales	Pontederiaceae	*Eichhornia crassipes*	AB	NA	Caruso *et al.*, 2013; Chang *et al.*, 2013
Cucurbitales	Cucurbitaceae	*Cucurbita pepo*	NA	W	Caruso *et al.*, 2013
Cucurbitales	Cucurbitaceae	*Mormodica charantia*	AV	R	Balasubramanian *et al.*, 2007
Cucurbitales	Cucurbitaceae	*Mormodica cochinchinensis*	AP	L	Wu *et al.*, 2011
Cyatheales	Cyatheaceae	*Cyathea kanehirae*	AB, IM	L	Yeh and Chen, 2009
Dipsacales	Caprifoliaceae	*Lonicera japonica*	AB, AV, IM	L	Ardò *et al.*, 2008 ; Direkbysarakom *et al.*, 2006
Dryopteridales	Dryopteridaceae	*Dryopteris crassirizhoma*	AP	NA	Lu *et al.*, 2012
Ericales	Primulaceae	*Aegiceras corniculatum*	AB	NA	Choudhury *et al.*, 2005
Ericales	Theaceae	*Camellia sinensis*	AB, AP, GP	NA	Sheikhzadeh *et al.*, 2011
Ericales	Lecythidaceae	*Cariniana legalis*	AB	NA	Castro *et al.*, 2008

Table 9.1 (Continued)

Order	Family	Species	Activities	Part used	Reference
Ericales	Balsaminaceae	*Impatiens biflora*	AB, AV	NA	Direkbysarakom *et al.*, 2004
Ericales	Primulaceae	*Lysimachia christinae*	AP	NA	Huang *et al.*, 2013
Ericales	Styracoceae	*Styrax japonica*	AB	S	Harikrishnan *et al.*, 2011g
Fabales	Fabaceae	*Albizia saman*	NA	NA	Caruso *et al.*, 2013
Fabales	Fabaceae	*Astragalus membranaceus*	AB, IM	L	Pan *et al.*, 2013
Fabales	Fabaceae	*Caesalpinia sappan*	AP	NA	Huang *et al.*, 2013
Fabales	Fabaceae	*Cassia alata*	AV	NA	Sivasankar *et al.*, 2015
Fabales	Fabaceae	*Cassia fistula*	AV	NA	Sivasankar *et al.*, 2015
Fabales	Fabaceae	*Cynometra iripa*	AB	NA	Choudhury *et al.*, 2005
Fabales	Fabaceae	*Falcataria moluccana*	NA	NA	Caruso *et al.*, 2013
Fabales	Fabaceae	*Gliricidia sepium*	NA	NA	Caruso *et al.*, 2014
Fabales	Fabaceae	*Glycine max*	NA	R	Caruso *et al.*, 2015
Fabales	Fabaceae	*Koompassia malaccensis*	NA	NA	Caruso *et al.*, 2016
Fabales	Fabaceae	*Leucaena leucocephala*	NA	L, R	Caruso *et al.*, 2017
Fabales	Fabaceae	*Leucaena glauca*	AP	W	Caruso *et al.*, 2013; Direkbysarakom *et al.*, 2004
Fabales	Fabaceae	*Lupinus perennis*	NA	NA	Awad and Austin, 2010
Fabales	Fabaceae	*Mimosa pudica*	AV	NA	Sivasankar *et al.*, 2015
Fabales	Fabaceae	*Mucuna pruriens*	AP	W	Ekanem *et al.*, 2004
Fabales	Fabaceae	*Parkia speciosa*	NA	L	Caruso *et al.*, 2013
Fabales	Fabaceae	*Psoralea corylifolia*	AP, GP	L	Ling *et al.*, 2003
Fabales	Fabaceae	*Senna alata*	AB, AV	NA	Caruso *et al.*, 2013
Fabales	Fabaceae	*Senna siamea*	NA	NA	Caruso *et al.*, 2013
Fabales	Fabaceae	*Sesbania grandiflora*	NA	NA	Caruso *et al.*, 2013
Fabales	Fabaceae	*Sophora alopercuroides*	AB, AP	NA	Yi *et al.*, 2012
Fabales	Fabaceae	*Sophora flavescens*	AB, AP	NA	Caruana *et al.*, 2012; Wu *et al.*, 2013
Fabales	Fabaceae	*Tamarindus indica*	NA	L, R	Caruso *et al.*, 2013
Fabales	Fabaceae	*Tephrosia purpurea*	NA	NA	Sivasankar *et al.*, 2015
Fabales	Fabaceae	*Trifolium pratense*	GP	S	Syahidah *et al.*, 2015

(Continued)

Table 9.1 (Continued)

Order	Family	Species	Activities	Part used	Reference
Fabales	Polygalaceae	*Polygala tenuifolia*	AP	NA	Lu *et al.*, 2012
Fabales	Quillajaceae	*Quillaja saponaria*	GP	NA	Francis *et al.*, 2005
Fagales	Betulaceae	*Alnus firma*	AB	NA	Harikrishnan *et al.*, 2011i
Gentianales	Apocynaceae	*Anathoda vasica*	AB, IM	L	Minomol, 2005
Gentianales	Apocynaceae	*Calotropis gigantea*	AB, IM	L	Olusola *et al.*, 2013
Gentianales	Apocynaceae	*Catharanthus roseus*	AV	L	Sivasankar *et al.*, 2015
Gentianales	Apocynaceae	*Daemia extensa*	AB	L	Jinish, 2002
Gentianales	Apocynaceae	*Plumeria rubra*	NA	NA	Caruso *et al.*, 2013
Gentianales	Rubiaceae	*Coffea arabica*	NA	NA	Abdel, 2015
Gentianales	Rubiaceae	*Morinda citrifolia*	NA	NA	Caruso *et al.*, 2013
Lamiales	Acanthaceae	*Andrographis paniculata*	AB, GP	NA	Caruso *et al.*, 2009; Rattanachaikunsopon and Phumkhachorn, 2009
Lamiales	Acanthaceae	*Clinacanthus nutans*	AV	W	Direkbysarakom *et al.*, 1998
Lamiales	Acanthaceae	*Hygrophila spinosa*	AB, IM	L	Raja *et al.*, 2012
Lamiales	Lamiaceae	*Leucas lavandulifolia*	NA	NA	Caruso *et al.*, 2013
Lamiales	Lamiaceae	*Mentha piperita*	NA	W	Abasali and Mohamad, 2010
Lamiales	Lamiaceae	*Ocimum americanum*	NA	NA	Sivasankar *et al.*, 2015
Lamiales	Lamiaceae	*Ocimum basilicum*	GP	W	Syahidah *et al.*, 2015
Lamiales	Lamiaceae	*Ocimum sanctum*	AB, IM, GP	NA	Logambal *et al.*, 2000; Pajaraj *et al.*, 2011
Lamiales	Lamiaceae	*Ocimum tenuiflorum*	NA	NA	Caruso *et al.*, 2013
Lamiales	Lamiaceae	*Origanum monites*	AF	W	Syahidah *et al.*, 2015
Lamiales	Lamiaceae	*Origanum heracleoticum*	AB	W	Zheng *et al.*, 2007
Lamiales	Lamiaceae	*Origanum minutiflorum*	AP	Fr	Karagouni *et al.*, 2005
Lamiales	Lamiaceae	*Origanum onites*	AF	S	Caruso *et al.*, 2013
Lamiales	Lamiaceae	*Origanum vulgare*	AB, GP	NA	Caruso *et al.*, 2013
Lamiales	Lamiaceae	*Prunella vulgaris*	AP, IM	R	Harikrishnan *et al.*, 2011d
Lamiales	Lamiaceae	*Rosmarinus officinalis*	AB, AP	NA	Abutbul *et al.*, 2004

Table 9.1 (Continued)

Order	Family	Species	Activities	Part used	Reference
Lamiales	Lamiaceae	*Satureja khuzistanica*	IM	NA	Khansari *et al.*, 2013
Lamiales	Lamiaceae	*Satureja bachtiarica*	AB	B	Pirbalouti *et al.*, 2011
Lamiales	Lamiaceae	*Satureja thymbra*	AF	B	Syahidah *et al.*, 2015
Lamiales	Lamiaceae	*Scutellaria baicalensis*	AB, IM	B	Harikrishnan *et al.*, 2012b; Pan *et al.*, 2013
Lamiales	Lamiaceae	*Plectranthus scutellarioides*	NA	W	Caruso *et al.*, 2013
Lamiales	Lamiaceae	*Tectona grandis*	NA	NA	Caruso *et al.*, 2013
Lamiales	Lamiaceae	*Thymbra spicata*	AF	L, B	Syahidah *et al.*, 2015
Lamiales	Lamiaceae	*Zataria multiflora*	AF	NA	Soltani *et al.*, 2010
Lamiales	Oleaceae	*Fructus forsythiae*	AB	NA	Pan *et al.*, 2013
Lamiales	Oleaceae	*Nyctanthes arbortristis*	AB, IM	NA	Kibubakaran *et al.*, 2010
Lamiales	Oleaceae	*Olea europea*	AV	NA	Micol *et al.*, 2005
Lamiales	Plantaginaceae	*Picrorhiza kurrooa*	AB, AV, IM	L	Raja *et al.*, 2012
Lamiales	Pedaliacae	*Sesamum indicum*	NA	L	Dada *et al.*, 2014
Lamiales	Verbenaceae	*Lantana camara*	AV	L, S, B	Balasubramanian *et al.*, 2007
Laurales	Lauraceae	*Cinnamomum cassia*	AB, AP	W	Ji *et al.*, 2012
Laurales	Lauraceae	*Cinnamomum verum*	AB, GP	NA	Talpur *et al.*, 2013
Laurales	Lauraceae	*Cinnamomum zeylanicum*	AB	L	Ahmad *et al.*, 2011
Laurales	Lauraceae	*Laurus nobilis*	AB, IM	L, B	Bilen and Bulut, 2010
Laurales	Lauraceae	*Lindera aggregata*	AP	NA	Ji *et al.*, 2012
Laurales	Siparunaceae	*Siparuna guianensis*	AB	NA	Castro *et al.*, 2008
Liliales	Melanthiaceae	*Paris polyphylla*	NA	NA	Wang *et al.*, 2010a
Magnoliales	Annonaceae	*Annona muricata*	AB	L	Caruso *et al.*, 2013
Magnoliales	Annonaceae	*Xylopia aethiopica*	NA	NA	Okeke *et al.*, 2001
Magnoliales	Magnoliaceae	*Magnolia officinalis*	AV, AF	NA	Caruana *et al.*, 2012; Huang *et al.*, 2015
Magnoliales	Myristicaceae	*Myristica fragans*	AB, IM, GP	L	Sivaram *et al.*, 2004
Magnoliales	Myristicaceae	*Virola sebifera*	AB	NA	Castro *et al.*, 2008
Malpighiales	Calophyllaceae	*Calophyllum inophyllum*	AV	NA	Sivasankar *et al.*, 2015

(Continued)

Table 9.1 (Continued)

Order	Family	Species	Activities	Part used	Reference
Malpighiales	Euphorbiaceae	*Acalypha indica*	AB, AV, IM	NA	Raja *et al.*, 2012
Malpighiales	Euphorbiaceae	*Acalypha australis*	AV	L	Direkbysarakom *et al.*, 2004
Malpighiales	Euphorbiaceae	*Actinostemon concolor*	AB	W	Castro *et al.*, 2008
Malpighiales	Euphorbiaceae	*Croton floribundus*	AB	NA	Castro *et al.*, 2008
Malpighiales	Euphorbiaceae	*Croton zambesicus*	AV	NA	Sivasankar *et al.*, 2015
Malpighiales	Euphorbiaceae	*Euphorbia antiquorum*	NA	NA	Caruso *et al.*, 2013
Malpighiales	Euphorbiaceae	*Euphorbia fishceriana*	AF, AP	W	Zhang *et al.*, 2014
Malpighiales	Euphorbiaceae	*Euphorbia hirta*	AB	NA	Huang *et al.*, 2015; Pratheepa and Sukumaran, 2011
Malpighiales	Euphorbiaceae	*Euphorbia plumerioides*	NA	NA	Caruso *et al.*, 2013
Malpighiales	Euphorbiaceae	*Euphorbia thymifolia*	AB	NA	Direkbysarakom *et al.*, 2004
Malpighiales	Euphorbiaceae	*Exoecaria agallocha*	AB	W	Dhayanithi *et al.*, 2012
Malpighiales	Euphorbiaceae	*Hura crepitans*	AV	L	Sivasankar *et al.*, 2015
Malpighiales	Euphorbiaceae	*Manihot esculenta*	NA	NA	Caruso *et al.*, 2013
Malpighiales	Euphorbiaceae	*Sapium sebiferum*	AV	NA	Direkbysarakom *et al.*, 2004
Malpighiales	Euphorbiaceae	*Tetracarpidium conophorum*	AB, IM, GP	Fr	Olusola *et al.*, 2013
Malpighiales	Hypericaceae	*Cratoxylum formosum*	AB, IM, GP	NA	Rattanachaikunsopon and Phumkhachorn, 2010c
Malpighiales	Phyllanthaceae	*Antidesma bunius*	NA	W	Caruso *et al.*, 2013
Malpighiales	Phyllanthaceae	*Phyllanthus acidus*	NA	L, F	Caruso *et al.*, 2013
Malpighiales	Phyllanthaceae	*Phyllanthus amarus*	AB, AV	L	Balasubramanian *et al.*, 2007
Malpighiales	Phyllanthaceae	*Phyllanthus niruri*	GP	L	Citarasu *et al.*, 2002
Malpighiales	Phyllanthaceae	*Phyllanthus debelis*	AB, AV	L, B, Fr	Sivasankar *et al.*, 2015
Malpighiales	Phyllanthaceae	*Phyllanthus emblica*	AV, IM	NA	Sivasankar *et al.*, 2015
Malpighiales	Phyllanthaceae	*Phyllanthus reticulatus*	AB, AV	W	Sivasankar *et al.*, 2015
Malpighiales	Phyllanthaceae	*Phyllanthus urinaria*	AB, AV	R, F, S	Caruso *et al.*, 2013

Table 9.1 (Continued)

Order	Family	Species	Activities	Part used	Reference
Malpighiales	Phyllanthaceae	*Sauropus androgynus*	GP	NA	Putra *et al.*, 2013
Malvales	Malvaceae	*Hibiscus rosa-sinensis*	NA	NA	Caruso *et al.*, 2013
microalgae		*Euglena viridis*	AB, IM	NA	Das, 2009
Mucorales	Mucoraceae	*Massa medicata*	AB, GP	NA	Ji *et al.*, 2007a,2007b
Myrtales	Combretaceae	*Terminalia bellerica*	AB	NA	Jinish, 2002
Myrtales	Combretaceae	*Terminalia cattapa*	AB, AP	S	Chitmanat *et al.*, 2005; Purivirojkul, 2012
Myrtales	Lythraceae	*Punica granatum*	AB, AV, AP, IM, GP	NA	Harikrishnan *et al.*, 2010e
Myrtales	Myrtaceae	*Calyptranthes clusiifolia*	AB	W	Castro *et al.*, 2008
Myrtales	Myrtaceae	*Myrcia tomentosa*	AB	NA	Castro *et al.*, 2008
Myrtales	Myrtaceae	*Psidium guajava*	AB, AV	NA	Pachanawan *et al.*, 2008
Myrtales	Myrtaceae	*Syzygium aromaticum*	NA	NA	Rattanachaikunsopon and Phumkhachorn, 2010; Abd El-Galil, 2012
Myrtales	Onagraceae	*Epilobium hirsutum*	AB	NA	Pakravan *et al.*, 2011
Myrtales	Onagraceae	*Oenothera biennis*	AB, AV	L, R	Shangliang *et al.*, 1990 (sriva)
Pinales	Pinaceae	*Pinus massoniana*	AB, AF, AP	L, R	Direkbysarakom *et al.*, 2004
Pinales	Pinaceae	*Pseudolarix kaempferi*	AP	NA	Ji *et al.*, 2012
Piperales	Aristolochiaceae	*Aristolochia indica*	AV	NA	Sivasankar *et al.*, 2015
Piperales	Piperaceae	*Piper betle*	AB, AF	NA	Caruso *et al.*, 2013
Piperales	Piperaceae	*Piper longum*	GP	NA	Citarasu *et al.*, 2002
Piperales	Piperaceae	*Piper guineense*	AP	S	Ekanem *et al.*, 2004
Piperales	Piperaceae	*Piper nigrum*	IM	R	Caruso *et al.*, 2013
Poales	Poaceae	*Cynodon dactylon*	AB, AV, AP, IM, GP	NA	Balasubramanian *et al.*, 2007, 2008a,2008b; Kaleeswaran *et al.*, 2011
Poales	Poaceae	*Oryza sativa*	NA	NA	Caruso *et al.*, 2013

(*Continued*)

Table 9.1 (Continued)

Order	Family	Species	Activities	Part used	Reference
Poales	Poaceae	*Panicum repens*	NA	R	Caruso *et al.*, 2014
Poales	Poaceae	*Setaria barbata*	NA	NA	Caruso *et al.*, 2015
Proteales	Nelumbonaceae	*Nelumbo nucifera*	NA	NA	Liu *et al.*, 2004; Shao *et al.*, 2004
Ranuncudales	Menispermaceae	*Tinospora cordifolia*	AB, IM	Fr	Alexander *et al.*, 2010; Sudhakaran *et al.*, 2006
Ranuncudales	Menispermaceae	*Tinospora crispa*	NA	W	Sivasankar *et al.*, 2015
Ranuncudales	Menispermaceae	*Tinospora tuberculata*	NA	NA	Caruso *et al.*, 2013
Ranuncudales	Papaveraceae	*Chelidonium majus*	AP	L	Yao *et al.*, 2011
Ranuncudales	Papaveraceae	*Macleaya microcarpa*	AP	NA	Wang *et al.*, 2010b
Ranuncudales	Ranunculaceae	*Cimifuga fetida*	AP	NA	Wu *et al.*, 2011
Ranuncudales	Ranunculoideae	*Nigella sativa*	NA	L, B, Fr	Dorucu *et al.*, 2009
Ranuncudales	Ranunculaceae	*Rhizoma cimigufae*	AP	NA	Wu *et al.*, 2011
Rosales	Moraceae	*Artocarpus altilis*	NA	W	Caruso *et al.*, 2013
Rosales	Moraceae	*Artocarpus heterophyllus*	NA	NA	Caruso *et al.*, 2014
Rosales	Moraceae	*Ficus benghalensis*	IM	Fr	Olusola *et al.*, 2013
Rosales	Moraceae	*Ficus septica*	AB	NA	Caruso *et al.*, 2013
Rosales	Moraceae	*Morus alba*	AV, AP	L	Sivasankar *et al.*, 2015
Rosales	Rosaceae	*Crataegi fructus*	AB, GP	NA	Ji *et al.*, 2007b; Takaoka *et al.*, 2011
Rosales	Rosaceae	*Eriobotrya japonica*	AB	NA	Kim *et al.*, 2011
Rosales	Rosaceae	*Prunus amygdalus*	AP	L	Wu *et al.*, 2011
Rosales	Urticaceae	*Urtica dioica*	AB, IM	L	Awad and Austin, 2010
Salviniales	Salviniaceae	*Salvinia adnata*	NA	NA	Caruso *et al.*, 2013
Santalales	Santalaceae	*Santalum album*	AP	NA	Tu *et al.*, 2013
Santalales	Santalaceae	*Viscum album*	AB, IM	NA	Park and Choi, 2012; Sharma *et al.*, 2010
Sapindales	Anacardiaceae	*Anacardium occidentale*	NA	NA	Caruso *et al.*, 2013
Sapindales	Anacardiaceae	*Cotinus coggyria*	GP	NA	Bilen *et al.*, 2011
Sapindales	Anacardiaceae	*Galla chinensis*	AV	NA	Direkbysarakom *et al.*, 2004
Sapindales	Anacardiaceae	*Mangifera indica*	AB, IM	NA	Awad and Austin, 2010; Awad *et al.*, 2011; Sahu *et al.*, 2007
Sapindales	Burseraceae	*Commiphora myrrha*	AP	L	Syahidah *et al.*, 2015

Table 9.1 (Continued)

Order	Family	Species	Activities	Part used	Reference
Sapindales	Meliaceae	*Azadirachta indica*	AB	NA	Talpur *et al.*, 2013
Sapindales	Meliaceae	*Dysoxylum gaudichaudianum*	NA	NA	Caruso *et al.*, 2013
Sapindales	Meliaceae	*Melia azedarach*	AV, AP	NA	Caruso *et al.*, 2013; Sivasankar *et al.*, 2015
Sapindales	Meliaceae	*Toona sinensis*	AB, IM	L	Wu *et al.*, 2010
Sapindales	Rutaceae	*Aegle marmelos*	AB, AV, AP	NA	Balasubramanian *et al.*, 2007; Pratheepa *et al.*, 2010
Sapindales	Rutaceae	*Murraya paniculata*	NA	W	Caruso *et al.*, 2013
Sapindales	Rutaceae	*Ruta graveolens*	AF	R	Caruso *et al.*, 2013; Hashemi-Karouei *et al.*, 2011
Sapindales	Rutaceae	*Zanthoxylum schinifolium*	AP, IM, GP	L	Harikrishnan *et al.*, 2010d
Sapindales	Simaroubaceae	*Brucea javanica*	NA	W	Wang *et al.*, 2011
Solanales	Convolvulaceae	*Cuscuta chinensis*	AP	R	Huang *et al.*, 2013
Solanales	Convolvulaceae	*Ipomoea aquatica*	NA	R	Caruso *et al.*, 2013
Solanales	Convolvulaceae	*Ipomomea batatas*	NA	R	Caruso *et al.*, 2013
Solanales	Convolvulaceae	*Merremia tomentosa*	AB	R	Castro *et al.*, 2008
Solanales	Solanaceae	*Brugmansia suaveolens*	AB	NA	Caruso *et al.*, 2013
Solanales	Solanaceae	*Capsicum frutescens*	AP	NA	Ling *et al.*, 2012
Solanales	Solanaceae	*Physalis angulata*	NA	NA	Caruso *et al.*, 2013
Solanales	Solanaceae	*Solanum nigurm*	NA	NA	Rajendiran *et al.*, 2008
Solanales	Solanaceae	*Solanum suratense*	AB	R	Jinish, 2002
Solanales	Solanaceae	*Solanum trilobatum*	AB, IM, GP	NA	Divyagnaneswari *et al.*, 2007
Solanales	Solanaceae	*Withania somnifera*	AB, AV, IM, GP	NA	Sharma *et al.*, 2010
Vitales	Vitaceae	*Cayrathia japonicus*	AV	NA	Direkbysarakom *et al.*, 2004
Vitales	Vitaceae	*Cissus quadrangularis*	GP	NA	Radhakrishnan *et al.*, 2014
Zingiberales	Zingiberaceae	*Curcuma longa*	AB, AF, IM	NA	Caruso *et al.*, 2013; Sahu *et al.*, 2008

(*Continued*)

Table 9.1 (Continued)

Order	Family	Species	Activities	Part used	Reference
Zingiberales	Zingiberaceae	*Curcuma mangga*	AB	NA	Caruso *et al.*, 2013
Zingiberales	Zingiberaceae	*Curcuma zanthorrhiza*	NA	NA	Caruso *et al.*, 2014
Zingiberales	Zingiberaceae	*Curcuma zeodaria*	AB, AF	NA	Caruso *et al.*, 2015
Zingiberales	Zingiberaceae	*Etlingera hemisphaerica*	NA	NA	Caruso *et al.*, 2016
Zingiberales	Musaceae	*Musa acuminata*	NA	NA	Caruso *et al.*, 2017
Zingiberales	Musaceae	*Musa balbisiana*	NA	NA	Caruso *et al.*, 2018
Zingiberales	Musaceae	*Musa paradisiace*	NA	NA	Caruso *et al.*, 2019
Zingiberales	Zingiberaceae	*Zingiber officinale*	AB, AV, AF, AP, IM, GP	NA	Dügenci *et al.*, 2003; Haghighi and Rohani, 2013; Nya and Austin, 2009
Algae	red	*Asparagopsis taxiformis*	AB, AF, AP	NA	Genovese *et al.*, 2012; Hutson *et al.*, 2012; Manilal *et al.*, 2012
Algae	brown	*Himanthalia elongata*	AB	NA	Cox *et al.*, 2010
Algae	brown	*Laminaria digitata*	AB	NA	Dubber and Harder, 2008
Algae	red	*Ceramium rubrum*	AB	NA	Dubber and Harder, 2009
Algae	red	*Gracilaria edulis*	AB	NA	Kolanjinathan *et al.*, 2009
Algae	red	*Gracilaria fisheri*	NA	NA	Harikrishnan *et al.*, 2011a
Algae	red	*Gracilaria tenuistipitata*	AB, AV	NA	Sirirustananun *et al.*, 2011
Algae	red	*Gelidium amansii*	AB, IM	NA	Fu *et al.*, 2007
Algae	brown	*Sargassum fusiforme*	AB, IM	NA	Huang *et al.*, 2006
Algae	brown	*Sargassum duplicatum*	AB, IM	NA	Yeh *et al.*, 2006
Algae	red	*Porphyridium cruentum*	AB	NA	Diaz-Rosales *et al.*, 2008
Algae	green	*Ulva sp.*	AP	NA	Hutson *et al.*, 2012
Mushroom		*Citrus paradisi*	AB	NA	Oladosu-Ayayi *et al.*, 2013
Mushroom		*Ganoderma lucidum*	AB, IM	NA	Olusola *et al.*, 2013
Mushroom		*Hericium erinaceum*	AP, IM	NA	Harikrishnan *et al.*, 2011b
Mushroom		*Inonotus obliquus*	AB	NA	Harikrishnan *et al.*, 2012a
Mushroom		*Volvariella volvacea*		NA	Caruso *et al.*, 2013

AV, antiviral; AB, antibacterial; AF, antifungal; AP, antiparasitic; F, flowers; Fr, fruit; GP, growth promoter; IM, immunostimulant; L, leaves; NA, not available; R, root; S, seeds; W, whole plant.

Most of the plants used both by fish farmers and in scientific studies for potential use in aquaculture correspond to plants widely used in traditional medicine. We identified over 250 plant species from 75 families and 32 orders, which have been used or reported as potentially interesting in aquaculture.

Plant Orders Most Frequently Used in Aquaculture

Plants from the order Lamiales (family Lamiaceae) were the most studied (12%), followed by the Fabales (family Fabaceae, 11%), Asterales (family Asteraceae, 10%) and Malpighiales (family Euphorbiaceae et Phyllanthaceae, 10%) (Figure 9.2).

Lamiales

The Lamiales order comprises about 20 families of dicotyledonous flowering plants (Allaby, 2012). Lamiaceae plants are frequently aromatic and include many culinary herbs such as basil (*Ocimum* sp.), mint (*Mentha* sp.), oregano (*Origanum* sp.), rosemary (*Rosmarinus officinalis*) and savory (*Satureja* sp.). Lamiaceae plants are widely used in traditional medicine for treatment of diseases such as colds, headaches, stomach disorders, inflammation and heart disease (Pattanayak *et al.*, 2010). Several essential oils have been reported to display antimicrobial, antispasmodic, carminative and antiviral activity (Mimica-Dukic and Bozin, 2008).

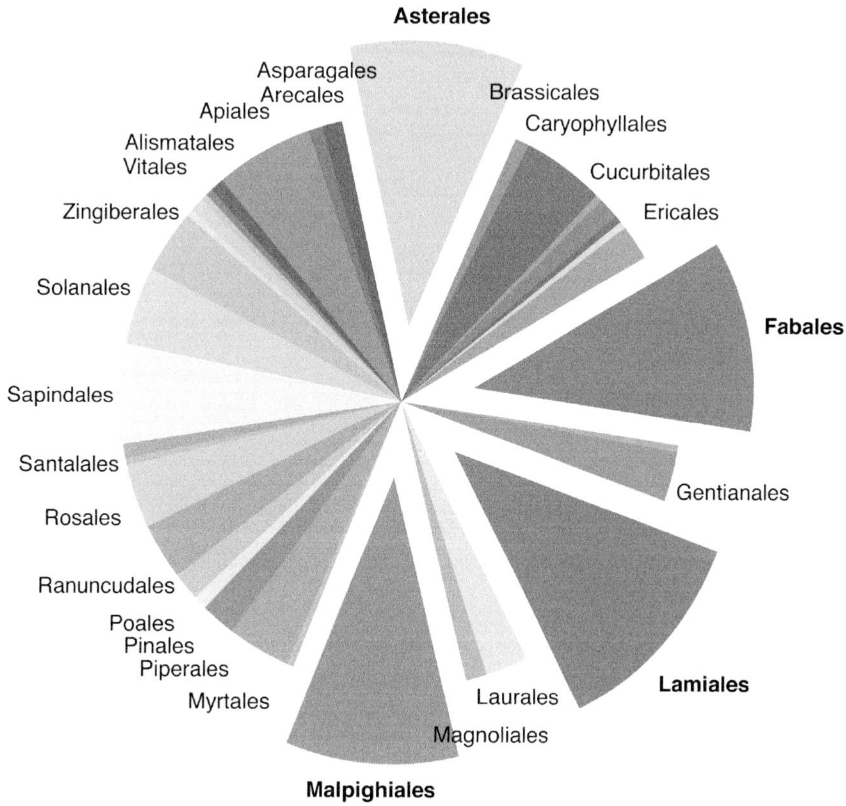

Figure 9.2 Orders of plants used in aquaculture. (*See plate section for the color representation of this figure.*)

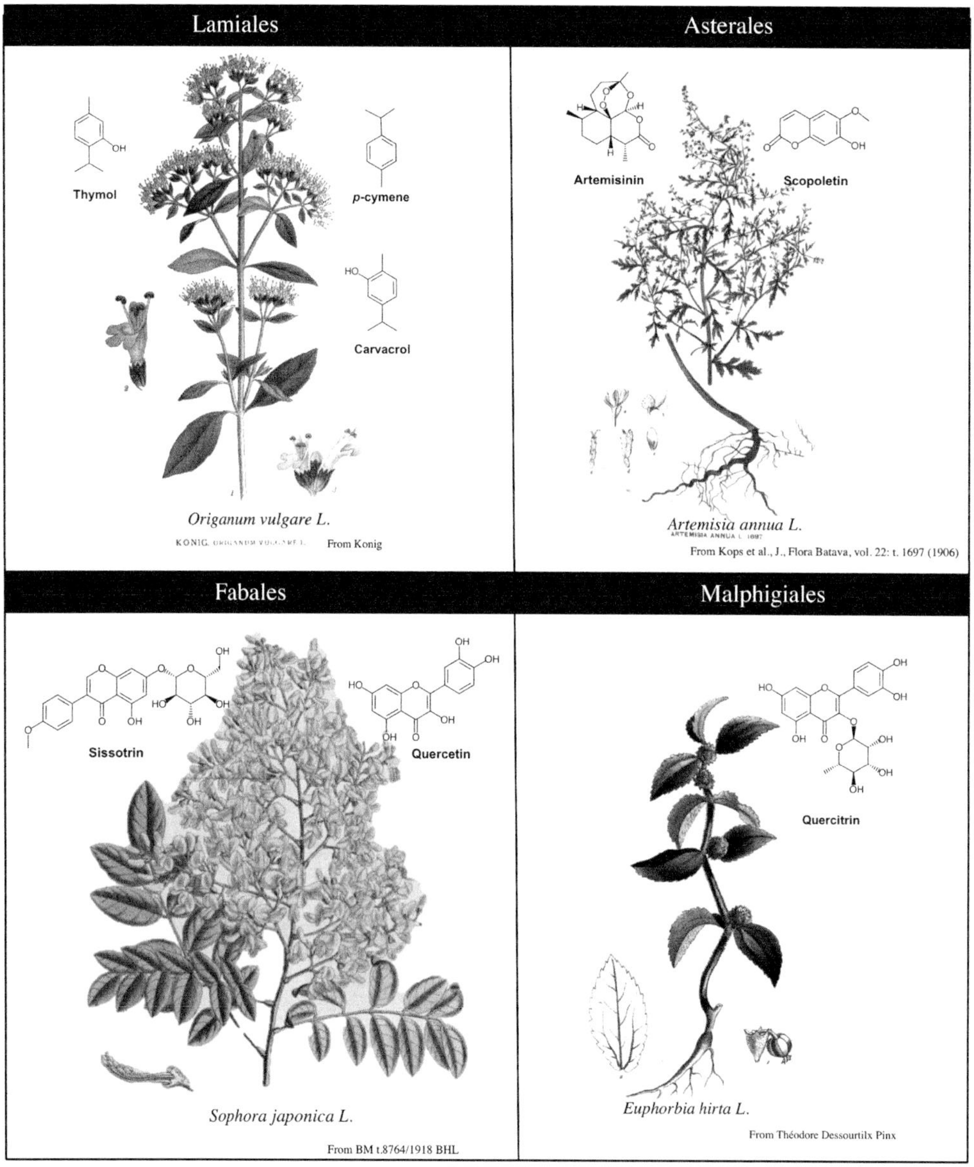

Figure 9.3 Plant examples and isolated molecules from the plant orders most used in aquaculture. (*See plate section for the color representation of this figure.*)

Lamiaceae plants contain a wide range of bioactive metabolites which include numerous monoterpenes and sesquiterpenes such as linalool, geraniol, eugenol, ocimene, carvacrol, p-cymene, thymol and myrcene and flavonoids like luteolin first isolated from *Salvia tomentosa* (Bower *et al.*, 2014; Malmir *et al.*, 2015; Mimica-Dukic and Bozin, 2008) (Figure 9.3). Plants from the family Lamiaceae also contain several bioactive fatty acids such as palmitic acid and myristic acid and phenolic actives such as rosmarinic acid (Pattanayak *et al.*, 2010). Rattanachaikunsopon and Phumkhachorn (2010) and Abd-El-Galil and Hashiem (2012) showed that antibacterial activity of carvacrol against *Edwarsiella tarda* and *Tenacibaculum maritimum* was enhanced when administered with cymene (see Figure 9.3). Gormez and Diler (2014) showed that essential oils of *Origanum onites* and *Thymbra spicata* were more bioactive against the fungus *Saprolegnia parasitica* than thymol or carvacrol alone. The latter studies indicate that synergistic effects between different bioactive compounds may exist and enhance plant bioactivity. Hao *et al.* (2012) found that palmitic acid was effective against the monogenean parasite *D. intermedium* in goldfish (*Carassius auratus*).

Fabales

The Fabales include the family Fabaceae, commonly known as the pea or bean family. The Fabaceae is the third largest plant family as it includes more than 12 000 plants (Allaby, 2012). Several plants from the family Fabaceae are used in traditional medicine for treatments against diarrhoea, parasite infections, inflammations, rheumatism and ulcers (Molares and Ladio, 2011). Several plants from the Fabaceae family (*Albizia saman, Falcataria moluccana, Gliricidia sepum, Koompassia malaccensis, Leucaena leucocephala, L. glauca, Parkia speciosa, Senna alata, S. siamea, Sesbania grandiflora* and *Tamarindus indica*) are used by Indonesian fish farmers to improve fish fitness and treat fish infections (Caruso *et al.*, 2013). Plants from the genus *Sophora* contain many phytoconstituents with pharmacological and therapeutic properties, including antioxidant, anticancer, antimicrobial, antiviral and anti-inflammatory (Abdelhady *et al.*, 2015). Several polyphenolic compounds have been identified in *Sophora japonica*, such as tamarixetin, sissotrin, rutin, gallic acid and quercetin (Abdelhady *et al.*, 2015) (see Figure 9.3). Liu *et al.* (2011) characterized the alkaloids matrine, oxymatrine, sophoridine, oxysophocarpine and sophocarpine from *Sophora flavescens*. Wu *et al.* (2013) showed that a diet supplemented with *Sophora flavescens* enhanced the non-specific immune system of Nile tilapia (*Oreochromis niloticus)* and increased disease resistance against *Streptococcus agalactiae.*

Asterales

Asterales is an order of dicotyledonous flowering plants that includes the large family Asteraceae, commonly known as the daisy family. The Asteraceae family contains more than 23 000 species; most members are herbaceous but a significant number are shrubs, vines or trees (Allaby, 2012).

Many *Artemisia* species are present in the Chinese pharmacopoeia, and they have been used as scholeretic, anti-inflammatory and diuretic agents in the treatment of diseases like epidemic hepatitis and fevers (Tang *et al.*, 1992). The use of *Artemisia annua* in Chinese traditional medicine was recorded before 168 BC, and in 1971 artemisinin, a sesquiterpene lactone with antimalarial properties, was isolated (Cávar *et al.*, 2012; Klayman, 1985). Artemisinin and its semi-synthetic derivatives are currently used worldwide for treatment against the malaria parasite *Plasmodium falciparum* (WHO, 2006) (see Figure 9.3). *Artemisia* plants also contain abundant monoterpenes (eucalyptol, germacrenes, camphor), coumarins (scopoletin), chlorogenic acids (quinic acid, caffeic acid) and flavonoids (luteolin, isovitexin) (Carbonara *et al.*, 2012; Cávar *et al.*, 2012; Efferth *et al.*, 2011; Juteau *et al.*, 2002) (see Figure 9.3). *Artemisia* sp. antibacterial and antiparasitic effects against aquaculture pathogens have also been studied. Ekanem and Brisibe (2010) showed the efficacy of ethanol extract of *Artemisia annua* against the monogenean parasite *Heterobranchus longifilis.* Huang *et al.* (2013) reported on the anthelminthic activity of *Artemisia argyi* against *D. intermedius* in goldfish. El-Deen and Mohamed (2009) demonstrated the efficacy of *Artemisia vulgaris* crude extracts against the ectoparasite *Trichodina* sp. and the bacterium *Aeromonas hydrophila* in Nile tilapia.

Aucklandia lappa is another plant from the Asteraceae family with numerous bioactivities and is widely used in traditional medicine for the treatment of asthma, rheumatism, coughs, tuberculosis and many other diseases. (Seo and Shin, 2015; Zhang *et al.*, 2014). *A. lappa* contains the sesquiterpene lactones costunolide, dehydrocostus lactone and alantolactone which are known to display multiple bioactivities (Li *et al.*, 2005; Seo and Shin, 2015). Xue-Gang *et al.* (2013) showed that *A. lappa* displayed antifungal activity against *Saprolegnia* sp. and *Achlya klebsiana*.

Other Asteraceae plants have been shown to display interesting bioactivities relevant to application in aquaculture. Oral administration of *Eclipta alba* in tilapia (*Oreochromis mossambicus*) enhanced non-specific immune parameters and reduced fish mortality when challenged with *A. hydrophila* (Christybapita *et al.*, 2007). A *Siegesbeckia glabrescens*-enriched diet displayed an immunomodulatory effect and increased disease resistance in kelp grouper (*Epinephelus bruneus*) (Harikrishnan *et al.*, 2012b). *Artemisia cina*, *Matricaria chamomilla* and *Tridax procumbens* promoted weight gain and enchanced non-specific immune responses in fish (Abdelhadi *et al.*, 2010; Sivasankar *et al.*, 2015). *Echinacea purpura* appeared to have immunostimulant, antibacterial and antifungal properties in fish (Aly and Mohamed, 2010; Caruana *et al.*, 2012).

Malpighiales

Malpighiales is a very diverse order, containing the flowering plant families Euphorbiaceae and Phyllanthaceae. Euphorbiaceae, the spurge family, is constituted mainly of herbs but also includes some shrubs and trees. The spurge family contains numerous species of medicinal plants such as different species from the genus *Euphorbia* or the irritant mangrove *Exoecaria agallocha* (Ernst et al., 2015). The study of the natural products of the *Euphorbia* species started in 1968 with the isolation of a tumour-promoting phorbol-12,13-diester from *Croton tiglium* L., and description of the antitumour activity of a diterpene isolated from *Euphorbia esula* L. in 1976 (Hecker, 1968; Kupchan, 1976). More recently, a diterpene drug (ingenol mebutate, Picato®) isolated from *Euphorbia peplus* was released for the treatment of actinic keratosis (Berman, 2012).

Euphorbia sp. contains several terpenes, such as the ingol-type diterpenes, euphorantins, flavonoids like quercitrin and tannins (Qi *et al.*, 2014, Trinh and Le, 2014) (see Figure 9.3). Different species of *Euphorbia* have displayed antibacterial, antiviral, antifungal and antiparastic activities against fish and shellfish pathogens (Direkbusarakom, 2004; Huang *et al.*, 2015; Zhang *et al.*, 2014).

The Phyllanthaceae family is a small (about 2000 species) but diverse family, which includes the genus *Phyllanthus*. *Phyllanthus* plants are well known for their potent medicinal activity and are used worldwide (Kumar *et al.*, 2015). Numerous bioactive phytochemicals have been isolated from *Phyllanthus* plants, including phyllanthin, phyltetralin, phyllangin, corilangin, gallic acid, methylgallate, and rhamnocitrin, protocatechuic acid, kaempferol 3-O-rutinoside, quercitrin and rutin (Fang *et al.*, 2008; Kumar *et al.*, 2015; Wei *et al.*, 2004). *Phyllanthus* possess a high antibacterial and antiviral potential against pathogens in aquaculture (Balasubramanian *et al.*, 2007; Punitha *et al.*, 2008; Sivasankar *et al.*, 2015).

Plant Species Most Widely Used in Aquaculture

The plant species that have displayed the highest potential for use in aquaculture are garlic (*Allium sativum*), pomegranate (*Punica granatum*), bermuda grass (*Cynodon dactylon*), Indian ginseng (*Whitania somnifera*) and ginger (*Zingiber officinale*).

Garlic (Asparagales, Amaryllidaceae) has been used by humans for over 7000 years for both culinary and medicinal purposes. Antibacterial, antiparasitic, antioxidant, immunostimulant and growth-promoting activities have been observed in fish and shellfish (Lee and Gao, 2012). Some studies have studied the effect of the pure garlic components allicin and ajoene in aquaculture and demonstrated their immunostimulant capacity and effectiveness against pathogenic fish protozoa *Spironucleus vortens*, *Ichthyophthirius multifiliis* and the bacteria *A. hydrophila* (Millet *et al.*, 2011; Nya *et al.*, 2010; Tanekhy and Fall, 2015).

Pomegranate (Myrtales, Lythraceae) has also been used for medical purposes since ancient times. Pomegranates contain numerous phytochemicals such as the bioactive polyphenol ellagitannins which exert antioxidant and anti-inflammatory effects. In aquaculture, studies have shown antibacterial, antiviral, antiparasitic, immunostimulant and growth-promoting activities (Harikrishnan *et al.*, 2010a,2010b; Pirbalouti *et al.*, 2011).

The chemical composition of Bermuda grass (Poales, Poaceae) includes phenolic compounds (gallic acid), tannins (cathechins), anthocyanins (cyanidin) and flavonoids (quercetin) (Khlifi *et al.*, 2013). *C. dactylon* displays antibacterial, antiviral, antiparasitic, immunostimulant and growth-promoting activities in fish and shellfish (Balasubramanian *et al.*, 2008a,2008b; Kaleeswaran *et al.*, 2011).

Indian ginseng (Solanales, Solanaceae) has been used for centuries in Ayurvedic medicine to increase longevity and vitality. Scientific research has shown antioxidant, anti-inflammatory, immune-modulating and antistress properties in the whole plant extract. *W. somnifera* biologically active chemical constituents include alkaloids (isopelletierine, anaferine), steroidal lactones (withanolides, withaferins) and saponins containing an additional acyl group (sitoindoside VII and VIII) (Mishra *et al.*, 2000). *W. somnifera* has antibacterial, antiviral, immunostimulant and growth-promoting activities in aquaculture (Sharma *et al.*, 2010; Talpur *et al.*, 2013; Yogeeswaran *et al.*, 2012).

Ginger (Zingiberales, Zingiberaceae) is a herbaceous perennial plant used for culinary and medicinal purposes. Ginger contains a mixture of zingerone, shogaols and gingerols as well as some sesquiterpenoids, with (-)-zingiberene as the main component (Ali *et al.*, 2008). Bioactivities include antioxidant, anti-inflammatory, antibacterial and apoptosis induction (Dugasani *et al.*, 2010; El-Ghorab *et al.*, 2010). In aquaculture, enrichment of diets with ginger has been shown to promote growth and immunostimulation as well as antibacterial, antiviral, antifungal and antiparasitic activities (Caruana *et al.*, 2012; Kanani *et al.*, 2014; Nya and Austin, 2009; Rajeswari *et al.*, 2012).

Analysis of Plant Bioactivity

Analysis of plant bioactivity showed that 36% of the plants studied presented antibacterial activity, whereas 17% had antiparasitic activity, 16% immunostimulant activity, 14% antiviral activity, 13% growth promoter and only 4% showed antifungal activity (Figure 9.4). Nevertheless, it should be taken into account that those proportions are biased by the number of studies performed to date on each targeted pathology; for example many more studies have been focused on antibacterial activities than antifungal activities.

Plant bioactivies were also analysed by plant order and we found that Asterales was the order with the highest number of bioactive plants (34), with nearly half of them displaying antibacterial activity (Figure 9.5). Lamiales and Malpighiales were the next two highest (33 and 32). The Lamiales order had the highest number of plants displaying immunostimulant activity (7) and antifungal activity (5), while the Malpighiales presented the highest antiviral activities (11) (see Figure 9.5).

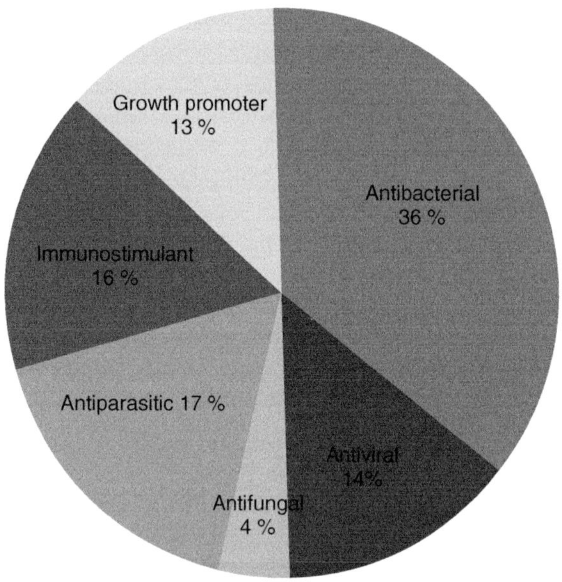

Figure 9.4 Plant bioactivities in aquaculture. (*See plate section for the color representation of this figure.*)

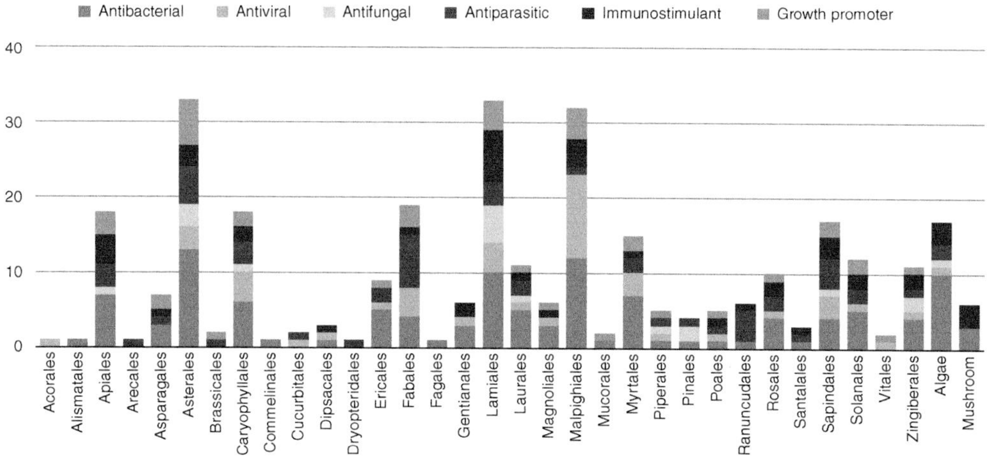

Figure 9.5 Bioactivities of plant orders in aquaculture. (*See plate section for the color representation of this figure.*)

Analysis of Plant Parts Used in Aquaculture

Most studies on the use of medicinal plants in aquaculture used plant leaves (37%), while 22% used the whole plant as powder, plant essential oil or extract. Root was also often used, at 18%, followed by seeds (8%), barks (6%), fruits (6%) and finally flowers (4%) (Figure 9.6).

Other Plants and Perspectives

Some algae and some mushrooms have also been studied for their potential application in aquaculture. Algae are considered to be a rich source of bioactive molecules ; most of the studied algae presented high antibacterial activities, and some also presented immunostimulant, antifungal, antiparasitic and antiviral activity (Choudhury *et al.*, 2005; Genovese

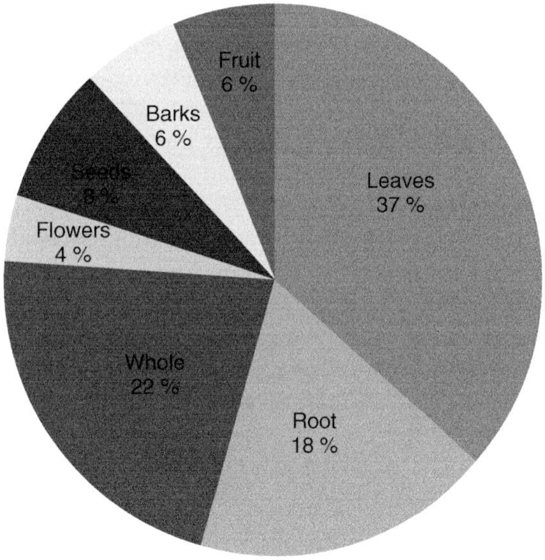

Figure 9.6 Parts of plants used in aquaculture. (*See plate section for the color representation of this figure.*)

et al., 2013 ; Hutson *et al.*, 2012; Sukoso *et al.*, 2012; Zbakh *et al.*, 2012). For example, the red alga *Asparagopsis taxiformis*, which is known to produce a high diversity of halogenated metabolites, displayed antibacterial, antifungal and antiparasitic activities against several fish pathogens (Genovese *et al.*, 2012, 2013). Also, *A. taxiformis* enhanced the immune system of *Penaeus monodon* and was highly efficient in the treatment of vibriosis in *P. monodon* (Manilal *et al.*, 2012, 2013). Also, studies like that of Mai *et al*, (2015) are starting to show interesting properties of other marine organisms such as sponges, which can inhibit quorum sensing of marine pathogenic bacteria such as *Vibrio harveyi*. Nevertheless, more research needs to be performed in this field, in order to establish the possibilities of application in aquaculture disease management.

Finally, there are numerous plants used in human medicine that have not yet been tested on aquaculture. For example, the gum rockrose (*Cistus ladanifer*, Cistaceae, Malvales) is a plant widely used in several Mediterranean countries which possesses anti-inflammatory, antibacterial and antioxidant activity (Ferreira *et al.*, 2012; Neves *et al.*, 2009). Dandelion (*Taraxacum officinale*, Asteraceae, Asterales) has long been used in the northern hemisphere for its diuretic, choleretic, anti-inflammatory, antioxidative, anticarcinogenic, analgesic, antihyperglycaemic, anticoagulatory and prebiotic effects (Schütz *et al.*, 2006).

Conclusion

Medicinal plants (including algae and mushrooms) present promising potential for use in aquaculture as a substitute for chemotherapy in the treatment of disease outbreaks. Ethnobotanical studies have been highly useful in the discovery of bioactive plants and natural products with interesting applications in aquaculture. However, there is still little knowledge on the mode of action of most bioactive plants, as well as the most suitable form for effective and safe administration. More research is needed to elucidate plant products and their modes of action (to establish the bioactive parts of the plant and the most suitable preparations), and to test plant effects on the organism's physiology in order to establish an appropriate treatment strategy (route of administration, dose and length). In addition, research in this field could also benefit greatly from the traditional knowledge of fish farmers who regularly use plants.

Finally, most studies have focused on the potential of terrestrial plants in aquaculture. Although these plants do offer interesting biological properties, they are not a natural component of either fish alimentation or the marine environment. Thus, continuous introduction of plant extracts and their bioactive compounds (through bath treatment or food diffusion) into the marine or freshwater environment could eventually cause environmental problems. Therefore, the use of bioactive algae and seaweeds from local natural environments where aquaculture is carried out could be a better alternative to avoid introduction of exogenous molecules into the environment. Algae are considered to be a rich source of original bioactive molecules which display multiple bioactivities. In aquaculture, several recent studies have showed the potential of algae for the treatment of pathogens or to improve fish fitness. However, they can also cause undesirable effects and toxicity in fish, so more research needs to be performed on the physiological effects of algae on fish and suitable dosing levels (Manilal *et al.*, 2010).

References

Abasali, H. and Mohamad, S. (2010) Immune response of common carp (*Cyprinus carpio*) fed with herbal immunostimulants diets. *Agricultural Journal*, **5**, 163–172.

Abd El-Galil, M.A.A. and Hashiem, M. (2012) Experimental infection of tenacibaculosis and a trial for treatment by plant extract carvacrol in surge wrasses fish (*Thalassoma Purpureum*). *Life Science Journal*, **9**, 442–447.

Abdel-Tawwab, M. (2012) The use of American ginseng (*Panax quinquefolium*) in practical diets for Nile tilapia (*Oreochromis niloticus*): growth performance and challenge with *Aeromonas hydrophila*. *Journal of Applied Aquaculture*, **24**, 366–376.

Abdel-Tawwab, M., Sharafeldin, K.M., Mosaad, M.N.M. and Ismaiel, N.E.M. (2015) Coffee bean in common carp, *Cyprinus carpio* L. diets: effect on growth performance, biochemical status, and resistance to waterborne zinc toxicity. *Aquaculture*, **448**, 207–213.

Abdelhadi, Y., Saleh, O. and Sakr, S. (2010) Study on the effect of wormseed plants; *Artemisia cina L.* and chamomile; *Matricaria chamomilla L.* on growth parameters and immune response of African catfish, *Clarias gariepinus*. *Journal of Fisheries International*, **5**, 1–7.

Abdelhady, M.I.S., Kamal, A.M., Othman, S.M., Mubarak, M.S. and Hadda, T.B. (2015) Total polyphenolic content, antioxidant, cytotoxic, antidiabetic activities, and polyphenolic compounds of *Sophora japonica* grown in Egypt. *Medicinal Chemistry Research*, **24**, 482–495.

Abutbul, S., Golan-Goldhirsh, A., Baranzani, O. and Zilberg, D. (2004) Use of *Rosmarinus officinalis* as a treatment against *Streptococcus iniae* in tilapia (*Oreochromis sp.*). *Aquaculture*, **238**, 97–105.

Ahmad, M.H. and Abdel-Tawwab, M. (2011) The use of caraway seed meal as a feed additive in fish diets: Growth performance, feed utilization, and whole-body composition of Nile tilapia, *Oreochromis niloticus* (L.) fingerlings. *Aquaculture*, **314**, 110–114.

Ahmad, M.H., El Mesallamy, A.M.D., Samir, F. and Zahran, F. (2011) Effect of cinnamon (*Cinnamomum zeylanicum*) on growth performance, feed utilization, whole-body composition, and resistance to *Aeromonas hydrophila* in Nile tilapia. *Journal of Applied Aquaculture*, **23**, 289–298.

Alexander, C.P., Kirubakaran, C.J.W. and Michael, R.D. (2010) Water soluble fraction of *Tinospora cordifolia* leaves enhanced the non-specific immune mechanisms and disease resistance in *Oreochromis mossambicus*. *Fish and Shellfish Immunology*, **29**, 765–772.

Ali, B.H., Blunden, G., Tanira, M.O. and Nemmar, A. (2008) Some phytochemical, pharmacological and toxicological properties of ginger (*Zingiber officinale* Roscoe): s review of recent research. *Food and Chemical Toxicology*, **46**, 409-420.

Alishahi, M., Ranjbar, M.M., Ghorbanpour, M., Peyghan, R., Mesbah, M. and Razi-jalali, M. (2010) Effects of dietary *Aloe vera* on some specific and nonspecific immunity in the common carp (*Cyprinus carpio*). *International Journal of Veterinary Research*, **4**, 189–195.

Allaby, M. (2012) *A Dictionary of Plant Sciences*. Oxford University Press, Oxford.

Aly, S.M. and Mohamed, M.F. (2010) *Echinacea purpurea* and *Allium sativum* as immunostimulants in fish culture using Nile tilapia (*Oreochromis niloticus*). *Journal of Animal Physiology and Animal Nutrition*, **94**, e31–39.

Aly, S.M., Atti, N.M.A. and Mohamed, M.F. (2008) Effect of garlic on the survival, growth, resistance and quality of *Oreochromis niloticus*. Presented at the 8th International Symposium on Tilapia in Aquaculture, pp.277–296.

Anderson, D.P. (1992) Immunostimulants, adjuvants, and vaccine carriers in fish: applications to aquaculture. *Annual Review of Fish Diseases*, **2**, 281–307.

Ardó, L., Yin, G., Xu, P., *et al.* (2008) Chinese herbs (*Astragalus membranaceus* and *Lonicera japonica*) and boron enhance the non-specific immune response of Nile tilapia (*Oreochromis niloticus*) and resistance against *Aeromonas hydrophila*. *Aquaculture*, **275**, 26–33.

Ashley, P.J. (2007) Fish welfare: current issues in aquaculture. *Applied Animal Behaviour Science, Fish Behavior and Welfare*, **104**, 199–235.

Ashraf, M.A. and Goda, S. (2008) Effect of dietary Ginseng herb (Ginsana© G115) supplementation on growth, feed utilization, and hematological indices of Nile Tilapia, *Oreochromis niloticus* (L.), fingerlings. *Journal of the World Aquaculture Society*, **39**, 205–214.

Awad, E. and Austin, B. (2010) Use of lupin, *Lupinus perennis*, mango, *Mangifera indica*, and stinging nettle, *Urtica dioica*, as feed additives to prevent *Aeromonas hydrophila* infection in rainbow trout, *Oncorhynchus mykiss* (Walbaum). *Journal of Fish Diseases*, **33**, 413–420.

Awad, E., Mitchell, W.J. and Austin, B. (2011) Effect of dietary supplements on cytokine gene expression in rainbow trout, *Oncorhynchus mykiss* (Walbaum). *Journal of Fish Diseases*, **34**, 629–634.

Ayyanar, M. and Ignacimuthu, S. (2011) Ethnobotanical survey of medicinal plants commonly used by Kani tribals in Tirunelveli hills of Western Ghats, India. *Journal of Ethnopharmacology*, **134**, 851–864.

Balasubramanian, G., Sarathi, M., Kumar, S.R. and Hameed, A.S.S. (2007) Screening the antiviral activity of Indian medicinal plants against white spot syndrome virus in shrimp. *Aquaculture*, **263**, 15–19.

Balasubramanian, G., Sarathi, M., Venkatesan, C., Thomas, J. and Sahul Hameed, A.S. (2008a) Oral administration of antiviral plant extract of *Cynodon dactylon* on a large scale production against White spot syndrome virus (WSSV) in *Penaeus monodon*. *Aquaculture*, **279**, 2–5.

Balasubramanian, G., Sarathi, M., Venkatesan, C., Thomas, J. and Sahul Hameed, A.S. (2008b) Studies on the immunomodulatory effect of extract of *Cynodon dactylon* in shrimp, *Penaeus monodon*, and its efficacy to protect the shrimp from white spot syndrome virus (WSSV). *Fish and Shellfish Immunology*, **25**, 820–828.

Banskota, A.H., Tezuka, Y., Le Tran, Q. and Kadota, S. (2003) Chemical constituents and biological activities of Vietnamese medicinal plants. *Current Topics in Medicinal Chemistry*, **3**, 227–248.

Berman, B. (2012) New developments in the treatment of actinic keratosis: focus on ingenol mebutate gel. *Clinical, Cosmetic and Investigational Dermatology*, **5**, 111–122.

Bhuvaneswari, R. and Balasundaram, C. (2006) Traditional Indian herbal extracts used in vitro against growth of the pathogenic bacteria – *Aeromonas hydrophila*. *Israeli Journal of Aquaculture – Bamidgeh*, **58**, 89–96.

Bilen, S. and Bulut, M. (2010) Effects of laurel (*Laurus nobilis*) on the non-specific immune responses of rainbow trout (*Oncorhynchus mykiss*, Walbaum). *Journal of Animal and Veterinary Advances*, **9**, 1275–1279.

Bilen, S., Bulut, M. and Bilen, A.M. (2011) Immunostimulant effects of *Cotinus coggyria* on rainbow trout (*Oncorhynchus mykiss*). *Fish and Shellfish Immunology*, **30**, 451–455.

Bondad-Reantaso, M.G., Subasinghe, R.P., Arthur, J.R., *et al.* (2005) Disease and health management in Asian aquaculture. From Science to Solutions, plenary lectures presented at the 20th Conference of the World Association for the Advancement of Veterinary Parasitology, **132**, 249–272.

Bower, A.M., Real Hernandez, L.M., Berhow, M.A. and de Mejia, E.G. (2014) Bioactive compounds from culinary herbs inhibit a molecular target for type 2 diabetes management, dipeptidyl peptidase IV. *Journal of Agricultural and Food Chemistry*, **62**, 6147–6158.

Cabello, F.C. (2006) Heavy use of prophylactic antibiotics in aquaculture: a growing problem for human and animal health and for the environment. *Environmental Microbiology*, **8**, 1137–1144.

Calixto, J.B. (2005) Twenty-five years of research on medicinal plants in Latin America: a personal view. *Journal of Ethnopharmacology*, **100**, 131–134.

Carbonara, T., Pascale, R., Argentieri, M.P., *et al.* (2012) Phytochemical analysis of a herbal tea from *Artemisia annua L. Journal of Pharmaceutical and Biomedical Analysis*, **62**, 79–86.

Caruana, S., Yoon, G.H., Freeman, M.A., Mackie, J.A. and Shinn, A.P. (2012) The efficacy of selected plant extracts and bioflavonoids in controlling infections of *Saprolegnia australis* (Saprolegniales; Oomycetes). *Aquaculture*, **358–359**, 146–154.

Caruso, D., Lusiastuti, A.M., Taukhid, Slembrouck, J., Komarudin, O. and Legendre, M. (2013) Traditional pharmacopeia in small scale freshwater fish farms in West Java, Indonesia: an ethnoveterinary approach. *Aquaculture*, **416–417**, 334–345.

Castro, S.B.R., Leal, C.A.G., Freire, F.R., Carvalho, D.A., Oliveira, D.F. and Figueiredo, H.C.P. (2008) Antibacterial activity of plant extracts from Brazil against fish pathogenic bacteria. *Brazilian Journal of Microbiology*, **39**, 756–760.

Ćavar, S., Maksimović, M., Vidic, D. and Parić, A. (2012) Chemical composition and antioxidant and antimicrobial activity of essential oil of *Artemisia annua L.* from Bosnia. *Industrial Crops and Products*, **37**, 479–485.

Chakrabarti, R., Srivastava, P.K., Verma, N. and Sharma, J. (2014) Effect of seeds of *Achyranthes aspera* on the immune responses and expression of some immune-related genes in carp *Catla catla*. *Fish and Shellfish Immunology*, **41**, 64–69.

Chakraborty, S.B. and Hancz, C. (2011) Application of phytochemicals as immunostimulant, antipathogenic and antistress agents in finfish culture. *Reviews in Aquaculture*, **3**, 103–119.

Chang, C.C., Tan, H.-C. and Cheng, W. (2013) Effects of dietary administration of water hyacinth (*Eichhornia crassipes*) extracts on the immune responses and disease resistance of giant freshwater prawn, *Macrobrachium rosenbergii*. *Fish and Shellfish Immunology*, **35**, 92–100.

Chaves, T.P., Santana, C.P., Véras, G., *et al.* (2013) Seasonal variation in the production of secondary metabolites and antimicrobial activity of two plant species used in Brazilian traditional medicine. *African Journal of Biotechnology*, **12**, 847–853.

Chitmanat, C., Tongdonmuan, K., Khanom, P., Pachontis, P. and Nunsong, W. (2005) Antiparasitic, antibacterial and antifungal activities derived from a *Terminalia catappa* solution against some tilapia (*Oreochromis niloticus*) pathogens. *Acta Horticulturae*, 179–182.

Choudhury, S., Sree, A., Mukherjee, S.C., Pattnaik, P. and Bapuji, M. (2005) In vitro antibacterial activity of extracts of selected marine algae and mangroves against fish pathogens. *Asian Fisheries Science*, **18**, 285–294.

Christybapita, D., Divyagnaneswari, M. and Michael, R.D. (2007) Oral administration of *Eclipta alba* leaf aqueous extract enhances the non-specific immune responses and disease resistance of *Oreochromis mossambicus*. *Fish and Shellfish Immunology*, **23**, 840–852.

Citarasu, T. (2010) Herbal biomedicines: a new opportunity for aquaculture industry. *Aquaculture International*, **18**, 403–414.

Citarasu, T., Sekar, R.R., Babu, M.M. and Marian, M.P. (2002) Developing *Artemia* enriched herbal diet for producing quality larvae in *Penaeus monodon*. *Asian Fisheries Science*, **15**, 21–32.

Cox, S., Abu-Ghannam, N. and Gupta, S. (2010) An assessment of the antioxidant and antimicrobial activity of six species of edible Irish seaweeds. *International Food Research Journal*, **17**, 205–220.

Dada, A.A. and Adeparusi, E.O. (2014) Dietary effects of two medicinal plants (*Sesamum indicum*) and (Croton zambesicus) on the reproductive indices in female African catfish (*Clarias gariepinus*) broodstock. *Egyptian Journal of Aquatic Research*, **38**, 269–273.

Das, B.K., Pradhan, J. and Sahu, S. (2009) The effect of *Euglena viridis* on immune response of rohu, *Labeo rohita* (Ham.). *Fish and Shellfish Immunology*, **26**, 871–876.

Davis, K.B., Griffin, B.R. and Gray, W.L. (2002) Effect of handling stress on susceptibility of channel catfish *Ictalurus punctatus* to *Ichthyophthirius multifiliis* and channel catfish virus infection. *Aquaculture*, **214**, 55–66.

Dhayanithi, N.B., Kumar, T.T.A. and Balasubramanian, T. (2012) Effect of *Excoecaria agallocha* leaves against *Aeromonas hydrophila* in marine ornamental fish, *Amphiprion sebae*. *Indian Journal of Geo-Marine Science*, **41**, 76–82.

Díaz-Rosales, P., Chabrillón, M., Abdala, R.T., Figueroa, F.L., Balebona, M.C. and Moriñigo, M.A. (2008) Effect of dietary administration of *Porphyridium cruentum* on the respiratory burst activity of sole, *Solea senegalensis* (Kaup), phagocytes. *Journal of Fish Diseases*, **31**, 489–495.

Direkbusarakom, S. (2004) Application of medicinal herbs to aquaculture in Asia. *Walailak Journal of Science and Technology*, **1**, 7–14.

Direkbusarakom, S., Herunsalee, A., Yoshimizu, M. and Ezura, Y. (1996) Antiviral activity of several Thai traditional herb extracts against fish pathogenic viruses. *Fish Pathology*, **31**, 209–213.

Direkbusarakom, S., Ruangpan, L., Ezura, Y. and Yoshimizu, M. (1998) Protective efficacy of *Clinacanthus nutans* on yellow-head disease in black tiger shrimp (*Penaeus monodon*). *Fish Pathology*, **33**, 401–404.

Divyagnaneswari, M., Christybapita, D. and Michael, R.D. (2007) Enhancement of nonspecific immunity and disease resistance in *Oreochromis mossambicus* by *Solanum trilobatum* leaf fractions. *Fish and Shellfish Immunology*, **23**, 249–259.

Dorucu, M., Ozesen Colak, S., Ispir, U., Altinterim, B. and Celayir, Y. (2009) The effect of black cumin seeds, Nigella sativa, on the immune response of rainbow trout, *Oncorhynchus mykiss*. *Mediterranean Aquaculture Journal*, **2**, 1–7.

Dubber, D. and Harder, T. (2008) Extracts of *Ceramium rubrum*, *Mastocarpus stellatus* and *Laminaria digitata* inhibit growth of marine fish pathogenic bacteria at ecologically realistic concentrations. *Aquaculture*, **274**, 196–200.

Dugasani, S., Pichika, M.R., Nadarajah, V.D., Balijepalli, M.K., Tandra, S. and Korlakunta, J.N. (2010) Comparative antioxidant and anti-inflammatory effects of [6]-gingerol, [8]-gingerol, [10]-gingerol and [6]-shogaol. *Journal of Ethnopharmacology*, **127**, 515–520.

Dügenci, S.K., Arda, N. and Candan, A. (2003) Some medicinal plants as immunostimulant for fish. *Journal of Ethnopharmacology*, **88**, 99–106.

Efferth, T., Herrmann, F., Tahrani, A. and Wink, M. (2011) Cytotoxic activity of secondary metabolites derived from *Artemisia annua L.* towards cancer cells in comparison to its designated active constituent artemisinin. *Phytomedicine*, **18**, 959–969.

Ekanem, A.P. and Brisibe, E.A. (2010) Effects of ethanol extract of *Artemisia annua L.* against monogenean parasites of *Heterobranchus longifilis*. *Parasitology Research*, **106**, 1135–1139.

Ekanem, A.P., Obiekezie, A., Kloas, W. and Knopf, K. (2004) Effects of crude extracts of *Mucuna pruriens* (Fabaceae) and *Carica papaya* (Caricaceae) against the protozoan fish *parasite Ichthyophthirius multifiliis*. *Parasitology Research*, **92**, 361–366.

Ekanem, A.P., Ekpo, I.A., Morah, F., Amanke, E. and Afangide, U. (2007) Acute toxicity of ethanol extracts from two ichthyotoxic plants *Adenia cissampeloides* (Passifloraceae) and *Blighia sapida* (Sapindaceae) to one week old *Heterobranchus longifilis* juveniles. *Nigerian Journal of Botany*, **20**, 157–161.

El-Deen, A.I.E. and Mohamed, R.A. (2009) Application of some medicinal plants to eliminate *Trichodina sp* in tilapia (*Oreochromis niloticus*). *Report and Opinion*, **1**, 1–5.

El-Ghorab, A.H., Nauman, M., Anjum, F.M., Hussain, S. and Nadeem, M. (2010) A comparative study on chemical composition and antioxidant activity of ginger (*Zingiber officinale*) and cumin (*Cuminum cyminum*). *Journal of Agricultural and Food Chemistry*, **58**, 8231–8237.

Ernst, M., Grace, O.M., Saslis-Lagoudakis, C.H., Nilsson, N., Simonsen, H.T. and Rønsted, N. (2015) Global medicinal uses of *Euphorbia L.* (Euphorbiaceae). *Journal of Ethnopharmacology*, **176**, 90–101.

Fang, S.H., Rao, Y.K. and Tzeng, Y.M. (2008) Anti-oxidant and inflammatory mediator's growth inhibitory effects of compounds isolated from *Phyllanthus urinaria*. *Journal of Ethnopharmacology*, **116**, 333–340.

Ferreira, S., Santos, J., Duarte, A., Queiroz, J.A. and Domingues, F.C. (2012) Screening of antimicrobial activity of *Cistus ladanifer* and *Arbutus unedo* extracts. *Natural Products Research*, **26**, 1557–1560.

Food and Agriculture Organization of the United Nations, Fisheries and Aquaculture Department (2014) *The State of World Fisheries and Aquaculture*. Food and Agriculture Organization of the United Nations, Rome.

Forwood, J.M., Harris, J.O. and Deveney, M.R. (2013) Efficacy of current and alternative bath treatments for *Lepidotrema bidyana* infecting silver perch, *Bidyanus bidyanus*. *Aquaculture*, **416–417**, 65–71.

Francis, G., Makkar, H.P.S. and Becker, K. (2005) *Quillaja* saponins – a natural growth promoter for fish. *Animal Feed Science and Technology*, **121**, 147–157.

Fu, Y.W., Hou, W.Y., Yeh, S.T., Li, C.H. and Chen, J.C. (2007) The immunostimulatory effects of hot-water extract of *Gelidium amansii* via immersion, injection and dietary administrations on white shrimp *Litopenaeus vannamei* and its resistance against *Vibrio alginolyticus*. *Fish and Shellfish Immunology*, **22**, 673–685.

Fu, Y., Zhang, Q., Xu, D.H., *et al.* (2014) Parasiticidal effects of *Morus alba* root bark extracts against *Ichthyophthirius multifiliis* infecting grass carp. *Diseases of Aquatic Organisms*, **108**, 129–136.

Genovese, G., Faggio, C., Gugliandolo, C., *et al.* (2012) In vitro evaluation of antibacterial activity of *Asparagopsis taxiformis* from the Straits of Messina against pathogens relevant in aquaculture. *Marine Environmental Research*, **73**, 1–6.

Genovese, G., Leitner, S., Minicante, S.A. and Lass-Flörl, C. (2013) The Mediterranean red alga *Asparagopsis taxiformis* has antifungal activity against *Aspergillus* species. *Mycoses*, **56**, 516–519.

Gormez, O. and Diler, O. (2014) In vitro antifungal activity of essential oils from *Tymbra, Origanum, Satureja* species and some pure compounds on the fish pathogenic fungus, *Saprolegnia parasitica*. *Aquaculture Research*, **45**, 1196–1201.

Gostner, J.M., Wrulich, O.A., Jenny, M., Fuchs, D. and Ueberall, F. (2012) An update on the strategies in multicomponent activity monitoring within the phytopharmaceutical field. *BMC Complementary and Alternative Medicine*, **12**, 18.

Haghighi, M. and Rohani, M.S. (2013) The effects of powdered ginger (*Zingiber officinale*) on the haematological and immunological parameters of rainbow trout *Oncorhynchus mykiss*. *Journal of Medicinal Plant and Herbal Therapy Research*, **1**, 8–12.

Hao, B., Liu, G.L., Hu, X.G. and Wang, G.X. (2012) Bioassay-guided isolation and identification of active compounds from *Semen pharbitidis* against *Dactylogyrus intermedius* (Monogenea) in goldfish (*Carassius auratus*). *Veterinary Parasitology*, **187**, 452–458.

Harikrishnan, R., Heo, J., Balasundaram, C., *et al.* (2010a) Effect of traditional Korean medicinal (TKM) triherbal extract on the innate immune system and disease resistance in *Paralichthys olivaceus* against *Uronema marinum*. *Veterinary Parasitology*, **170**, 1–7.

Harikrishnan, R., Heo, J., Balasundaram, C., *et al.* (2010b) Effect of *Punica granatum* solvent extracts on immune system and disease resistance in *Paralichthys olivaceus* against lymphocystis disease virus (LDV). *Fish and Shellfish Immunology*, **29**, 668–673.

Harikrishnan, R., Balasundaram, C., Kim, M.C., Kim, J.S., Han, Y.J. and Heo, M.S. (2010c) Effect of a mixed herb-enriched diet on the innate immune response and disease resistance of *Paralichthys olivaceus* against *Philasterides dicentrarchi* infection. *Journal of Aquatic Animal Health*, **22**, 235–243.

Harikrishnan, R., Balasundaram, C. and Heo, M.S. (2011a) Impact of plant products on innate and adaptive immune system of cultured finfish and shellfish. *Aquaculture*, **317**, 1–15.

Harikrishnan, R., Kim, J.S., Kim, M.C., Balasundaram, C. and Heo, M.S. (2011b) *Kalopanax pictus* as feed additive controls bacterial and parasitic infections in kelp grouper, *Epinephelus bruneus*. *Fish and Shellfish Immunology*, **31**, 801–807.

Harikrishnan, R., Kim, J.S., Kim, M.C., Balasundaram, C. and Heo, M.S. (2011c) *Lactuca indica* extract as feed additive enhances immunological parameters and disease resistance in *Epinephelus bruneus* to *Streptococcus iniae*. *Aquaculture*, **318**, 43–47.

Harikrishnan, R., Kim, J.S., Kim, M.C., Balasundaram, C. and Heo, M.S. (2011d) *Styrax japonica* supplementation diet enhances the innate immune response in *Epinephelus bruneus* against bacterial and protozoan infections. *Experimental Parasitology*, **129**, 260–265.

Harikrishnan, R., Kim, M.C., Kim, J.S., Kim, D.H., Hong, S.H. and Heo, M.S. (2011e) *Alnus firma* supplementation diet on haematology and innate immune response in olive flounder against *Tenacibaculum maritimum*. *Bulletin of the Veterinary Institute in Pulawy*, **55**, 649–655.

Harikrishnan, R., Kim, J.S., Kim, M.C., Balasundaram, C. and Heo, M.S. (2011f) *Prunella vulgaris* enhances the non-specific immune response and disease resistance of *Paralichthys olivaceus* against *Uronema marinum*. *Aquaculture*, **318**, 61–66.

Harikrishnan, R., Balasundaram, C. and Heo, M.S. (2012a) Effect of *Inonotus obliquus* enriched diet on hematology, immune response, and disease protection in kelp grouper, *Epinephelus bruneus* against *Vibrio harveyi*. *Aquaculture*, **344–349**, 48–53.

Harikrishnan, R., Kim, D.H., Hong, S.H., Mariappan, P., Balasundaram, C. and Heo, M.S. (2012b) Non-specific immune response and disease resistance induced by *Siegesbeckia glabrescens* against *Vibrio parahaemolyticus* in *Epinephelus bruneus*. *Fish and Shellfish Immunology*, **33**, 359–364.

Harikrishnan, R., Kim, J.S., Kim, M.C., *et al.* (2012c) Effect of dietary supplementation with *Suaeda maritima* on blood physiology, innate immune response, and disease resistance in olive flounder against *Miamiensis avidus*. *Experimental Parasitology*, **131**, 195–203.

Hashemi, K.S.M., Sadeghpour, H.M. and Gholampour, A.I. (2012) Isolation of Saprolegnia and the influence of root ethanolic extract of *Ruta graveolens* on *Saprolegnia. Spp* growth. *International Journal of Bioscience, Biochemistry and Bioinformatics*, **2**, 64–67.

Hecker, E. (1968) Cocarcinogenic principles from the seed oil of *Croton tiglium* and from other Euphorbiaceae. *Cancer Research*, **28**, 2338–2348.

Hoareau, L. and DaSilva, E.J. (1999) Medicinal plants: a re-emerging health aid. *Electronic Journal of Biotechnology*, **2**, 56–70.

Hoseinifar, S.H., Khalili, M., Rufchaei, R., *et al.* (2015) Effects of date palm fruit extracts on skin mucosal immunity, immune related genes expression and growth performance of common carp (*Cyprinus carpio*) fry. *Fish and Shellfish Immunology*, **47**, 706–711.

Huang, A.G., Yi, Y.L., Ling, F., *et al.* (2013) Screening of plant extracts for anthelmintic activity against *Dactylogyrus intermedius* (Monogenea) in goldfish (*Carassius auratus*). *Parasitology Research*, **112**, 4065–4072.

Huang, X., Zhou, H. and Zhang, H. (2006) The effect of *Sargassum fusiforme* polysaccharide extracts on vibriosis resistance and immune activity of the shrimp, *Fenneropenaeus chinensis*. *Fish and Shellfish Immunology*, **20**, 750–757.

Huang, X.L., Liu, R.J., Whyte, S., *et al.* (2015) *The in vitro* antifungal activity of 30 Chinese herb extracts to *Saprolegnia sp*. *Journal of Applied Ichtyology*, **31**, 681–686.

Hutson, K.S., Mata, L., Paul, N.A. and de Nys, R. (2012) Seaweed extracts as a natural control against the monogenean ectoparasite, *Neobenedenia sp*., infecting farmed barramundi (*Lates calcarifer*). *International Journal of Parasitology*, **42**, 1135–1141.

Iguchi, K., Ogawa, K., Nagae, M. and Ito, F. (2003) The influence of rearing density on stress response and disease susceptibility of ayu (*Plecoglossus altivelis*). *Aquaculture*, **220**, 515–523.

Innocent, X., Aly-Fathima, M.S. and Dhanalakshmi (2011) Studies on the immunostimulant activity of *Coriandrum sativum* and resistance to *Aeromonas hydrophila* in *Catla catla*. *Journal of Applied Pharmaceutical Science*, **1**, 132–135.

Ji, J., Lu, C., Kang, Y., Wang, G.X. and Chen, P. (2012) Screening of 42 medicinal plants for in vivo anthelmintic activity against *Dactylogyrus intermedius* (Monogenea) in goldfish (*Carassius auratus*). *Parasitology Research*, **111**, 97–104.

Ji, S.C., Jeong, G.S., Gwang-Soon, I., Lee, S.W., Yoo, J.H. and Takii, K. (2007a) Dietary medicinal herbs improve growth performance, fatty acid utilization, and stress recovery of Japanese flounder. *Fisheries Science*, **73**, 70–76.

Ji, S.C., Takaoka, O., Jeong G.S., *et al.* (2007b) Dietary medicinal herbs improve growth and some non-specific immunity of red sea bream *Pagrus major*. *Fisheries Science*, **73**, 63–69.

Jiang, J. and Wu, Z. (2004) Influences of traditional Chinese medicine on non-specific immunity of Jian Carp (*Cyprinus carpio* var. Jian). *Fish and Shellfish Immunology*, **16**, 185–191.

Jinish, L.J.G. (2002) Ayurvedic phytotherapeutics against *Vibrio* infections in grouper, *Epinephelus tauvina*, MSc dissertation, M.S. University, Tirunelveli, Tamil Nadu, India.

Juteau, F., Masotti, V., Bessière, J.M., Dherbomez, M. and Viano, J. (2002) Antibacterial and antioxidant activities of *Artemisia annua* essential oil. *Fitoterapia*, **73**, 532–535.

Kaleeswaran, B., Ilavenil, S. and Ravikumar, S. (2011) Dietary supplementation with *Cynodon dactylon* (L.) enhances innate immunity and disease resistance of Indian major carp, *Catla catla* (Ham.). *Fish and Shellfish Immunology*, **31**, 953–962.

Kaminskyy, V., Kulachkovskyy, O. and Stoika, R. (2008) A decisive role of mitochondria in defining rate and intensity of apoptosis induction by different alkaloids. *Toxicology Letters*, **177**, 168–181.

Kanani, H.G., Nobahar, Z., Kakoolaki, S. and Jafarian, H. (2014) Effect of ginger- and garlic-supplemented diet on growth performance, some hematological parameters and immune responses in juvenile *Huso huso*. *Fish Physiology and Biochemistry*, **40**, 481–490.

Kanjana, K., Radtanatip, T., Asuvapongpatana, S., Withyachumnarnkul, B. and Wongprasert, K. (2011) Solvent extracts of the red seaweed *Gracilaria fisheri* prevent *Vibrio harveyi* infections in the black tiger shrimp *Penaeus monodon*. *Fish and Shellfish Immunology*, **30**, 389–396.

Karagouni, E., Athanassopoulou, F., Lytra, A., Komis, C. and Dotsika, E. (2005) Antiparasitic and immunomodulatory effect of innovative treatments against *Myxobolus sp.* infection in *Diplodus puntazzo*. *Veterinary Parasitology*, **134**, 215–228.

Kavitha, C., Ramesh, M., Kumaran, S.S. and Lakshmi, S.A. (2012) Toxicity of *Moringa oleifera* seed extract on some hematological and biochemical profiles in a freshwater fish, *Cyprinus carpio*. *Experimental and Toxicologic Pathology*, **64**, 681–687.

Kemény-Beke, A., Aradi, J., Damjanovich, J., *et al.* (2006) Apoptotic response of uveal melanoma cells upon treatment with chelidonine, sanguinarine and chelerythrine. *Cancer Letters*, **237**, 67–75.

Khansari, A., Yavari, V., Alishahi, M., *et al.* (2013) Effects of *Oliviera decumbens* and *Satureja khuzestanica* extract on some immunological and haematological parameters of *Cyprinus carpio*. *Comparative Clinical Pathology*, **22**, 339–342.

Khlifi, D., Hayouni, E.A., Valentin, A., *et al.* (2013) LC–MS analysis, anticancer, antioxidant and antimalarial activities of *Cynodon dactylon L.* extracts. *Industrial Crops and Products*, **45**, 240–247.

Kim, J.S., Harikrishnan, R., Kim, M.C., *et al.* (2011) Enhancement of *Eriobotrya japonica* extracts on non-specific immune response and disease resistance in kelp grouper *Epinephelus bruneus* against *Vibrio carchariae*. *Fish and Shellfish Immunology*, **31**, 1193–1200.

Kim, K.H., Hwang, Y.J. and Bai, S.C. (1999) Resistance to *Vibrio alginolyticus* in juvenile rockfish (*Sebastes schlegeli*) fed diets containing different doses of aloe. *Aquaculture*, **180**, 13–21.

Kirubakaran, C.J.W., C.P. Alexander, and Michael, R.D. (2010) Enhancement of non-specific immune responses and disease resistance on oral administration of *Nyctanthes arbortristis* seed extract in *Oreochromis mossambicus* (Peters). *Aquaculture Research*, **41**, 1630–1639.

Klayman, D.L. (1985) Qinghaosu (artemisinin): an antimalarial drug from China. *Science*, **228**, 1049–1055.

Kolanjinathan, K., Ganesh, P. and Govindarajan, M. (2009) Antibacterial activity of ethanol extracts of seaweeds against fish bacterial pathogens. *European Reviews in Medicine and Pharmacology Sciences*, **13**, 173–177.

Krogdahl, A., Penn, M., Thorsen, J., Refstie, S. and Bakke, A.M. (2010) Important antinutrients in plant feedstuffs for aquaculture: an update on recent findings regarding responses in salmonids. *Aquaculture Research*, **41**, 333–344.

Kumar, S., Raman, R.P., Pandey, P.K., Mohanty, S., Kumar, A. and Kumar, K. (2013) Effect of orally administered azadirachtin on non-specific immune parameters of goldfish *Carassius auratus* (Linn. 1758) and resistance against *Aeromonas hydrophila*. *Fish and Shellfish Immunology*, **34**, 564–573.

Kumar, S., Chandra, P., Bajpai, V., *et al.* (2015) Rapid qualitative and quantitative analysis of bioactive compounds from *Phyllanthus amarus* using LC/MS/MS techniques. *Industrial Crops and Products*, **69**, 143–152.

Kupchan, S.M., Uchida, I., Branfman, A.R., Dailey, R.G. and Fei, B.Y. (1976) Antileukemic principles isolated from euphorbiaceae plants. *Science*, **191**, 571–572.

Lee, J.Y. and Gao, Y. (2012) Review of the application of garlic, *Allium sativum*, in aquaculture. *Journal of the World Aquaculture Society*, **43**, 447–458.

Li, A., Sun, A. and Liu, R. (2005) Preparative isolation and purification of costunolide and dehydrocostuslactone from *Aucklandia lappa* Decne by high-speed counter-current chromatography. *Journal of Chromatography A*, **1076**, 193–197.

Ling, F., Wang, J.G., Lu, C., Wang, G.X., Lui, Y.H. and Gong, X.N. (2012) Effects of aqueous extract of *Capsicum frutescens* (Solanaceae) against the fish ectoparasite *Ichthyophthirius multifiliis*. *Parasitology Research*, **111**, 841–848.

Ling, F., Lu, C., Tu, X., *et al.* (2013) Antiprotozoal screening of traditional medicinal plants: evaluation of crude extract of *Psoralea corylifolia* against *Ichthyophthirius multifiliis*. *Parasitology Research*, **112**, 2231–2240.

Liu, C., Tsai, W., Lin, Y., Liao, J., Chen, C. and Kuo, Y. (2004) The extracts from *Nelumbo nucifera* suppress cell cycle progression, cytokine genes expression, and cell proliferation in human peripheral blood mononuclear cells. *Life Science*, **75**, 699–716.

Liu, G., Dong, J., Wang, H., Hashi, Y. and Chen, S. (2011) Characterization of alkaloids in *Sophora flavescens* Ait. by high-performance liquid chromatography–electrospray ionization tandem mass spectrometry. *Journal of Pharmaceutical and Biomedical Analysis*, **54**, 1065–1072.

Logambal, S.M., Venkatalakshmi, S. and Michael, R.D. (2000) Immunostimulatory effect of leaf extract of *Ocimum sanctum* Linn. in *Oreochromis mossambicus* (Peters). *Hydrobiologia*, **430**, 113–120.

Lu, C., Zhang, H.Y., Ji, J. and Wang, G.X. (2012) *In vivo* anthelmintic activity of *Dryopteris crassirhizoma*, *Kochia scoparia*, and *Polygala tenuifolia* against *Dactylogyrus intermedius* (Monogenea) in goldfish (*Carassius auratus*). *Parasitology Research*, **110**, 1085–1090.

Mai, T., Tintillier, F., Lucasson, A., *et al.* (2015) Quorum sensing inhibitors from Leucette chagonensis Dendy, 1863. *Letters in Applied Microbiology*, **61**, 311–317.

Malikova, J., Zdarilova, A. and Hlobilkova, A. (2006) Effects of sanguinarine and chelerythrine on the cell cycle and apoptosis. *Biomedical Papers of the Medical Faculty of the University Palacky, Olomouc, Czech Republic*, **150**, 5–12.

Malmir, M., Gohari, A.R., Saeidnia, S. and Silva, O. (2015) A new bioactive monoterpene-flavonoid from *Satureja khuzistanica*. *Fitoterapia*, **105**, 107–112.

Manilal, A., Selvin, J., Kiran, G. K., *et al.* (2009) Antimicrobial potential and seasonality of red algae collected from the southwest coast of India tested against shrimp, human and phytopathogens. *Annals of Microbiology*, **59**, 207–219.

Manilal, A., Sujith, S., Sabarathnam, B., *et al.* (2010) Bioactivity of the red algae *Asparagopsis taxiformis* collected from the southwestern coast of India. *Brazilian Journal of Oceanography*, **58**, 93–100.

Manilal, A., Selvin, J. and Georges, S. (2012) In vivo therapeutic potentiality of red seaweed, *Asparagopsis* (Bonnemaisoniales, Rhodophyta) in the treatment of vibriosis in *Penaeus monodon* Fabricius. *Saudi Journal of Biological Science*, **19**, 165–175.

Manilal, A., Selvin, J. and Sugathan, S. (2013) Immuno-modulatory efficacy of Indian red algae, *Asparagopsis taxiformis*, in *Penaeus monodon*. *Journal of Applied Aquaculture*, **25**, 81–93.

Martins, M.L., Moraes, F.R., Miyazaki, D.M.Y., *et al.* (2002) Alternative treatment for *Anacanthorus penilabiatus* (Monogenea: Dactylogyridae) infection in cultivated pacu, *Piaractus mesopotamicus* (Osteichthyes: Characidae) in Brazil and its haematological effects. *Parasite*, **9**, 175–180.

Micol, V., Caturla, N., Perez-Fons, L., Mas, V., Perez, L. and Estepa, A. (2005) The olive leaf extract exhibits antiviral activity against viral haemorrhagic septicaemia rhabdovirus (VHSV). *Antiviral Research*, **66**, 129–136.

Militz, T.A., Southgate, P.C., Carton, A.G. and Hutson, K.S. (2013) Dietary supplementation of garlic (*Allium sativum*) to prevent monogenean infection in aquaculture. *Aquaculture*, **408–409**, 95–99.

Millet, C.O.M., Lloyd, D., Williams, C., *et al.* (2011) Effect of garlic and allium-derived products on the growth and metabolism of *Spironucleus vortens*. *Experimental Parasitology*, **127**, 490–499.

Mimica-Dukic, N. and Bozin, B. (2008) *Mentha L.* species (Lamiaceae) as promising sources of bioactive secondary metabolites. *Current Pharmaceutical Design*, **14**, 3141–3150.

Minomol, M. (2005) Culture of Gold fish *Carassius auratus* using medicinal plants having immunostimulant characteristics. MPhil dissertation, MS University, Tamil Nadu, India.

Miranda, C.D. and Zemelman, R. (2002) Antimicrobial multiresistance in bacteria isolated from freshwater Chilean salmon farms. *Science of the Total Environment*, **293**, 207–218.

Mishra, L.C., Singh, B.B. and Dagenais, S. (2000) Scientific basis for the therapeutic use of *Withania somnifera* (ashwagandha): a review. *Alternative Medicine Review*, **5**, 334–346.

Molares, S. and Ladio, A. (2011) The usefulness of edible and medicinal Fabaceae in Argentine and Chilean Patagonia: environmental availability and other sources of supply. *Evidence-Based Complementary and Alternative Medicine*, **2012**, e901918.

Neves, J.M., Matos, C., Moutinho, C., Queiroz, G. and Gomes, L.R. (2009) Ethnopharmacological notes about ancient uses of medicinal plants in Trás-os-Montes (northern of Portugal). *Journal of Ethnopharmacology*, **124**, 270–283.

Nya, E.J. and Austin, B. (2009) Use of dietary ginger, *Zingiber officinale Roscoe*, as an immunostimulant to *control Aeromonas hydrophila* infections in rainbow trout, *Oncorhynchus mykiss* (Walbaum). *Journal of Fish Diseases*, **32**, 971–977.

Nya, E.J., Dawood, Z. and Austin, B. (2010) The garlic component, allicin, prevents disease caused by *Aeromonas hydrophila* in rainbow trout, *Oncorhynchus mykiss* (Walbaum). *Journal of Fish Diseases*, **33**, 293–300.

Okeke, M.I., Iroegbu, C.U., Jideofor, C.O., Okoli, A. and Esimone, C.O. (2001) Antimicrobial activity of ethanol extracts of two indigenous Nigerian spices. *Journal of Herbs, Spices and Medicinal Plants*, **8**, 39–48.

Oladosu-Ayayi, R.N., George, F.O.A., Obasa, S.O. and Bankole, M.O. (2013) Effects of some plant extracts on some biological parameters of catfish *Clarias gariepinus* (Burchell, 1822). *Journal of Fisheries and Aquatic Science*, **8**, 142–147.

Olusola, S.E., Emikpe, B.O. and Olaifa, F.E. (2013) The potentials of medicinal plants extracts as bio-antimicrobial in aquaculture. *International Journal of Medicinal Aromatic Plants*, **3**, 404–412.

Pachanawan, A., Phumkhachorn, P. and Rattanachaikunsopon, P. (2008) Potential of *Psidium guajava* supplemented fish diets in controlling *Aeromonas hydrophila* infection in tilapia (*Oreochromis niloticus*). *Journal of Bioscience and Bioengineering*, **5**, 419–424.

Pakravan, S., Hajimoradloo, A. and Ghorbani, R. (2012) Effect of dietary willow herb, *Epilobium hirsutum* extract on growth performance, body composition, haematological parameters and *Aeromonas hydrophila* challenge on common carp, *Cyprinus carpio*. *Aquaculture Research*, **43**, 861–869.

Pan, T.S., Yan, M.C., Chen, S.B. and Wang, X.P. (2013) Effects of ten traditional chinese herbs on immune response and disease resistance of *Sciaenops ocellatus* (Actinopterygii: Perciformes: Sciaenidae). *Acta Ichthyologica Piscatoria*, **43**, 41–49.

Park, K.H. and Choi, S.H. (2012) The effect of mistletoe, *Viscum album coloratum*, extract on innate immune response of Nile tilapia (*Oreochromis niloticus*). *Fish and Shellfish Immunology*, **32**, 1016–1021.

Pasnik, D.J., Evans, J.J., Panangala, V.S., Klesius, P.H., Shelby, R.A. and Shoemaker, C.A. (2005) Antigenicity of *Streptococcus agalactiae* extracellular products and vaccine efficacy. *Journal of Fish Diseases*, **28**, 205–212.

Pattanayak, P., Behera, P., Das, D. and Panda, S.K. (2010) *Ocimum sanctum Linn.* A reservoir plant for therapeutic applications: an overview. *Pharmacognosy Review*, **4**, 95–105.

Pavaraj, M., Balasubram, V., Baskaran, S. and Ramasamy, P. (2011) Development of immunity by extract of medicinal plant *Ocimum sanctum* on common carp *Cyprinus carpio (L.)*. *Research Journal of Immunology*, **4**, 12–18.

Petrovska, B.B. (2012) Historical review of medicinal plants' usage. *Pharmacognosy Review*, **6**, 1–5.

Philchenkov, A., Kaminskyy, V., Zavelevich, M. and Stoika, R. (2008) Apoptogenic activity of two benzophenanthridine alkaloids from *Chelidonium majus* L. does not correlate with their DNA damaging effects. *Toxicology In Vitro*, **22**, 287–295.

Pirbalouti, G., Broujeni, N., Momeni, M., Poor, M. and Hamedi, B. (2011) Antibacterial activity of Iranian medicinal plants against *Streptococcus iniae* isolated from rainbow trout (*Oncorhynchus mykiss*). *Archives of Biological Science*, **63**, 59–66.

Pratheepa, V. and Sukumaran, N. (2011) Specific and nonspecific immunostimulation study of *Euphorbia hirta* on *Pseudomonas fluorescens*-infected *Cyprinus carpio*. *Pharmaceutical Biology*, **48**, 484–491.

Pratheepa, V., Ramesh, S. and Sukumaran, N. (2010) Immunomodulatory effect of *Aegle marmelos* leaf extract on freshwater fish *Cyprinus carpio* infected by bacterial pathogen *Aeromonas hydrophila*. *Pharmaceutical Biology*, **48**, 1224–123.

Punitha, S.M.J., Babu, M.M., Sivaram, V., *et al.* (2008) Immunostimulating influence of herbal biomedicines on nonspecific immunity in Grouper *Epinephelus tauvina* juvenile against *Vibrio harveyi* infection. *Aquaculture International*, **16**, 511–523.

Purivirojkul, W. (2012) Potential application of extracts from Indian almond (*Terminalia catappa* Linn.) leaves in Siamese fighting fish (*Betta splendens* Regan) culture. *Communications in Agricultural Applied Biological Sciences*, **77**, 439–448.

Putra, A.A.S. Santoso, U., Lee, M.C. and Nan, F.H. (2013) Effects of dietary katuk leaf extract on growth performance, feeding behavior and water quality of grouper *Epinephelus coioides*. *Aceh International Journal of Science and Technology*, **2**.

Qi, W.Y., Zhang, W.Y., Shen, Y., Leng, Y., Gao, K. and Yue, J.M. (2014) Ingol-type diterpenes from *Euphorbia antiquorum* with mouse 11β-hydroxysteroid dehydrogenase type 1 inhibition activity. *Journal of Natural Products*, **77**, 1452–1458.

Radhakrishnan, S., Bhavan, P.S., Seenivasan, C., Shanthi, R. and Poongodi, R. (2014) Influence of medicinal herbs (*Alteranthera sessilis, Eclipta alba* and *Cissus quadrangularis*) on growth and biochemical parameters of the freshwater prawn *Macrobrachium rosenbergii*. *Aquaculture International*, **22**, 551–572.

Raja Rajeswari, P., Velmurugan, S., Babu, M.M., Dhas, S.A., Kesavan, K. and Citarasu, T. (2012) A study on the influence of selected Indian herbal active principles on enhancing the immune system in *Fenneropenaeus indicus* against *Vibrio harveyi* infection. *Aquaculture International*, **20**, 1009–1020.

Rajendiran, A., Natarjan, E. and Subramanian, P. (2008) Control of *Aeromonas hydrophila* infection in spotted snakehead *Channa punctatus*, by *Solanum nigrum* L., a medicinal plant. *Journal of the World Aquaculture Society*, **39**, 375–383.

Rajeswari, P.R., Velmurugan, S., Babu, M.M., Dhas, S.A., Kesavan, K. and Citarasu, T. (2012) A study on the influence of selected Indian herbal active principles on enhancing the immune system in *Fenneropenaeus indicus* against *Vibrio harveyi* infection. *Aquaculture International*, **20**, 1009–1020.

Rattanachaikunsopon, P. and Phumkhachorn, P. (2009a) Potential of Chinese chive oil as a natural antimicrobial for controlling *Flavobacterium columnare* infection in Nile tilapia *Oreochromis niloticus*. *Fisheries Science*, **75**, 1431.

Rattanachaikunsopon, P. and Phumkhachorn, P. (2009b) Prophylactic effect of *Andrographis paniculata* extracts against *Streptococcus agalactiae* infection in Nile tilapia (*Oreochromis niloticus*). *Journal of Bioscience and Bioengineering*, **107**, 579–582.

Rattanachaikunsopon, P. and Phumkhachorn, P. (2010a) Assessment of synergistic efficacy of carvacrol and cymene against *Edwardsiella tarda* in vitro and in Tilapia (*Oreochromis niloticus*). *African Journal of Microbiology Research*, **4**, 420–425.

Rattanachaikunsopon, P. and Phumkhachorn, P. (2010b) Effect of *Cratoxylum formosum* on innate immune response and disease resistance against *Streptococcus agalactiae* in tilapia *Oreochromis niloticus*. *Fisheries Science*, **76**, 653–659.

Reverter, M., Bontemps, N., Lecchini, D., Banaigs, B. and Sasal, P. (2014) Use of plant extracts in fish aquaculture as an alternative to chemotherapy: current status and future perspectives. *Aquaculture*, **433**, 50–61.

Rico, A., Phu, T.M., Satapornvanit, K., *et al.* (2013) Use of veterinary medicines, feed additives and probiotics in four major internationally traded aquaculture species farmed in Asia. *Aquaculture*, **412–413**, 231–243.

Romero Ormazábal, J.M., Feijoó, C.G. and Navarrete Wallace, P.A. (2012) Antibiotics in aquacul ture – use, abuse and alternatives, in *Health and Environment in Aquaculture* (eds E.D. Carvalho, J.S. David and R.J. Silva), InTech, Croatia, p. 159.

Roomiani, L., Soltani, M., Akhondzadeh Basti, A., Mahmoodi, A., Taheri , Mirghaed, A. and Yadollahi, F. (2013) Evaluation of the chemical composition and in vitro antimicrobial activity of *Rosmarinus officinalis, Zataria multiflora, Anethum graveolens* and *Eucalyptus globulus* against *Streptococcus iniae*; the cause of zoonotic disease in farmed fish. *Iranian Journal of Fish Science*, **12**, 702–716.

Sahu, S., Das, B.K., Pradhan, J., Mohapatra, B.C., Mishra, B.K. and Sarangi, N. (2007) Effect of *Mangifera indica* kernel as a feed additive on immunity and resistance to *Aeromonas hydrophila* in *Labeo rohita* in fingerlings. *Fish and Shellfish Immunology*, **23**, 109–118.

Sahu, S., Das, B.K., Mishra, B.K. and Pradhan, J. (2008) Effect of dietary *Curcuma longa* on enzymatic and immunological profiles of rohu, Labeo rohita (Ham.), infected with *Aeromonas hydrophila*. *Aquaculture Research*, **39**, 1720–1730.

Sakai, M. (1999) Current research status of fish immunostimulants. *Aquaculture*, **172**, 63–92.

Sambasivam, S., Karpagam, G., Chandran, R. and Khan, S.A. (2003) Toxicity of leaf extract of yellow oleander *Thevetia nerifolia* on Tilapia. *Journal of Environmental Biology*, **24**, 201–204.

Schütz, K., Carle, R. and Schieber, A. (2006) Taraxacum – a review on its phytochemical and pharmacological profile. *Journal of Ethnopharmacology*, **107**, 313–323.

Seo, C.S. and Shin, H.K. (2015) Simultaneous determination of three sesquiterpene lactones in *Aucklandia lappa Decne* by high-performance liquid chromatography. *Pharmacognosy Magazine*, **11**, 562–566.

Seyfried, E.E., Newton, R.J., Iv, K.F.R., Pedersen, J.A. and McMahon, K.D. (2010) Occurrence of tetracycline resistance genes in aquaculture facilities with varying use of oxytetracycline. *Microbial Ecology*, **59**, 799–807.

Shangliang, T., Hetrick, F.M., Roberson, B.S. and Baya, A. (1990) The antibacterial and antiviral activity of herbal extracts for fish pathogens. *Journal of Ocean University of Qingdao*, **02**.

Shao, B., Xu, W., Dai, H., Tu, P., Li, Z. and Gao, X. (2004) A study on the immune receptors for polysaccharides from the roots of *Astragalus membranaceus*, a Chinese medicinal herb. *Biochemical and Biophysial Research Communications*, **320**, 1103–1111.

Sharma, A., Deo, A.D., Tandel Riteshkumar, S., Chanu, T.I. and Das, A. (2010) Effect of *Withania somnifera* (L. Dunal) root as a feed additive on immunological parameters and disease resistance to *Aeromonas hydrophila* in *Labeo rohita* (Hamilton) fingerlings. *Fish and Shellfish Immunology*, **29**, 508–512.

Sheikhzadeh, N., Nofouzi, K., Delazar, A. and Oushani, A.K. (2011) Immunomodulatory effects of decaffeinated green tea (*Camellia sinensis*) on the immune system of rainbow trout (Oncorhynchus mykiss). *Fish and Shellfish Immunology*, **31**, 1268–1269.

Sirirustananun, N., Chen, J.C., Lin, Y.C., *et al.* (2011) Dietary administration of a *Gracilaria tenuistipitata* extract enhances the immune response and resistance against *Vibrio alginolyticus* and white spot syndrome virus in the white shrimp *Litopenaeus vannamei*. *Fish and Shellfish Immunology*, **31**, 848–855.

Sivaram, V., Babu, M.M., Immanuel, G., Murugadass, S., Citarasu, T. and Marian, M. (2004) Growth and immune response of juvenil greasy groupers (*Epinephelus tauvina*) fed with herbal antibacterial active principle supplemented diets against *Vibrio harveyi* infections. *Aquaculture*, **237**, 9–20.

Sivasankar, L., Santhiya, A.V. and Kanaga, V. (2015) A review on plants and herbal extracts against viral diseases in aquaculture. *Journal of Medicinal Plants Studies*, **3**, 75–79.

Slaninová, I., Táborská, E., Bochoráková, H. and Slanina, J. (2001) Interaction of benzo[c]phenanthridine and protoberberine alkaloids with animal and yeast cells. *Cell Biology and Toxicology*, **17**, 51–63.

Soltani, M., Sheikhzadeh, N., Ebrahimzadeh-Mousavi, H.A. and Zargar, A. (2010) Effects of *Zataria multiflora* essential oil on innate immune responses of common carp (*Cyprinus carpio*). *Journal of Fisheries and Aquatic Science*, **5**, 191–199.

Srivastava, J., Chandra, H., Nautiyal, A.R. and Kalra, S.J.S. (2014) Antimicrobial resistance (AMR) and plant-derived antimicrobials (PDAms) as an alternative drug line to control infections. *3 Biotech*, **4**, 451–460.

Sudhakaran, D.S., Srirekha, P., Devasree, L.D., Premsingh, S. and Michael, R.D. (2006) Immunostimulatory effect of *Tinospora cordifolia* Miers leaf extract in *Oreochromis mossambicus*. *Indian Journal of Experimental Biology*, **44**, 726–732.

Sukoso, Nursyam, H., Sy, S.R. and Sormin, R.B.D. (2012) Study antibacterial and cytotoxic activities of seaweed *Porphyra* sp. extract. *International Journal of Current Research*, **4**, 141–143.

Syahidah, A., Saad, C.R., Daud, H.M. and Abdelhadi, Y.M. (2015) Status and potential of herbal applications in aquaculture: a review. *Iranian Journal of Fisheries Sciences*, **14**, 27–44.

Takaoka, O., Ji, S.C., Ishimaru, K., *et al.* (2011) Effect of rotifer enrichment with herbal extracts on growth and resistance of red sea bream, *Pagrus major* (Temminck & Schlegel) larvae against *Vibrio anguillarum*. *Aquaculture Research*, **42**, 1824–1829.

Talpur, A.D., Ikhwanuddin, M. and Ambok Bolong, A.M. (2013) Nutritional effects of ginger (*Zingiber officinale Roscoe*) on immune response of Asian sea bass, *Lates calcarifer* (Bloch) and disease resistance against *Vibrio harveyi*. *Aquaculture*, **400–401**, 46–52.

Tanekhy, M. and Fall, J. (2015) Expression of innate immunity genes in kuruma shrimp *Marsupenaeus japonicus* after in vivo stimulation with garlic extract (allicin). *Veterinární Medicína*, **60**, 39–47.

Tang, W. and Eisenbrand, G. (1992) *Chinese Drugs of Plant Origin*, Springer Verlag, Berlin.

Trinh, Q. and Le, L. (2014) An investigation of antidiabetic activities of bioactive compounds in *Euphorbia hirta Linn* using molecular docking and pharmacophore. *Medicinal Chemistry Research*, **23**, 2033–2045.

Tu, X., Ling, F., Huang, A., Zhang, Q. and Wang, G. (2013) Anthelmintic efficacy of *Santalum album* (Santalaceae) against monogenean infections in goldfish. *Parasitology Research*, **112**, 2839–2845.

Umeda, N., Nibe, H., Hara, T. and Hirazawa, N. (2006) Effects of various treatments on hatching of eggs and viability of oncomiracidia of the monogenean *Pseudodactylogyrus anguillae* and *Pseudodactylogyrus bini*. *Aquaculture*, **253**, 148–153.

Van Hai, N. (2015) The use of medicinal plants as immunostimulants in aquaculture: a review. *Aquaculture*, **446**, 88–96.

Vasudeva Rao, Y., Das, B.K., Jyotyrmayee, P. and Chakrabarti, R. (2006) Effect of *Achyranthes aspera* on the immunity and survival of *Labeo rohita* infected with *Aeromonas hydrophila*. *Fish and Shellfish Immunology*, **20**, 263–273.

Walterová, D., Ulrichová, J., Válka, I., *et al.* (1995) Benzo[c]phenanthridine alkaloids sanguinarine and chelerythrine: biological activities and dental care applications. *Biomedical Papers of the Medical Faculty of the University Palacky, Olomouc, Czech Republic*, **139**, 7–16.

Wang, G.X., Han, J., Zhao, L.W., Jiang, D.X., Liu, Y.T. and Liu, X.L. (2010a) Anthelmintic activity of steroidal saponins from *Paris polyphylla*. *Phytomedicine*, **17**, 1102–1105.

Wang, G.X., Zhou, Z., Jiang, D.X., *et al.* (2010b) *In vivo* anthelmintic activity of five alkaloids from *Macleaya microcarpa* (Maxim) Fedde against *Dactylogyrus intermedius* in *Carassius auratus*. *Veterinary Parasitology*, **171**, 305–313.

Wang, Q.K., Chen, C.X., Guo, Y.J., *et al.* (2011) Dietary polysaccharide from *Angelica sinensis* enhanced cellular defence responses and disease resistance of grouper *Epinephelus malabaricus*. *Aquaculture International*, **19**, 945–956.

Wang, Y., Wu, Z.F., Wang, G.X., *et al.* (2011) *In vivo* anthelmintic activity of bruceine A and bruceine D from *Brucea javanica* against *Dactylogyrus intermedius* (Monogenea) in goldfish (*Carassius auratus*). *Veterinary Parasitology*, **177**, 127–133.

Wei, L.S., Musa, N., Sengm, C.T., Wee, W. and Shazili, N.A.M. (2008) Antimicrobial properties of tropical plants against 12 pathogenic bacteria isolated from aquatic organisms. *African Journal of Biotechnology*, **7**, 2275–2278.

Wei, W.X., Pan, Y.J., Zhang, H., Lin, C.W. and Wei, T.Y. (2004) Two new compounds from *Phyllanthus niruri*. *Chemistry of Natural Compounds*, **40**, 460–464.

Whittington, I.D. (2012) *Benedenia seriolae* and *Neobenedenia species*, in *Fish Parasites: Pathobiology and Protection* (eds P.T.K. Woo and K. Buchmann), CABI, Wallingford, pp. 225–244.

Won, K.M., Kim, P.K., Lee, S.H. and Park, S.I. (2008) Effect of the residuum extract of Siberian ginseng *Eleutherococcus senticosus* on non-specific immunity in olive flounder *Paralichthys olivaceus*. *Fisheries Science*, **74**, 635–641.

World Health Organization (2006) *WHO Briefing on Malaria Treatment Guidelines and Artemisinin Monotherapies*, WHO, Geneva.

Wu, C.C., Liu, C.H., Chang, Y.P. and Hsieh, S.L. (2010) Effects of hot-water extract of *Toona sinensis* on immune response and resistance to *Aeromonas hydrophila* in *Oreochromis mossambicus*. *Fish and Shellfish Immunology*, **29**, 258–263.

Wu, Y.R., Gong, Q.F., Fang, H., Liang, W.W., Chen, M. and He, R.J. (2013) Effect of *Sophora flavescens* on non-specific immune response of tilapia (GIFT *Oreochromis niloticus*) and disease resistance against *Streptococcus agalactiae*. *Fish and Shellfish Immunology*, **34**, 220–227.

Wu, Z.F., Zhu, B., Wang, Y., Lu, C. and Wang, G.X. (2011) In vivo evaluation of anthelmintic potential of medicinal plant extracts against *Dactylogyrus intermedius* (Monogenea) in goldfish (*Carassius auratus*). *Parasitology Research*, **108**, 1557–1563.

Xie, J., Liu, B., Zhou, Q., *et al.* (2008) Effects of anthraquinone extract from rhubarb *Rheum officinale* Bail on the crowding stress response and growth of common carp *Cyprinus carpio* var. Jian. *Aquaculture*, **281**, 5–11.

Xue-Gang, H., Lei, L., Cheng, C., Kun, H., Xian-Le, Y. and Gao-Xue, W. (2013) In vitro screening of Chinese medicinal plants for antifungal activity against *Saprolegnia* sp. and *Achlya klebsiana*. *North American Journal of Aquaculture*, **75**, 468–473.

Yao, J.Y., Zhou, Z.M., Pan, X., *et al.* (2011) *In vivo* anthelmintic activity of chelidonine from *Chelidonium majus* L. against *Dactylogyrus intermedius* in *Carassius auratus*. *Parasitology Research*, **109**, 1465–1469.

Yeh, S.T., Lee, C.S. and Chen, J.C. (2006) Administration of hot-water extract of brown seaweed *Sargassum duplicatum* via immersion and injection enhances the immune resistance of white shrimp *Litopenaeus vannamei*. *Fish and Shellfish Immunology*, **20**, 332–345.

Yi, Y.L., Lu, C., Hu, X.G., Ling, F. and Wang, G.X. (2012) Antiprotozoal activity of medicinal plants against *Ichthyophthirius multifiliis* in goldfish (*Carassius auratus*). *Parasitology Research*, **111**, 1771–1778.

Yogeeswaran, A., Velmurugan, S., Punitha, S.M.J., *et al.* (2012) Protection of *Penaeus monodon* against white spot syndrome virus by inactivated vaccine with herbal immunostimulants. *Fish and Shellfish Immunology*, **32**, 1058–1067.

Yoshida, T., Kruger, R. and Inglis, V. (1995) Augmentation of non-specific protection in African catfish, *Clarias gariepinus* (Burchell), by the long-term oral administration of immunostimulants. *Journal of Fish Diseases*, **18**, 195–198.

Yuan, C., Li, D., Chen, W., *et al.* (2007) Administration of a herbal immunoregulation mixture enhances some immune parameters in carp (*Cyprinus carpio*). *Fish Physiology and Biochemistry*, **33**, 93–101.

Zbakh, H., Chiheb, H., Bouziane, H., Sánchez, V.M. and Riadi, H. (2012) Antibacterial activity of benthic marine algae extracts from the mediterranean coast of Morocco. *Journal of Microbiology, Biotechnology and Food Science*, **2**, 219–228.

Zhang, J., Hu, X., Gao, W., *et al.* (2014) Pharmacokinetic study on costunolide and dehydrocostuslactone after oral administration of traditional medicine *Aucklandia lappa Decne.* by LC/MS/MS. *Journal of Ethnopharmacology*, **151**, 191–197.

Zheng, Z.I., Tan, J.Y.W., Liu, H.Y., Zhou, X.H., Xiang, X. and Wang K.Y. (2009) Evaluation of oregano essential oil (*Origanum heracleoticum* L.) on growth, antioxidant effect and resistance against *Aeromonas hydrophila* in channel catfish (*Ictalurus punctatus*). *Aquaculture*, **292**, 214–218.

10

Antibiotics and Disinfectants

Brian Austin

Institute of Aquaculture, University of Stirling, Stirling, Scotland, UK

Introduction

A diverse range of compounds, including antibiotics and disinfectants, are used in aquaculture (Gräslund *et al.*, 2003; Tonguthai, 2000), although there has been a move away from the use of medically important compounds, notably antibiotics, and chemicals for which health risks have been identified. In the case of antibiotics, the reasons stem from concerns about the acquisition and transfer of resistance to human and veterinary pathogens, the accumulation of tissue residues and their implications for human health (including issues with allergies) (Meek *et al.*, 2015), and environmental issues such as interference with the natural microflora (Cabello, 2006). Use of some chemicals has been discontinued for health and environmental reasons; an example is malachite green, which used to be a favoured and successful broad-spectrum treatment for fungal and protozoan infections, but has been linked to potential toxicity, carcinogenicity, mutagenity and teratogenicity issues (Mitrowska and Posyniak, 2005). A wide range of medically and veterinary inhibitory compounds have been used in aquaculture. Although the use of such compounds in aquaculture has generally declined, many products are still employed, although aquaculturists need to be careful as the presence of antibiotics in fish tissues would most likely lead to the imposition of trade restrictions in many countries.

The use of antimicrobial compounds in aquaculture started with Gutsell (1946), who recognized the role of sulfonamides for the control of furunculosis. This started the heyday of antimicrobial use, and the lack of interest in alternative means of disease control, until issues with resistance started affecting disease control. Rucker *et al.* (1951) identified sulfadiazine as an effective therapeutant for bacterial kidney disease (BKD). Then, potentiated sulfonamides – using trimethoprim as the potentiator – were developed, and are still used commercially in aquaculture. After the sulfonamides, the range of antibiotic-like compounds increased quickly to include chloramphenicol (a medically important antibiotic for the control of typhoid fever) (Wold, 1950), oxytetracycline (this remains a widely used antibiotic in aquaculture) (Snieszko and Griffin, 1951), kanamycin (Conroy, 1961), nifurprazine (Shiraki *et al.*, 1970), oxolinic acid (Endo *et al.*, 1973), sodium nifurstyrenate (Kashiwagi *et al.*, 1977a,b), flumequine (Michel *et al.*, 1980) and enrofloxacin (= Baytril) (Bragg and Todd, 1988).

Diagnosis and Control of Diseases of Fish and Shellfish, First Edition. Edited by Brian Austin and Aweeda Newaj-Fyzul.

Antibiotics

The preferred method of application of antibiotics to aquatic animals is orally on feed (Table 10.1). The provisos are that the fish are actively feeding (this is not always the case as inappetance is a feature of numerous diseases) and the compound is palatable. With this method, the compounds are mixed with feed, possibly in the presence of a binder, and administered to the animals at a predetermined dose over a number of days. The first decision is whether the medicated diet should be given over the full feeding period or restricted to one or two feeds per days; normal feed would be administered for the remainder of each day. Generally, medicated feed tends to be stable (McCracken and Fidgeon, 1977), and if sensible feeding regimes are adopted then there will be minimal waste, that is, the animals will consume all the diet and therefore release of the bioactive compounds into the environment will be minimized, although there will be some leaching during the feeding process. Examples of the dosages of commonly used compounds are included in Table 10.2.

Bioencapsulation of the inhibitory compounds has been researched (Duis *et al.*, 1995), including the use of *Artemia* nauplii, which have been used with a range of products, including sulfamethoxazole and trimethoprim (Touraki *et al.*, 1996). Application to sea bass larvae followed by *Vibrio anguillarum* challenge led to enhanced survival (Touraki *et al.*, 1996). Bioencapsulation may be effective in allowing the bioactive compounds to survive passage through the stomach to the intestine where uptake across the wall and into the main body of the host will occur. Also, bioactive compounds may be protected in liposomes, which may target the compounds to particular organs.

Chemotherapy Regimes

Bacterial Kidney Disease (BKD)

Some success has been achieved with erythromycin, which was dosed at 100 mg of drug/kg body weight of fish/day for 21 days (Wolf and Dunbar, 1959), penicillin (Decew, 1972) and enrofloxacin (Hsu *et al.*, 1994). In feeding trials using 20 mg of enrofloxacin/kg body

Table 10.1 Application of antimicrobial compounds to aquatic animals.

Method	Comments
Oral/bioencapsulation	Need palatable products
Injection	Feasible for large and/or valuable (pet) fish; requires anaesthesia and is therefore slow
Topical	Used for treatment of surface lesions, such as ulcers, on valuable/pet fish
Likely to result in environmental concerns:	
Bath	Need for fairly lengthy exposure to dilute solution/suspension of the compound in water; concern about disposal of used compound
Dip	Brief immersion in high concentration of compound; concern about disposal of used compound
Flush	Brief exposure to fish; the compound is flushed through the aquaculture facility by the water flow, leading to concerns about environmental pollution

Table 10.2 Methods of administering commonly used antimicrobial compounds.

Antimicrobial compound	Diseases controlled	Method(s) of administration
Antibiotics/antimicrobial compounds		
Amoxicillin	Furunculosis, gill disease	60–80 mg/kg body weight/day for 10 days
Doxycycline	Streptococcosis	20 mg/kg body weight/day for an unspecified duration
Enrofloxacin	BKD, furunculosis	10 or 20 mg/kg body weight/day for 10 days
Erythromycin	BKD, streptococcosis	25–100 mg/kg body weight/day for 4–21 days 20 mg of erythromycin/kg of brood stock by injection
Florfenicol	Furunculosis	10 mg/kg body weight/day for 10 days
Flumequine	Furunculosis, enteric redmouth, vibriosis	6 mg/kg of fish/day for 6 days
Furanace	Coldwater disease, columnaris, fin/tail rot, gill disease, haemorrhagic septicaemia, vibriosis	a) 2–4 mg/kg of fish/day for 3–5 days b) 0.5–1 mg/L water for 5-10 min, as a bath
Furazolidone	Carp erythrodermatitis, furunculosis, vibriosis	25–75 mg/kg of fish/day for up to 20 days
Oxolinic acid	Columnaris, enteric redmouth, furunculosis, haemorrhagic septicaemia, vibriosis	a) 10 mg/kg of fish/day for 10 days b) 1 mg/L of water, as a bath for 24 h (recommended for columnaris)
Oxytetracycline	*Acinetobacter* disease, coldwater disease, columnaris, edwardsiellosis, emphysematous putrefactive disease, enteric redmouth, enteric septicaemia, fin rot, furunculosis, gaffkemia, gill disease, haemorrhagic septicaemia, saltwater columnaris, streptococcosis, ulcer disease	50–75 mg/kg of fish/day for 10 days (doses of 300 mg/kg of fish/day for indefinite periods are used to treat rainbow trout fry syndrome)
Potentiated sulfonamide	Enteric redmouth, furunculosis, haemorrhagic septicaemia, vibriosis	30 mg/kg of fish/day for 10 days
Sulfonamides (sulfisoxazole, sulfamerazine, sulfamethazine)	BKD, coldwater disease, columnaris, enteric redmouth, furunculosis, haemorrhagic septicaemia, mycobacteriosis, nocardiosis, vibriosis	100–200 mg/kg/day for 10–20 days
Vancomycin	Gaffkemia	25 mg/kg of lobster by injection through the carapace
Disinfectants		
Acriflavine	Columnaris	5–25 mg/L in water for up to several days; 5–10 mg/L for 24 h (aquarium fish). 100 mg/L for 3–5 sec (eggs)

(*continued*)

Table 10.2 (Continued)

Antimicrobial compound	Diseases controlled	Method(s) of administration
Benzalkonium chloride	Fin/tail rot, gill disease, shrimp diseases	1–2, or 200 mg/L of water for 1 h or 20–30 min, respectively
Chloramine B or T	Fin/tail rot, gill disease	18–20 mg/L of water at pH 7.5–8.0 for 2–3 days
Copper sulfate	*Aeromonas* septicaemia, fin/tail rot; shrimp diseases; protozoans	1% of total alkalinity; bath for 18 h; 40–50 mg/L for 20–30 min (protozoans); 0.5 mg/L for filamentous bacteria on shrimp
Formalin	Fin/tail rot; ciliates; monogeneans, shrimp diseases	25–30 mg/L for 15–60 min
Iodophors/iodine	*Acinetobacter* disease, BKD, flavobacteriosis, furunculosis, haemorr-hagic septicaemia, mycobacteriosis, IPN	25–200 mg of available iodine/L water for 5–15 min; 1–5 g/m^3 as a disinfectant for hatcheries and ponds; 50 mg of free iodine/L for 6 min to inactivate viruses
Lime	*Staphylococcus aureus*	250 mg/L of pond water every 4th day
Potassium permanganate	*A. hydrophila, Staphylococcus aureus*, columnaris, external monogeneans	1–5 mg/L for 5–10 min (may be used at 500 mg/L as a dip for aquarium fish
Quaternary ammonium compounds	Viral and bacterial pathogens	Hand sanitizer; disinfects plastic surfaces
Aqua Des Liquid[a)]	Bacteria, parasites, viruses (IPN)	1:200 (bacteria), 1:200 (viruses)
Steri 7 Xtra[b)]	Bacteria and viruses (Koi herpes virus)	1:20 for disinfecting nets
Ultraviolet light	Vegetative bacterial cells	3.4 mJ/cm^2
Vanoquat[c)]	Bacteria	Use at 1:100
Virasure[d)]	IPN, ISA, VHS, salmonid alphavirus, BKD, ERM, RTFS, furunculosis, winter ulcer disease, nocardiosis, mycobacteriosis, *Pasteurella* sp.	0.5% (bacteria and viruses; IPN); 4% for fungi; for surface disinfection use at 1% for bacteria and viruses, 4% for fungi with a contact time of 30 min

a) 5% peracteric acid, 20% hydrogen peroxide, acetic acid and some minor components.
b) 0.147% (w/w) didecyldimethylammonium chloride, 0.086% (w/w) benzalkonium chloride, 0.0854% (w/w) polyhexamethylene biguanide.
c) Alkyl dimethyl benzyl ammonium chloride, C_{12}-15 alcohol ethoxylate (7EO).
d) 30–50% pentapotassium bis(peroxymonosulfate)bis(sulfate), 10–25% malic acid, 5–10% sodium alkyl olefin sulfonates, 2.5–5% sulfamic acid, 2.5–5% NaCl.

BKD, bacterial kidney disease; ERM, enteric redmouth, IPN, infectious pancreatic necrosis; ISA, infectious salmon anaemia; RTFS, rainbow trout fry syndrome; VHS, viral haemorrhagic septicaemia.

weight/day for 10 days, there was reduced mortality – 43% and 72% mortality among the treated groups compared to 93% and 100% among the controls (Hsu *et al.*, 1994). Erythromycin, which was injected at a dose of 20 mg erythromycin/kg of broodstock, was effective at preventing vertical transmission of the pathogen (Brown *et al.*, 1990; Evelyn *et al.*, 1986; Lee and Evelyn 1994). Erythromycin phosphate, at 1–2 mg/L for 30 minutes, may be used for water hardening of eggs (Klontz, 1978). At best, antimicrobial compounds keep mortality rates of BKD under control, but clinical disease is likely to return upon cessation of treatment.

Chryseobacterium scophthalmum

Furazolidone was effective at controlling mortality in turbot when injected intraperitoneally at 50 mg/kg body weight of fish or by immersion in 50 mg/L for 30 minutes daily for 10 days (Mudarris and Austin, 1989).

Coldwater Disease/Rainbow Trout Fry Syndrome (RTFS)

Oxytetracycline (Winton *et al.*, 1983), sulfonamides (Amend *et al.*, 1965) and furanace (Holt *et al.*, 1975) have been recommended. For example, infected fry were dosed with furanace at 0.5 μg/mL for one hour on every third day.

Coldwater Vibriosis

Oxolinic acid has been used successfully to control mortality.

Columnaris

Therapeutic regimes have included the following:

- oxytetracycline fed at 50–100 mg/kg body weight/day for 10 days (Ferguson, 1977)
- oxolinic acid used orally at 10 mg/kg body weight/day for 10 days (Soltani *et al.*, 1995)
- sulfadiazine, sulfamerazine or sulfamethiazine, fed at 220 mg/kg body weight/day for 10 days (Wolf and Snieszko, 1963).

For external infections, oxytetracycline or chlortetracycline was used as a bath containing 26–60 mg/L for one hour (Wood, 1968).

Edwardsiellosis (*Edwardsiella ictaluri*)

Oxytetracycline fed at 2.5 g/45.4 kg of fish/day for 4–5 days reduced disease (Hawke, 1979).

Edwardsiellosis (*E. tarda*)

Feeding oxytetracycline at 55 mg g/kg body weight/day for 10 days has been successful, with mortality reducing within two days of initiating chemotherapy, although recovery is slow and survivors may exhibit scarring (Meyer and Bullock, 1973).

Enteric Redmouth (ERM)

Early success was achieved by feeding sulfamerazine (200 mg/kg body weight/day for three days) (Klontz and Huddleston, 1976; Rucker, 1966), followed by oxytetracycline (50 mg/kg body weight/day for three days). Bullock *et al.* (1983) reported the effectiveness of feeding sulfadimethoxime and ormetroprim (50 mg/kg body weight/day for five days). Bosse and Post (1983) favoured sulfadiazine and trimethoprim at only 1 mg/kg body weight/day for 14 days. Also, Bosse and Post recommended feeding with tiamulin at 5 mg/kg body weight/day for 14 days. Rodgers and Austin (1982) reported the benefit of using oxolinic acid, which was fed at 10 mg/kg body weight/day for 10 days.

Flavobacteriosis

Oxytetracycline was regarded as allowing some control of the disease (Acuigrup, 1980).

Flavobacterium johnsoniae

Oxolinic acid was suggested for chemotherapy (Carson *et al.*, 1993).

Francisellosis

Florfenicol is effective for the treatment of tilapia when dosed orally at 15 mg/kg body weight/day for 10 days (Soto *et al.*, 2010).

Furunculosis; Carp Erythrodermatitis; Goldfish Ulcer Disease

A wide range of compounds have been used with varying degrees of success, including:

- sulfamerazine dosed orally at 22 g/100 kg of fish/day (Snieszko, 1958a)
- oxytetracycline fed at 5–7 g/100 kg of fish/day (Snieszko, 1958a)
- florfenicol administered orally at 10 mg/kg body weight/day for 10 days (Nordmo *et al.*, 1994; Samuelsen *et al.*, 1998)
- enrofloxacin fed at 10 mg/kg body weight/day for 10 days (Hsu *et al.*, 1995)
- difloxacin, fed at 5 mg/kg body weight for five or 10 days, and 1.25 or 2.5 mg/kg body weight for 10 days (Elston *et al.*, 1995).

Enrofloxacin, which was administered as a single injection containing 5 mg enrofloxacin/kg of fish, has been effective with atypical *Aeromonas salmonicida* infections in tom cod (Williams *et al.*, 1997). External infections involving *A. salmonicida* were controlled by feeding 77 mg oxytetracycline/kg body weight/day for 10 days with mortality ceasing within four days of initiating treatment (Cipriano *et al.*, 1996).

Gaffkemia

Oxyetracycline (Bayer and Daniel, 1987) and vancomycin (Stewart and Arie, 1974; Stewart *et al.*, 2004) have been proposed for the control of gaffkemia caused by *Aerococcus viridans* subsp. *homari* in lobsters. Injection of 25 mg of vancomycin/kg of lobster was successful in controlling disease during the early stages of infection when bacterial numbers in the haemolymph were $<3 \times 10^4$/mL (Stewart and Arie, 1974).

Lactococcosis and Streptococcosis

Erythromycin, fed at 25 mg/kg body weight/day for 4–7 days, controlled streptococcosis in yellowtail (Kitao, 1982)., Similarly, doxycycline, dosed at 20 mg/kg body weight/day for an unspecified duration (Nakamura, 1982), josamycin (30 mg/kg body weight/day for three days or 20 mg/kg body weight/day for five days) (Kusuda and Takemaru, 1987; Takemaru and Kusuda, 1988) and sodium nifurstyrenate (50 mg/kg body weight/day for 3–5 days) (Kashiwagi *et al.*, 1977,1977) were successful. The fluoroquinolone enrofloxacin, fed at 5 or 10 mg/kg body weight/day for 10 days, led to a rapid reduction of mortality to 11% and 17% of treated fish compared to 55% and 40% of untreated controls, respectively (Stoffregen *et al.*, 1996). Also, amoxicillin was effective when fed at 80 mg/kg of fish/day for 12 days when mortality rates dropped from 96% to 6% in the experimental group of blue tilapia (Darwish and Hobbs, 2005).

Motile *Aeromonas* Septicaemia (*Aeromonas hydrophila*)

Oxytetracycline (Meyer, 1964) and enrofloxacin (Bragg and Todd, 1988) have been used successfully. It is noteworthy that enrofloxacin is effective even at low dosages, with the minimum inhibitory concentration reported as 0.002 µg/mL (Bragg and Todd, 1988).

Mycobacteriosis

It is controversial whether or not fish with mycobacteriosis should be destroyed. However, the use of chloramine B or T administered as a bath at 10 mg/L of tank water for 24 hours, after which the water should be changed, has been suggested (van Duijn, 1981).

Nocardiosis

It has been suggested that infected (pet) fish may be treated with sulfisoxazole fed at 2 mg/g of food, with an improvement being noticeable after 10 days of treatment although chemotherapy should be continued for 21 days (van Duijn, 1981).

Pasteurellosis

Fosfomycin fed at 40 mg/ kg body weight/day for five days has shown promise (Sano *et al.*, 1994).

Plesiomonas shigelloides

Potentiated sulfonamide comprising sulfadiazine (administered orally at 200 mg/kg of body weight/day for 10 days) and trimethoprim (dosed at 50 mg/kg body weight/day for 10 days) reduced mortality rates (Cruz *et al.*, 1986).

Rickettsiosis

Oxytetracycline has been used effectively for chemotherapy (Chern and Chao, 1994).

Sekiten byo; Red Spot

Nalidixic acid, oxolinic acid and piromidic acid have been suggested for chemotherapy (Jo, 1978).

Sporocytophaga sp.

Control was achieved using oxytetracycline or chlortetracycline, at 1 mg/L for one hour (Wood, 1968).

Staphylococcus aureus

Early mortality rates were controlled by bathing in potassium permanganate (1 ml/L) for 5–10 minutes. In addition, pond water was disinfected with 250 mg/L of lime and 1 mg/L of potassium permanganate every fourth day (Shah and Tyagi, 1986).

Staphylococcus epidermidis

Wang *et al.* (1996) suggested that erythromycin, fed at 20 mg/kg body weight/day for 10 days, was effective.

Tenacibaculum maritimum

Sodium nifurstyrenate applied orally (30 mg/kg body weight/day for four days) or by bathing (0.5 µg/µL for one hour) reduced mortality in yellowtail from 100% to 60.5% (Baxa *et al.*, 1988). Also, trimethoprim and amoxicillin (fed at 80 mg/kg body weight) have been recommended (Soltani *et al.*, 1995).

Vibriosis (*Vibrio anguillarum; V. ordalii*)
Furanace, nitrofurazone, oxolinic acid, oxytetracycline and sulfamerazine have been used successfully as feed additives.

Vibrio alginolyticus
Chloramphenicol, which was fed at 50 mg /kg body weight/day for an unspecified period, and nitrofurantoin (immersed in 50 mg/L of water for one hour) reduced mortality (Colorni *et al.*, 1981).

Vibrio harveyi
Oral oxytetracycline (Saeed, 1995) and immersion in nifurpirinol (0.1 mg/L for an unspecified period) (Kraxberger-Beatty *et al.*, 1990) have been recommended.

Vibrio pelagius
Feeding with oxytetracycline reduced mortality (Angulo *et al.*, 1992).

Vibrio splendidus
Flumequine was successful when used orally (Angulo *et al.*, 1994).

Disinfectants

There is an extensive literature pointing to the success of physical (e.g. temperature increases, ultraviolet light) and chemical agents for use in disinfection. Certainly, a wide range of chemicals have been used, including benzalkonium chloride, chloramine B and T, chlorine, formalin, hydrogen peroxide and iodophors and ozone for water, surfaces and/or equipment disinfection. In a comparison of iodophor, formalin, hydrogen peroxide and bronopol, bluefin sea bream fertilized eggs (14–16 hours after fertilization) were disinfected most effectively in terms of a reduction in bacterial numbers with the first mentioned (at 75 and 100 mg/L for four minutes). Moreover, there was the least effect on egg hatching and larval survival. However, immersion of lake sturgeon eggs in 50 mg of iodine/L for 30 minutes resulted in a substantial decline (average of 57.8%), but not complete elimination in viable bacterial numbers (Chalupnicki *et al.*, 2015). Formalin (100 and 150 mg/L) was second best, hydrogen peroxide less so, and bronopol the most disappointing (El-Dakour *et al.*, 2015). Ozone has been used successfully to disinfect fish eggs. Thus, Atlantic cod eggs were not adversely affected for up to 30 days post hatch by ozone at a dose of <3.0 mg/L for 90 seconds. Similarly, rainbow trout and Atlantic salmon eggs did not display any harmful effects on the subsequent larvae (Fry *et al.*, 2015).

Changes in salinity may adversely affect pathogens and parasites. Sato *et al.* (1982) used chlorine to disinfect water, and thus control infection by *Citrobacter freundii*. Newer developments include an electrochemical system using a honeycombed platinum-coated titanium electrode in which cell suspensions of *V. alginolyticus*, *V. anguillarum*, *E. tarda* and *Lactococcus garvieae* were inactivated in sea water within three hours (Tanaka *et al.*, 2013).

Soaking nets used to collect zebrafish in sodium hypochlorite for 30 minutes and in potassium peroxymonosulfate with sodium chloride for five or 30 minutes was effective for disinfection (Collymore *et al.*, 2014).

Disinfectant Regimes

Aeromonas Septicaemia; Fin/Tail Rot

Copper sulfate was effective for channel catfish when dosed at 1% of total alkalinity as a continuous bath for 18 hours (Bebak *et al.*, 2012).

Amoebic Gill Disease (AGD) and Sea Lice

Bathing salmon in fresh water is an effective control measure for AGD and sea lice (Powell *et al.*, 2015).

Bacterial Gill Disease

Chloramine T has been used successfully at 12 mg/L to control mortality attributed to bacterial gill disease (Bowker *et al.*, 2015).

Bacterial Kidney Disease

Egg disinfection with iodophors dosed at 25–100 mg/L for five minutes has been effective at reducing transmission of the disease although (egg) internal populations of the pathogen were not eliminated (Evelyn *et al.*, 1984). Fish farm water may be disinfected with 0.05 mg of free chlorine/L , which inactivated renibacterial cells in 18 seconds (Pascho *et al.*, 1995).

Botulism

Disinfection involves moving of stock to clean facilities, draining the ponds and removing sediment/detritus followed by the application of slaked lime at 1.6 kg/m^2 which needs to be worked well into the bottom of the ponds, left not less than seven days, and the pond then returned to use (Cann and Taylor, 1982).

Citrobacter freundii

Success was achieved using chlorine for water disinfection (Sato *et al.*, 1982).

Coldwater Disease

Increasing water temperature to 28 °C from 18 °C for three days controlled cold-water disease in ayu (Sugahara *et al.*, 2010), with a correlation to protective immunity, which was induced in the warmer waters (Sugahara and Eguchi, 2012).

Columnaris

Suggestions have included:

- a 30-second dip in 8% (w/v) sodium chloride cleared up an infection in rainbow trout fingerlings within a few days
- arsenic, cadmium, copper, lead and selenium mixture used at 1–3 μg/L for one day (MacFarlane *et al.*, 1986)
- copper sulfate – 1:2000 dilution for a 1–2-minute dip (Snieszko, 1958b)
- pyridylmercuric acetate 2 mg/L for one hour (Snieszko, 1958b)
- diquat 1–2 mg/L for 30–60 minutes (McCarthy, 1975)
- quaternary ammonium compounds 2 mg/L for one hour (McCarthy, 1975).

Chloramine T has been used successfully at 12 mg/L to control mortality (Bowker *et al.*, 2015).

Columnaris and *Ichthyobodo necator* – Concurrent Infections

Use of copper sulfate, dosed at 2.1 mg/L at 24-hour intervals on three consecutive days, led to significantly enhanced survival (73%, compared to 41.5% of controls) of channel catfish. Moreover, the populations of pathogens and parasites were significantly reduced. In comparison, potassium permanganate was less successful in terms of mortality and pathogen/parasite numbers (Farmer *et al.*, 2014).

Crayfish Plague

Thirty milligrams of Proxitane (peracetic acid)/L and 3 g of Virkon (potassium peroxymonosulfate), sodium dodecylbenzenesulfonate, sulfamic acid and inorganic buffers)/L but not hydrogen peroxide were effective against *Aphanomyces astaci* spores in both clean and dirty conditions (Jussila *et al.*, 2014). Mortality was reduced following bathing in chloramine T, hydrogen peroxide and potassium permanganate, but not copper sulfate and hydrogen peroxide (Bowker *et al.*, 2013; Thomas-Jinu and Goodwin, 2004). Also, sodium chloride baths may reduce mortality (Suomalainen *et al.*, 2005).

Flavobacterium johnsoniae

Acriflavine has been suggested (Carson *et al.*, 1993).

Gyrodactylus salaris

The parasite was eliminated from Atlantic salmon parr by 6–8 days following exposure to sodium hypochlorite-enriched water, containing 50 g chlorine/L. A lower dose of 18 g chlorine/L also led to elimination of the parasite after 6–8 days (Hagen *et al.*, 2014).

Infectious Haematopoietic Necrosis (IHN)

Infectious haematopoietic necrosis was inactivated rapidly at pH 3.0, and in iodine and sodium hypochlorite, but not completely with formalin (Torgersen and Håstein, 1995).

Infectious Pancreatic Necrosis (IPN)

Infectious pancreatic necrosis virus (IPNV) was inactivated, that is, >99.9% inactivation within five minutes, in acids and alkalis, oxygen-releasing products and halogens, but not quaternary ammonium compounds. In distilled water, 0.1 mg sodium hypochlorite/L inactivated IPNV within one minute (Torgersen and Håstein, 1995), 25 mg sodium hypochlorite/L inactivated 10^5 tissue culture infective dose (TCID)/mL of IPNV in 30 minutes but 40 mg/L was needed to inactivate 10^7 TCID/mL, also in 30 minutes. However, it was realized that the presence of organic material necessitated higher amounts of disinfectant to ensure inactivation of the virus (Desautels and MacKelvie, 1975).

Mycobacteriosis

For mycobacteriosis, 25 mg/L of povidone-iodine for five minutes was effective for disinfecting zebrafish embryos, but not so hydrogen peroxide or unbuffered chlorine bleach (Chang *et al.*, 2015).

Pseudomonas fluorescens

Immersion in 1–2 mg benzalkonium chloride/L water/1 hour or in 0.5–1 mg furanace/L water/5–10 minutes has been suggested.

Sporocytophaga sp.

Control was achieved using pyridylmercuric acetate and ethylmercuric phosphate, at 1 mg/L for one hour (Wood, 1968), and a two-minute dip in 1:2000 copper sulfate, which was repeated on three consecutive days (Anderson and Conroy, 1969).

Conclusion

Whereas many compounds have historically been used in aquaculture, growing concern about resistance, tissue residues and environmental damage is likely to result in even greater restrictions on their use in the future.

References

Acuigrup (1980) Flavobacteriosis in coho salmon (*Oncorhynchus kisutch*), in *Fish Diseases, Third COPRAQ Session* (ed. W. Ahne), Springer-Verlag, Berlin, pp.212–217.

Amend, D.F., Fryer, J.L. and Pilcher, K.S. (1965) Production trials utilizing sulfonamide drugs for the control of 'cold–water' disease in juvenile coho salmon. *Research Briefs, Fish Commission of Oregon*, **11**, 14–17.

Anderson, J.I.W. and Conroy, D.A. (1969) Myxobacteria as fish pathogens. *Journal of Applied Bacteriology*, **32**, 30–39.

Angulo, L., Lopez, J.E., Lema, C. and Vicente, J.A. (1992) *Vibrio pelagius* associated with mortalities in farmed turbot, *Scophthalmus maximus. Thalassas*, **10**, 129–133.

Angulo, L., Lopez, J.E., Vicente, J.A. and Saborido, A.M. (1994) Haemorrhagic areas in the mouth of farmed turbot, *Scophthalmus maximus* (L.). *Journal of Fish Diseases*, **17**, 163–169.

Baxa, D.V., Kawai, K. and Kusuda, R. (1988) Chemotherapy of *Flexibacter maritimus* infection. *Reports of the USA Marine Biological Institute, Kochi University*, **10**, 9–14.

Bayer, R.C. and Daniel, P.C. (1987) Safety and efficacy of oxytetracycline for control of gaffkemia in the American lobster *(Homarus americanus). Fisheries Research*, **5**, 71–81.

Bebak, J., Garcia, J.C. and Darwish, A. (2012) Effect of copper sulfate on *Aeromonas hydrophila* infection in channel catfish fingerlings. *North American Journal of Aquacultur*, **74**, 494–498.

Bosse, M.P. and Post, G. (1983) Tribrissen and tiamulin for control of enteric redmouth disease. *Journal of Fish Diseases*, **6**, 27–32.

Bowker, J.D., Carty, D., Trushenski, J.T., Bowman, M.P., Wandelear, N. and Matthews, M. (2013) Controlling mortality caused by external columnaris in largemouth bass and bluegill with chloramine-T and hydrogen peroxide. *North American Journal of Aquaculture*, **75**, 342–351.

Bowker, J.D., Carty, D.G., Trushenski, J.T., Glover, D.C. and Bowman, M.P. (2015) Considerations for consistently applying flow-through Chloramine-T treatments to hatchery raceways. *North American Journal of Aquaculture*, **77**, 524–531.

Bragg, R.R. and Todd, J.M. (1988) *In vitro* sensitivity to Baytril of some bacteria pathogenic to fish. *Bulletin of the European Association of Fish Pathologists*, **8**, 5.

Brown, L.L., Albright, L.J. and Evelyn, T.P.T. (1990) Control of vertical transmission of *Renibacterium salmoninarum* by injection of antibiotics into maturing female coho salmon *Oncorhynchus kisutch. Diseases of Aquatic Organisms*, **9**, 127–131.

Bullock, G.L., Maestrone, G., Starliper, C. and Schill, B. (1983) Potentiated sulfonamide therapy of enteric redmouth disease. *Canadian Journal of Fisheries and Aquatic Sciences*, **40**, 101–102.

Cabello, F.C. (2006) Heavy use of prophylactic antibiotics in aquaculture: a growing problem for human and animal health and for the environment. *Environmental Microbiology*, **8**, 1137–1144.

Cann, D. C. and Taylor, L. Y. (1982) An outbreak of botulism in rainbow trout, *Salmo gairdneri* Richardson, farmed in Britain. *Journal of Fish Diseases*, **5**, 393–399.

Carson, J., Schmidtke, L.M. and Munday, B.L. (1993) *Cytophaga johnsonae*: a putative skin pathogen of juvenile farmed barramundi, *Lates calcarifer* Bloch. *Journal of Fish Diseases*, **16**, 209–218.

Chalupnicki, M., Dittman, D., Starliper, C.E. and Iwanowicz, D.D. (2015) Efficacy of iodine for disinfection of lake sturgeon eggs from the St. Lawrence River, New York. *North American Journal of Aquaculture*, **77**, 82–89.

Chang, C.T., Colicino, E.G., DiPaola, E.J., Al-Hasnawi, H.J. and Whipps, C.M. (2015) Evaluating the effectiveness of common disinfectants at preventing the propagation of *Mycobacterium* spp. isolated from zebrafish. *Comparative Biochemistry and Physiology C Toxicology and Pharmacology*, **178**, 45–50.

Chern, R.S. and Chao, C.B. (1994) Outbreaks of disease caused by rickettsia-like organism in cultured tilapias in Taiwan. *Fish Pathology*, **29**, 61–71.

Cipriano, R.C., Ford, L.A., Starliper, C.E., Teska, J.D., Nelson, J.T. and Jensen, B.N. (1996) Control of external *Aeromonas salmonicida*: topical disinfection of salmonids with chloramine T. *Journal of Aquatic Animal Health*, **8**, 52–57.

Collymore, C., Porelli, G., Lieggi, C. and Lipman, N.S. (2014). Evaluation of 5 cleaning and disinfection methods for nets Used to collect zebrafish (*Danio rerio*). *Journal of the American Association for Laboratory Animal Science*, **53**, 657–660.

Colorni, A., Paperna, I. and Gordin, H. (1981) Bacterial infections in gilthead sea bream *Sparus aurata* cultured in Elat. *Aquaculture*, **23**, 257–267.

Conroy, D.A. (1961) Estudio in vitro de la Accion de la Kanamicina sobre bacterias patogenas para los peces. *Microbiología Española*, **14**, 147–155.

Cruz, J.M., Saraiva, A., Eiras, J.C., Branco, R. and Sousa, J.C. (1986) An outbreak of *Plesiomonas shigelloides* in farmed rainbow trout, *Salmo gairdneri* Richardson, in Portugal. *Bulletin of the European Association of Fish Pathologists*, **6**, 20–22.

Darwish, A.M. and Hobbs, M.S. (2005) Laboratory efficacy of amoxicillin for the control of *Streptoococcus iniae* infection in blue tilapia. *Journal of Aquatic Animal Health*, **17**, 197–202.

Decew, M.G. (1972) Antibiotic toxicity, efficacy and teratogenicity in adult spring chinook salmon *(Oncorhynchus tschawytscha). Journal of the Fisheries Research Board of Canada*, **29**, 1513–1517.

Desautels, D. and MacKelvie, R.M. (1975) Practical aspects of survival and destruction of infectious pancreatic necrosis virus. *Journal of the Fisheries Research Board of Canada*, **32**, 523–531.

Duis, K., Hammer, C., Beveridge, M.C.M., Inglis, V. and Braum, E. (1995) Delivery of quinolone antibacterials to turbot, *Scophthalmus maximus* (L.), via bioencapsulation: quantification and efficacy trial. *Journal of Fish Diseases*, **18**, 229–238.

El-Dakour, S., Saheb, A.I. and Al-Abdul, K. (2015) Effects of commonly used disinfectants on bacterial load, hatchability and survival of bluefin sea bream (*Sparidentex hasta*) eggs. *Aquaculture Research*, **46**, 1281–1291.

Elston, R., Drum, A.S. and Bunnell, P.R. (1995) Efficacy of orally administered difloxacin for the treatment of Atlantic salmon held in seawater. *Journal of Aquatic Animal Health*, **7**, 22–28.

Endo, T., Ogishima, K., Hayasaki, H., Kaneko, S. and Ohshima, S. (1973) Application of oxolinic acid as a chemotherapeutic agent for treating infectious diseases in fish. I. Antibacterial activity, chemotherapeutic effect and pharmacokinetic effect of oxolinic acid in fish. *Bulletin of the Japanese Society of Scientific Fisheries*, **3**, 165–171.

Evelyn, T.P.T., Ketcheson, J.E. and Prosperi-Porta, L. (1984) Further evidence for the presence of *Renibacterium salmoninarum* in salmonid eggs and for the failure of povidine-iodine to reduce the intra-ovum infection in water-hardened eggs. *Journal of Fish Diseases*, **7**, 173–182.

Evelyn, T.P.T., Ketcheson, J.E. and Prosperi-Porta, L. (1986) Use of erythromycin as a means of preventing vertical transmission of *Renibacterium salmoninarum*. *Diseases of Aquatic Organisms*, **2**, 7–11.

Farmer, B.D., Straus, D.L., Mitchell, A.J., Beck, B.H., Fuller, S.A. and Barnett, L.M. (2014) Comparative effects of copper sulfate or potassium permanganate on channel catfish concurrently infected with *Flavobacterium columnare* and *Ichthyobodo necator*. *Journal of Applied Aquaculture*, **26**, 71–83.

Ferguson, H.W. (1977) Columnaris disease in rainbow trout *(Salmo gairdneri)* in Northern Ireland. *Veterinary Record*, **101**, 55–56.

Fry, J., Casanova, J.P., Hamoutene, D., Lush, L., Walsh, A. and Couturier, C. (2015) The impact of egg ozonation on hatching success, larval growth, and survival of Atlantic cod, Atlantic salmon, and rainbow trout. *Journal of Aquatic Animal Health*, **27**, 57–64.

Gräslund, S., Holmström, K. and Wahlström, A. (2003) A field survey of chemicals and biological products used in shrimp farming. *Marine Pollution Bulletin*, **46**, 81–90.

Gutsell, J. (1946) Sulfa drugs and the treatment of furunculosis in trout. *Science*, **104**, 85–86.

Hagen, A.G., Hytterod, S. and Olstad, K. (2014) Low concentrations of sodium hypochlorite affect population dynamics in *Gyrodactylus salaris* (Malmberg, 1957): practical guidelines for the treatment of the Atlantic salmon, *Salmo salar* L. parasite. *Journal of Fish Diseases*, **37**, 1003–1011.

Hawke, J.P. (1979) A bacterium associated with disease of pond cultured channel catfish, *Ictalurus punctatus*. *Journal of the Fisheries Research Board of Canada*, **36**, 1508–1512.

Holt, R.A., Conrad, J.F. and Fryer, J.L. (1975) Furanace for control of *Cytophaga psychrophila* the causal agent of cold-water disease in coho salmon. *Progressive Fish Culturist*, **37**, 137–139.

Hsu, H.M., Wooster, G.A. and Bowser, P.R. (1994) Efficacy of enrofloxacin for the treatment of salmonids with bacterial kidney disease, caused by *Renibacterium salmoninarum*. *Journal of Aquatic Animal Health*, **3**, 220–223.

Hsu, H.M., Bowser, P.R., Schachte, J.H. Jr, Scarlett, J.M. and Babish, J.G. (1995) Winter field trials of enrofloxacin for the control of *Aeromonas salmonicida* infection in salmonids. *Journal of the World Aquaculture Society*, **26**, 307–314.

Jo, Y. (1978) Therapeutic experiments on red spot disease. *Fish Pathology*, **13**, 41–42.

Jussila, J., Toljamo, A., Makkonen, J., Kukkonen, H. and Kokko, H. (2014) Practical disinfection chemicals for fishing and crayfishing gear against crayfish plague transfer. *Knowledge and Management of Aquatic Ecosystems*, **413**, 02P1–02P8.

Kashiwagi, S., Sugimoto, N., Watanabe, K., Ohta, S. and Kusuda, R. (1977a) Chemotherapeutic studies on sodium nifurstyrenate against *Streptococcus* infection in cultured yellowtails – I. *In vitro* studies on sensitivity and bacteriocidal effect. *Fish Pathology*, **12**, 11–14.

Kashiwagi, S., Sugimoto, N., Ohta, S. and Kusuda, R. (1977b) Chemotherapeutical studies on sodium nifurstyrenate against *Streptococcus* infection in cultured yellowtail – II. Effect of sodium nifurstyrenate against experimental streptococcal infection. *Fish Pathology*, **12**, 157–162.

Kitao, T. (1982) Erythromycin – the application to streptococcal infection in yellowtails. *Fish Pathology*, **17**, 77–85.

Klontz, G. (1978) Prevention of bacterial kidney disease in adult and juvenile salmonids. *Proceedings of the Joint 3rd Biennial Fish Health Section and 9th Annual Midwest Fish Disease Workshops*, Kansas City, 11–14.

Klontz, G.W. and Huddleston, T.R. (1976) *Control of Enteric Redmouth Disease. A Twelve Month Activity Report on Contract 10690004 DEMO–1014*, University of Idaho, Moscow.

Kraxberger-Beatty, T., McGarey, D.J., Grier, H.J. and Lim, D.V. (1990) *Vibrio harveyi*, an opportunistic pathogen of common snook, *Centropomus undecimalis* (Block), held in captivity. *Journal of Fish Diseases*, **13**, 557–560.

Kusuda, R. and Takemaru, I. (1987) Efficacy of josamycin against experimental streptococcal infection in cultured yellowtail. *Nippon Suisan Gakkaishi*, **53**, 1519–1523.

Lee, E.G.H. and Evelyn, T.P.T. (1994) Prevention of vertical transmission of the bacterial kidney disease agent *Renibacterium salmoninarum* by broodstock injection with erythromycin. *Diseases of Aquatic Organisms*, **18**, 1–4.

MacFarlane, R.D., Bullock, G.L. and McLaughlin, J.J.A. (1986) Effects of five metals on susceptibility of striped bass to *Flexibacter columnaris*. *Transactions of the American Fisheries Society*, **115**, 227–231.

McCarthy, D.H. (1975) Columnaris disease. *Journal of the Institute of Fisheries Management*, **6**, 44–47.

McCracken, A. and Fidgeon, S. (1977) The effect of storage on drugs incorporated into pelleted fish food. *Journal of Applied Bacteriology*, **42**, 289–290.

Meek, R.W., Vyas, H. and Piddock, L.J.V. (2015) Nonmedical uses of antibiotics: time to restrict their use? *PLOS Biology*, **13**, e1002266.

Meyer, F.P. (1964) Field treatments of *Aeromonas liquefaciens* infections in golden shiners. *Progressive Fish Culturist*, **26**, 33–35.

Meyer, F.P. and Bullock, G.L. (1973) *Edwardsiella tarda*, a new pathogen of channel catfish *(Ictalurus punctatus)*. *Applied Microbiology*, **25**, 155–156.

Michel, C., Gerard, J.P., Fourbet, B., Collas, R. and Chevalier, R. (1980) Emploi de la flumequine contre la furunculose des salmonides; essais therapeutiques et perspectives pratiques. *Bulletin Français de Pisciculture*, **52**, 154–162.

Mitrowska, K. and Posyniak, A. (2005) Malachite green: pharmacological and toxicological aspects and residue control. *Medycyna Weterynaryjna*, **61**, 742–745.

Mudarris, M. and Austin, B. (1989) Systemic disease in turbot *Scophthalmus maximus* caused by a previously unrecognised *Cytophaga*-like bacterium. *Diseases of Aquatic Organisms*, **6**, 161–166.

Nakamura, Y. (1982) Doxycycline. *Fish Pathology*, **17**, 67–76.

Nordmo, R., Varma, K.J., Sutherland, I.H. and Brokken, E.S. (1994) Florfenicol in Atlantic salmon, *Salmo salar* L.: field evaluation of efficacy against furunculosis in Norway. *Journal of Fish Diseases*, **17**, 239–244.

Pascho, R.J., Landolt, M.L. and Ongerth, J.E. (1995) Inactivation of *Renibacterium salmoninarum* by free chlorine. *Aquaculture*, **131**, 165–175.

Powell, M.D., Reynolds, P. and Kristensen, T. (2015) Freshwater treatment of amoebic gill disease and sea-lice in seawater salmon production: considerations of water chemistry and fish welfare in Norway. *Aquaculture*, **448**, 18–28.

Rodgers, C.J. and Austin, B. (1982) Oxolinic acid for control of enteric redmouth disease in rainbow trout. *Veterinary Record*, **112**, 83.

Rucker, R.R. (1966) Redmouth disease of rainbow trout *(Salmo gairdneri)*. *Bulletin de l'Office International des Epizooties*, **65**, 825–830.

Rucker, R.R., Bernier, A.F., Whipple, W.J. and Burrows, R.E. (1951) Sulfadiazine for kidney disease. *Progressive Fish Culturist*, **13**, 135–137.

Saeed, M.O. (1995) Association of *Vibrio harveyi* with mortalities in cultured marine fish in Kuwait. *Aquaculture*, **136**, 21–29.

Samuelsen, O.B., Hjeltnes, B. and Glette, J. (1998) Efficacy of orally administered florfenicol in the treatment of furunculosis in Atlantic salmon. *Journal of Aquatic Animal Health*, **10**, 56–61.

Sano, M., Nakano, H., Kimura, T. and Kusuda, R. (1994) Therapeutic effect of fosfomycin on experimentally induced pseudotuberculosis in yellowtail. *Fish Pathology*, **29**, 187–192.

Sato, N., Yamane, N. and Kawamura, T. (1982) Systemic *Citrobacter freundii* infection among sunfish *Mola mola* in Matsushima aquarium. *Bulletin of the Japanese Society of Scientific Fisheries*, **48**, 1551–1557.

Shah, K.L. and Tyagi, B.C. (1986) An eye disease in silver carp, *Hypophthalmichthys molitrix*, held in tropical ponds, associated with the bacterium *Staphylococcus aureus*. *Aquaculture*, **55**, 1–4.

Shiraki, K., Miyamoto, F., Sato, T., Sonezaki, I. and Sano, K. (1970) Studies on a new chemotherapeutic agent nifurprazine (HB-115) against infectious diseases. Part 1. *Fish Pathology*, **4**, 130–137.

Snieszko, S.F. (1958a) *Fish Furunculosis*. Fishery Leaflet 467. United States Fish and Wildlife Service, Washington, D.C.

Snieszko, S.F. (1958b) *Columnaris Disease of Fishes*. Fishery Leaflet 46. United States Fish and Wildlife Service, Washington, D.C.

Snieszko, S.F. and Griffin, P.J. (1951) Successful treatment of ulcer disease in brook trout with terramycin. *Science*, **112**, 717–718.

Soltani, M., Shanker, S. and Munday, B.L. (1995) Chemotherapy of *Cytophaga/Flexibacter*-like bacteria (CFLB) infections in fish: studies validating clinical efficacies of selected antimicrobials. *Journal of Fish Diseases*, **18**, 555–565.

Soto, E., Endris, R.G. and Hawke, J.P. (2010) *In vitro* and *in vivo* efficacy of florfenicol for treatment of *Francisella asiatica* infection of tilapia. *Antimicrobial Agents and Chemotherapy*, **54**, 4664–4670.

Stewart, J.E. and Arie, B. (1974) Effectiveness of vancomycin against gaffkemia, bacterial disease of lobsters (genus *Homarus*). *Journal of the Fisheries Research Board of Canada*, **31**, 1873–1879.

Stewart, J.E., Arie, B. and Marks, L.J. (2004) Induced resistance to infection of lobsters *Homarus americanus* by *Aerococcus viridans* (var.) homari, the bacterium causing gaffkemia. *Diseases of Aquatic Organisms*, **62**, 197–204.

Stoffregen, D.A., Backman, S.C., Perham, R.E., Bowser, P.R. and Babish, J.G. (1996) Initial disease report of *Streptococcus iniae* infection in hybrid striped (sunshine) bass and successful therapeutic intervention with the fluoroquinolone antibacterial enrofloxacin. *Journal of the World Aquaculture Society*, **27**, 420–434.

Sugahara, K. and Eguchi, M. (2012) The use of warmed water treatment to induce protective immunity against the bacterial cold-water disease pathogen *Flavobacterium psychrophilum* in ayu (*Plecoglossus altivelis*). *Fish and Shellfish Immunology*, **32**, 489–493.

Sugahara, K., Fujiwara-Nagata, E. and Eguchi, M. (2010) Dynamics of the bacterial cold-water disease pathogen, *Flavobacterium psychrophilum*, in infected fish organs and rearing water after warmed water treatment. *Fish Pathology*, **45**, 58–65.

Suomalainen, L.R., Tiirola, M. and Valtonen, E.T. (2005) Treatment of columnaris disease of rainbow trout: low pH and salt as possible tools. *Diseases of Aquatic Organisms*, **65**, 115–120.

Takemaru, I. and Kusuda, R. (1988) Chemotherapeutic effect of josamycin against natural streptococcal infection in cultured yellowtail. *Bulletin of the Japanese Society of Scientific Fisheries*, **54**, 1849.

Tanaka, T., Shimoda, M., Shionoiri, N., et al. (2013) Electrochemical disinfection of fish pathogens in seawater without the production of a lethal concentration of chlorine using a flow reactor. *Journal of Bioscience and Bioengineering*, **116**, 480–484.

Thomas-Jinu, S. and Goodwin, A.E. (2004) Acute columnaris infection in channel catfish, *Ictalurus punctatus* (Rafinesque): efficacy of practical treatment for warmwater aquaculture ponds. *Journal of Fish Diseases*, **27**, 23–28.

Tonguthai, K. (2000) *The use of chemicals in aquaculture in Thailand, in* Use of Chemicals in Aquaculture in Asia: Proceedings of the Meeting on the Use of Chemicals in Aquaculture in Asia (eds J.R. Arthur, C.R. Lavilla-Pitogo and R.P. Subasinghe), 20–22 May 1996, Tigbauan, Iloilo, Philippines, pp. 207–220.

Torgersen, Y. and Håstein, T. (1995) Disinfection in aquaculture. *Scientific and Technical Review of the Office International des Epizooties*, **14**, 419–434.

Touraki, M., Mourelatos, S., Karamanlidou, G., Kalaitzopoulou, S. and Kastritsis, C. (1996) Bioencapsulation of chemotherapeutics in *Artemia* as a means of prevention and treatment of infectious disease in marine fish fry. *Aquacultural Engineering*, **15**, 133–147.

Van Duijn, C. (1981) Tuberculosis in fishes. *Journal of Small Animal Practice*, **22**, 391–411.

Wang, W.S., Chang, Y.C., Shieh, M.T. and Lin, C.C. (1996) *Staphylococcus epidermidis* and cestode infection of cultured grass carp *(Ctenopharyngodon idella)* in Taiwan. *Reports on Fish Disease Research*, **17**, 57–63.

Williams, P.J., Courtenay, S.C. and Vardy, C. (1997) Use of enrofloxacin to control atypical *Aeromonas salmonicida* in Atlantic tom cod. *Journal of Aquatic Animal Health*, **9**, 216–222.

Winton, J.R., Rohovec, J.S. and Fryer, J.L. (1983) Bacterial and viral diseases of cultured salmonids in the Pacific Northwest, in *Bacterial and Viral Diseases of Fish: Molecular Studies* (ed. J.H. Crosa), University of Washington, pp.1–20.

Wold, A. (1950) A promising drug … chloromycetin. *Aquarium*, September.

Wolf, K. and Dunbar, C.E. (1959) Test of 34 therapeutic agents for control of kidney disease in trout. *Transactions of the American Fisheries Society*, **88**, 117–124.

Wolf, K. and Snieszko, S.F. (1963) Uses of antibiotics and other antimicrobials in therapy of diseases of fishes. *Antimicrobial Agents and Chemotherapy*, **161**, 597–603.

Wood, J.W. (1968) *Diseases of Pacific Salmon: Their Prevention and Treatment*, State of Washington Department of Fisheries, Hatchery Division.

11

Management Techniques and Disease Control

Aweeda Newaj-Fyzul[1] *and Brian Austin*[2]

[1] *University of the West Indies, Trinidad and Agriquatics, Chaguanas, Trinidad*
[2] *Institute of Aquaculture, University of Stirling, Stirling, Scotland, UK*

Cleanliness is next to godliness (ancient Babylonian and Hebrew religious texts; John Wesley, 1778)

Introduction

Although there have been tremendous developments in understanding and controlling disease of aquatic animals, it is worth remembering that much may be achieved at the farm management level. It is appropriate to consider the age-old adage that prevention is better than cure but within the context that natural may well be better. Specifically, there is anecdotal evidence that sites which are scrupulous in hygiene practices and try to generate virtual gnotobiotic (germ-free) conditions are likely to suffer as many disease episodes as other establishments. An explanation is that ultra-hygiene removes the protective microflora, allowing potential pathogens to proliferate and instigate disease conditions. Nevertheless, there is much that may be done by improved management practices to reduce the risk of disease, starting with regular observation to spot the initial signs of trouble. The sooner a disease situation is recognized, the better the chance of control and minimizing the impact on the business. In short, there needs to be a quick response to unusual signs that may suggest the start of a disease cycle.

Disinfection

There needs to be a disinfectant policy for equipment that enters the fish-holding facilities, such as nets, fish size grading machinery, protective footwear, notably boots, and vehicles (particles on the tyres) that enter and leave the site. Disinfectants need to be replaced regularly as the presence of organic matter will often decrease effectiveness. Used disinfectants need to be disposed of sensibly, and not just discarded into the water course.

Diagnosis and Control of Diseases of Fish and Shellfish, First Edition. Edited by Brian Austin and Aweeda Newaj-Fyzul.

Hygiene

Attention to hygiene issues will considerably reduce the risk of disease. Specifically, uneaten fish food and moribund/dead fish should be removed promptly from the fish-holding facilities; corpses should be incinerated or buried in quicklime so that there is no chance of seepage from pits draining into the fish facilities. The emphasis is on the prompt removal of dead/moribund stock as it may need only one diseased individual to act as a reservoir of infection for the rest of the animals. The presence of decaying fish around the outlets to the holding facilities is not concomitant with good management practice.

Acquisition of New Stock

Whereas it is desirable to aim for self-sufficiency in the production cycle from eggs to broodstock, it is appreciated that in many cases this would be a utopian dream. Therefore, it is essential that imported stock are disease free. This means that the buyer needs to have confidence in the seller, and preferably see evidence of meaningful health certificates signed by competent authorities. Acquired stock should be kept in quarantine for several weeks after acquisition, with regular monitoring to ensure the absence of disease, and to minimize the risk of infecting the rest of the stock. Eggs need to be disinfected on arrival.

Boxes and the water used to transport stock should be disinfected thoroughly before disposal. Incineration of cardboard boxes should be considered. There should be evidence that fish transporters were thoroughly disinfected before the collection of stock. Upon arrival at the new site, the vehicle's wheels should be disinfected before and after the delivery process. Where feasible, the water used to transport the fish should be discharged in such a way as to minimize the risk of contaminating the receiving sites, preferably after disinfection.

Stocking Levels

Although it is tempting to increase stocking levels as a means of improving production, the opposite may well achieve the desired goals, that is, reduced stocking levels leads to higher production quantities (M'balaka *et al.*, 2012). Reducing the stocking density when water temperatures are high may reduce the incidence of some diseases, such as columnaris (Suomalainen *et al.*, 2005). Enhanced stocking levels may increase the stress to the fish by greater competition for feed and oxygen – levels of which could decline – and by deterioration of water quality resulting from the build-up of faeces, uneaten food and increased microbial populations, some components of which may be pathogenic

Water Flow and Aeration

Water flow may be influenced by blockages to pipework and cages, and by summer droughts. In the case of cage sites, water flow may be adversely affected if biofouling communities develop and block the holes in nets/cages. As far as possible, an adequate water flow needs to be maintained; oxygen levels should be checked, and if appropriate, aeration or oxygen added to the water. High microbial populations may develop in slow-running water, and may contribute to reduced oxygen levels in the water, as well as being a source of pathogens (for humans as well as fish!). A reduction in oxygen may lead to a concomitant increase in nitrogen levels, especially as ammonium salts. If algal blooms develop, their collapse could result in the release of toxic materials into the water within the fish-holding facilities. Regular observation is needed to ensure that inflow pipes are not blocked by debris. Increasing water temperatures may be troublesome during summer, and if feasible, water chillers could be considered for use, particularly in confined areas, such as hatcheries. Alternatively, shading of the fish-holding facilities in sunny weather would protect the fish from direct sunlight, and have a cooling effect.

Feed/Feeding Regimes

Feed should be kept in a clean, cool, dry location and used before the expiry date. Personal observation suggests that with dampness, mould and bacteria may develop in the feed. If this feed is then used, the micro-organisms may be transferred to the recipient fish if they consume the diet. Feed needs to be protected from vermin as rats may be infected with *Leptospira*, which could pose a risk of leptospirosis in humans (Gil *et al.*, 1985). When feeding, care should be taken to prevent overfeeding, which could lead to the build-up of uneaten feed in the fish-holding facilities. Such feed could lead to the development of high microbial populations in the water.

Vermin

Rodents need to be controlled across the aquaculture site to prevent the threat of disease, such as leptospirosis, and damage to infrastructure, for example cables, caused by gnawing. Although not regarded as vermin, efforts need to be made to reduce the impact of predatory birds and otters, which will take or injure stock, and could transmit disease.

References

Gil, O.N., Coghlan, J.D. and Calder, I.M. (1985) The risk of leptospirosis in United Kingdom fish farm workers. Results from a 1981 serological survey. *Journal of Hygiene (London)*, **94**, 81–86.

M'balaka, M., Kassam, D. and Rusuwa, B. (2012) The effect of stocking density on the growth and survival of improved and unimproved strains of *Oreochromis shiranus*. *Egyptian Journal of Aquatic Research*, **38**, 205–211.

Suomalainen, L.R., Tiirola, M. and Valtonen, E.T. (2005) Influence of rearing conditions on *Flavobacterium columnare* infection of rainbow trout, *Oncorhynchus mykiss* (Walbaum). *Journal of Fish Diseases*, **28**, 271–278.

12

Conclusions

Brian Austin[1] *and Aweeda Newaj-Fyzul*[2]

[1] *Institute of Aquaculture, University of Stirling, Stirling, Scotland, UK*
[2] *University of the West Indies, Trinidad and Agriquatics, Chaguanas, Trinidad*

There has been a continual increase in the list of fish and shellfish pathogens and parasites described in the scientific literature, and it is predicted that this trend will continue. One scenario is that an increase will reflect the movement of pathogens from one host to another, with the second having greater susceptibility to infection (= less resistance). The movement of live fish is considered to be the greatest source of transfer of pathogens from one area to another, even where there is 100% testing of broodstock and health certification before movement from one country to another. Unfortunately, such testing is non-existent in the movement of ornamental fish around the world. In the case of the bacteria, some of the increase has led from the description of new species and reclassification of others. For example, the number of fish/shellfish pathogenic vibrios has proliferated. Fortunately, there have been dramatic improvements in diagnosis, from the initial emphasis on phenotype before the 1970s, to serology and now molecular methods, notably sequencing of the 16S rRNA gene, which have become widespread not only for diagnostics but also in vaccinology and the study of pathogenic mechanisms.

With the availability of whole-genome sequencing, new information will emerge with relevance to the understanding of pathogenicity and candidates for vaccine development. Molecular biology has enabled culture-independent approaches to blossom. It must be remembered that identification of organisms via either culture and biochemical testing or molecular methods still does not confirm the organism identified is the responsible pathogen for the disease. Only by using the principle of Koch's postulates will isolates be confirmed as pathogens. Let us hope that the next major breakthrough will be the availability of field kits permitting the rapid and accurate diagnosis of disease. Serology has gone a long way to allowing rapid field diagnosis, for example with the development of enzyme-linked immunosorbent assays, but there is an issue of speed, and the specificity of antisera leading to the inability to recognize more than one disease simultaneously. This is now being addressed with new technologies such as reverse line blot hybridization, a system which can detect multiple pathogens at the same time. The one causing the disease, however, would still remain speculative.

The tendency to study only single isolates – particularly of bacterial pathogens – is of concern. Are the single isolates representative of the species as a whole? Are they still actively pathogenic or have they become attenuated laboratory cultures? With the recognition of *Candidatus* (Fehr *et al.*, 2013), there has been a realization that not all species are culturable, the

Diagnosis and Control of Diseases of Fish and Shellfish, First Edition. Edited by Brian Austin and Aweeda Newaj-Fyzul.

reasons for which are complex. Is there a lack of suitable methods or does it reflect the state of the cell, for example damaged or senescent?

The development of effective disease control strategies must continue. Already, there has been progress in genetic manipulation techniques for the development of effective vaccines. We may expect continued interest in non-specific immunostimulants, natural plant products, prebiotics and probiotics. Developments will hopefully be matched with a continual reduction in use of medically important anti-infective (microbial?) agents.

The reasons for the occurrence of disease continue to concern society. It is clear that pollution may be an underlying factor in many outbreaks of disease, particularly of wild animal stocks (Leonardi *et al.*, 2009; Pippy and Hare, 1969; Stentiford *et al.*, 2014). However, there is a lack of clarity on the role of pollution and the health of aquatic animals (Bucke, 1991, 1997; Abdel-Moneim, 2014), although studies point to the impact of pollutants on health, particularly in well-studied areas, notably the Great Lakes and the North Sea. Survey work, especially in the North Sea, has tried to correlate disease with pollution (Dethlefsen and Watermann, 1980, Dethlefsen *et al.*, 1987, 2000; Vethaak and ap Rheinallt, 1992). As an oversimplification, fish have been caught and the incidence of disease recorded, with the general conclusion that a higher incidence of diseased animals occur in the polluted rather than clean sites (Dethlefsen *et al.*, 2000), although the effects of migration on the incidence of fish disease need consideration (Bucke *et al.*, 1992; Jacquez *et al.*, 1994; Vethaak *et al.*, 1992). Nevertheless, pollution has been linked to fin and tail rot (Vatsos and Angelidis, 2011; Vethaak, 1992; Vethaak *et al.*, 1996), gill disease and hyperplasia (Kirk and Lewis 1993; Vatsos and Angelidis, 2011) and skin disease/ulceration (Rodjuk *et al.*, 2012; Vethaak, 1992; Vethaak and Jol, 1996). Stressors (= pollutants) have been reported to include heavy metals, particularly chromium (Prabakaran *et al.*, 2006; Rødsaether *et al.*, 1977), hydrocarbons (Khan, 1987; Song *et al.*, 2008; Stentiford *et al.*, 2014), nitrogenous compounds such as ammonia (Kirk and Lewis, 1993) and nitrites (Hanson and Grizzle, 1985), pesticides (Voigt, 1994), sewage (Austin and Stobie, 1992; Dudley *et al.*, 1980; Siddall *et al.*, 1994), organic pollutants (Grawinski and Antychowicz, 2001) and as yet unspecified pollutants (Vethaak and Jol, 1996). The effect on the host includes immunosuppression (Klesius and Shoemaker, 2003) leading to increased susceptibility to infection (Arkoosh *et al.*, 1998).

Some fish and shellfish parasites and pathogens may occasionally cause disease in humans. Although comparatively rare, incidents may generate adverse publicity for the fish and shellfish industries, with examples including infections by *V. parahaemolyticus* (food-borne infection) (Numata *et al.*, 2000) and *V. vulnificus* (wound and food-borne infections) (Miyoshi *et al.*, 2014) and parasites, including *Anisakis simplex* (herring worm) (Faeste *et al.*, 2015) and *Diphyllobothrium latum* (fish tapeworm) (Esteban *et al.*, 2014).

We may predict that disease will continue to plague aquatic animals with new and 'known' pathogens emerging regularly as opportunities arise.

References

Abdel-Moneim, A.M. (2014) Histopathological and ultrastructural perturbations in tilapia liver as potential indicators of pollution in Lake Al-Asfar, Saudi Arabia. *Environmental Science and Pollution Research*, **21**, 4387–4396.

Arkoosh, M.R., Casillas, E., Huffman, P., et al. (1998) Increased susceptibility of juvenile chinook salmon from a contaminated estuary to *Vibrio anguillarum. Transactions of the American Fisheries Society*, **127**, 360–374.

Austin, B. and Stobie, M. (1992) Recovery of *Serratia plymuthica* and presumptive *Pseudomonas pseudoalcaligenes* from skin lesions in rainbow trout, *Oncorhynchus mykiss* (Walbaum), otherwise infected with enteric redmouth. *Journal of Fish Diseases*, **15**, 541–543.

Bucke, D. (1991) Current approaches to the study of pollution-related diseases of fish. *Bulletin of the European Association of Fish Pathologists*, **11**, 46–53.

Bucke, D. (1997) Facts and myths regarding pollution and fish health. *Bulletin of the European Association of Fish Pathologists*, **17**, 191–196.

Bucke, D., Vethaak, A.D. and Lang, T. (1992) Quantitative assessment of melanomacrophage centres (MMCs) in dab *Limanda limanda* as indicators of pollution effects on the non-specific immune system. *Marine Progress Series*, **91**, 193–196.

Dethlefsen, V. and Watermann, B. (1980) Epidermal papilloma of North Sea dab, *Limanda limanda*: histology, epidemiology and relation to dumping from TiO_2 industry. *ICES Special Meeting on Diseases of Commercially Important Marine Fish and Shellfish*, **8**, 1–30.

Dethlefsen, V. Watermann, B. and Hoppenheit, M. (1987) Diseases of North Sea dab (*Limanda limanda* L.) in relation to biological and chemical parameters. *Archive für Fishereiwissenschaft*, **37**, 101–237.

Dethlefsen, V., Lang, T. and Koves, P. (2000) Regional patterns in prevalence of principal external diseases of dab *Limanda limanda* in the North Sea and adjacent areas 1992–1997. *Diseases of Aquatic Organisms*, **42**, 119–132.

Dudley, D.J., Guentzel, M.N., Ibarra, M.J., Moore, B.E. and Sagik, B.P. (1980) Enumeration of potentially pathogenic bacteria from sewage sludges. *Applied and Environmental Microbiology*, **39**, 118–126.

Esteban, J.G., Muñoz-Antoli, C., Borras, M., Colomina, J. and Toledo, R. (2014) Human infection by a "fish tapeworm" *Diphyllobothrium latum*, in a non-endemic country. *Infection*, **42**, 191–194.

Faeste, C.K., Plassen, C., Lovberg, K.E., Moen, A. and Egaas, E. (2015) Detection of proteins from the fish parasite *Anisakis simplex* in Norwegian farmed salmon and processed fish products. *Food Analytical Methods*, **8**, 1390–1402.

Fehr, A., Walther, E., Schmidt-Posthaus, H., et al. (2013) *Candidatus syngnamydia venezia*, a novel member of the phylum Chlamydiae from the broad nosed pipefish, *Syngnathus typhle. PLoS One*, **8**, e0070853.

Grawinski, E. and Antychowicz, J. (2001) The pathogenicity of *Serratia plymuthica* for salmonid fish. *Medycyna Weterynaryjna*, **57**, 187–189.

Hanson, L.A. and Grizzle, J.M. (1985) Nitrite-induced predisposition of channel catfish to bacterial diseases. *Progressive Fish Culturist*, **47**, 98–101.

Jacquez, G.M., Ziskowski, J. and Rolfe, F.J. (1994) Criteria for the evaluation of alternative environmental monitoring variables: theory and an application using winter flounder (*Pleuronectes americanus*) and Dover sole *(Microstomus pacificus). Environmental Monitoring and Assessment*, **30**, 275–290.

Khan, R.A. (1987) Crude oil and parasites of fish. *Parasitology Today*, **3**, 99–100.

Kirk, R.S. and Lewis, J.W. (1993) An evaluation of pollutant induced changes in the gills of rainbow trout using scanning electron microscopy. *Environmental Technology*, **14**, 577–585.

Klesius, P.H. and Shoemaker, C.A. (2003) The disease continuum model: bi-directional response between stress and infection linked by neuroimmune change, in *Biosecurity in Aquaculture*

Production Systems: Exclusion of Pathogens and Other Undesirables (eds C.S. Lee and P.J. O'Bryen), World Aquaculture Society, Baton Rouge, pp.13–14.

Leonardi, M., Vera, J. and Tarifeno, E. (2009) Diseases of the Chilean flounder *Paralichthys adspersus* (Steindachner, 1867) as biomarkers of marine coastal pollution near the Itata River (Chile). Part I: *in situ* macroscopic lesions. *Archives of Environmental Contamination and Toxicology*, **56**, 536–545.

Miyoshi, S.I., Ikehara, H., Kumagai, M., Mizuno, T., Kawase, T. and Maehara, Y. (2014) Defensive effects of human intestinal antimicrobial peptides against infectious diseases caused by *Vibrio mimicus* and *V. vulnificus*. *Biocontrol Science*, **19**, 199–203.

Numata, N., Ushimizu, M., Ohtomo, M., et al. (2000) The use of colony hybridization in the isolation of thermostable direct hemolysin-producing *Vibrio parahaemolyticus* from foods implicated in an incidence of food poisoning. *Japanese Journal of Infectious Diseases*, **53**, 75–77.

Pippy, J.H.C. and Hare, G.M. (1969) Relationship of river pollution to bacterial infection in salmon (*Salmo salar*) and suckers (*Catostomus commersoni*). *Transactions of the American Fisheries Society*, **98**, 685–690.

Prabakaran, M., Binuramesh, C., Steinhagen, D. and Michael, R.D. (2006) Immune response and disease resistance of *Oreochromis mossambicus* to *Aeromonas hydrophila* after exposure to hexavalent chromium. *Diseases of Aquatic Organisms*, **68**, 189–196.

Rodjuk, G.N., Chukalova, N.N., Shenderyuk, V.V., Bakholdina, L.P., Chernysheva, N.L. and Sayadov, S.O. (2012) Prevalence of skin ulceration in cod (*Gadus morhua callarias* L.) under anthropogenic contamination in the southeastern part of the Baltic Sea. *Inland Water Biology*, **5**, 133–139.

Rødsaether, M.C., Olafsen, J., Raa, J., Myhre, K. and Steen, J.B. (1977) Copper as an initiating factor of vibriosis (*Vibrio anguillarum*) in eel (*Anguilla anguilla*). *Journal of Fish Biology*, **10**, 17–21.

Siddall, R., Pike, A.W. and McVicar, A.H. (1994) Parasites of flatfish in relation to sewage dumping. *Journal of Fish Biology*, **45**, 193–209.

Song, J.Y., Nakayama, K., Murakami, Y., et al. (2008) Does heavy oil pollution induce bacterial diseases in Japanese flounder *Paralichthys olivaceus*? *Marine Pollution Bulletin*, **57**, 6–12.

Stentiford, G.D., Massoud, M.S., Al-Enezi, M. and Lyons B.P. (2014) Histopathological survey of potential biomarkers for the assessment of contaminant related biological effects in species of fish and shellfish collected from Kuwait Bay, Arabian Gulf. *Marine Environmental Research*, **98**, 60–67.

Vatsos, I.N. and Angelidis, P. (2011) Water quality and fish diseases. *Journal of the Hellenic Veterinary Medical Society*, **61**, 40–48.

Vethaak, A.D. (1992) Diseases of flounder (*Platichthys flesus* L.) in the Dutch Wadden Sea, and their relation to stress factors. *Netherlands Journal of Sea Research*, **29**, 257–272.

Vethaak, A.D. and ap Rheinallt, T. (1992) Fish disease as a monitor for marine pollution: the case of the North Sea. *Reviews in Fish Biology and Fisheries*, **2**, 1–32.

Vethaak, A.D. and Jol, J.G. (1996) Diseases of flounder *Platichthys flesus* in Dutch coastal and estuarine waters, with particular reference to environmental stress factors. 1. Epizootiology of gross lesions. *Diseases of Aquatic Organisms*, **26**, 81–97.

Vethaak, A.D., Bucke, D., Lang, T., Wester, P., Johl, J. and Carr, M. (1992) Fish disease monitoring along a pollution transect: a case study using dab *Limanda limanda* in the German Bight, North Sea. *Marine Ecology Progress Series*, **91**, 173–192.

Vethaak, A.D., Jol, J.G., Meijboom, A., et al. (1996) Skin and liver diseases induced in flounder (*Platichthys flesus*) after long-term exposure to contaminated sediments in large-scale mesocosms. *Environmental Health Perspectives*, **104**, 1218–1229.

Voigt, H.R. (1994) Fish surveys in the Vaike Vain Strait between the islands of Saaremaa and Muhu, western Estonia. *Proceedings of the Estonian Academy of Science and Ecology*, **4**, 128–135.

Index

Diagnosis and Control of Diseases of Fish and Shellfish, First Edition. Edited by Brian Austin and Aweeda Newaj-Fyzul.